SCHOOL PSYCHOLOGY FOR THE 21ST CENTURY

SCHOOL PSYCHOLOGY
for the 21st Century

FOUNDATIONS AND PRACTICES

SECOND EDITION

Kenneth W. Merrell
Ruth A. Ervin
Gretchen Gimpel Peacock

THE GUILFORD PRESS
New York   London

© 2012 The Guilford Press
A Division of Guilford Publications, Inc.
72 Spring Street, New York, NY 10012
www.guilford.com

Printed in the United States of America

This book is printed on acid-free paper.

Last digit is print number: 9 8 7 6 5 4

Library of Congress Cataloging-in-Publication Data
Merrell, Kenneth W.
  School psychology for the 21st century : foundations and practices / Kenneth W. Merrell,
Ruth A. Ervin, Gretchen Gimpel Peacock. — 2nd ed.
    p. cm.
  Includes bibliographical references and index.
  ISBN 978-1-60918-752-1 (hardcover : alk. paper)
  1. School psychology—United States. I. Ervin, Ruth A.   II. Gimpel Peacock,
Gretchen.   III. Title.
  LB1027.55.M47 2012
  371.7′13—dc23
                                                    2011029475

About the Authors

Kenneth W. Merrell, PhD, was Professor of School Psychology and Director of the Oregon Resiliency Project at the University of Oregon. For 25 years, Dr. Merrell's influential teaching and research focused on social–emotional assessment and intervention for at-risk children and adolescents and social–emotional learning in schools. He published over 90 peer-reviewed journal articles; several books and nationally normed assessment instruments; and the *Strong Kids* programs, a comprehensive social and emotional learning curriculum. Dr. Merrell was the Founding Editor of The Guilford Practical Intervention in the Schools Series. He was a Fellow of the Division of School Psychology (Division 16) and the Society of Clinical Child and Adolescent Psychology (Division 53) of the American Psychological Association. In 2011 he received the Senior Scientist Award from Division 16, the Division's highest honor for excellence in science, and the Outstanding Contributions to Training Award from the National Association of School Psychologists.

Sadly, Dr. Merrell passed away on August 19, 2011, at the age of 53 after a year-long battle with cancer. Although no longer present in person, his contributions to the field of school psychology will continue to live on in his published works, in the many students he mentored over the course of his career, and through the manner in which he touched the lives of his colleagues on both a professional and personal level.

Ruth A. Ervin, PhD, is Associate Professor of School Psychology and Special Education at the University of British Columbia, Vancouver, Canada. Her professional teaching and research interests lie within the domains of promoting systems-level change to address research-to-practice gaps in school settings; collaborative consultation with school personnel, parents, and other service providers for the prevention and treatment of emotional and/or behavioral disorders such as attention-deficit/hyperactivity disorder and oppositional defiant disorder via a data-driven, solution-oriented problem-solving approach; and linking assessment to intervention to promote academic performance and socially significant outcomes for school-age children. Emphasis in Dr. Ervin's work has been placed on systems-level change and the merging of research and practice agendas to support school personnel in the timely provision of primary, secondary, and tertiary prevention efforts to address student needs.

Gretchen Gimpel Peacock, PhD, is Professor of Psychology at Utah State University, where she is on the program faculty of the specialist-level school psychology program and the PhD program in clinical, counseling, and school psychology, and where she serves as head of the Department of Psychology. She regularly supervises practicum students in the departmental clinic. Dr. Gimpel Peacock is a licensed psychologist and educator-licensed school psychologist. Her publications and professional presentations are in the area of child behavior problems and family issues as related to child behaviors as well as professional issues in school psychology. Dr. Gimpel Peacock serves on the editorial advisory boards of several school psychology-related journals.

Preface

The field of school psychology continues to be at a critical juncture. Until recently considered to be a young field, school psychology is now showing signs of maturity. We believe the field has moved into a new era in which it is beginning to fulfill its potential to significantly affect the education and mental health needs of children, adolescents, and their families in a positive way and to become a key player in the advancement of American education. But let's face it: Growing up is hard. Arriving at a point at which maturity exists almost inevitably involves at least some of these four C's: confusion, chaos, compromises, and changes. The arrival of school psychology at this crossroads coincided to a great extent with the move from the 20th to the 21st century. Two of the seminal occurrences of this transition were a special issue of *School Psychology Review* (Vol. 29, No. 4, 2000) titled "School Psychology in the 21st Century" and the 2002 Future of School Psychology Conference, which was held in Indianapolis and simultaneously webcast. A quick scan of the content of these two projects indicates an emerging consensus regarding the maturation of school psychology from a philosophically based to a scientifically based profession and the need for maps or an overall vision to help it make the successful transition beyond the crossroads. The common understanding that emerged from these efforts, which helped serve as a stimulus for the first edition of this volume, was that school psychology is moving out of its decades-long struggle for identity, and beginning to marshal its vast resources into a rich vision for helping to solve the enormous challenges of promoting the education and mental health of young people in our complex society and troubled times. In a twist on the 19th-century German philosopher Friedrich Nietzsche's famous statement "out of chaos comes order," one of the presentations at the 2002 Future conference was a panel discussion entitled "From Chaos Comes Resolutions." This presentation (and its great title) summarized much of our view about where school psychology is as a field and what needs to happen for the field to successfully get past the crossroads:

1. Our focus should be increasingly on *context and systems*, and not just individuals.
2. We should focus primarily on diagnosing competence and the conditions that

enable and support it, not solely on the description and categorization of pathology.

3. School psychologists should direct their efforts toward helping *all* students, not just those who have been referred because of serious problems.

4. Our practices and decision-making processes must be *outcome focused* and *data based*.

Not coincidentally, the title of this volume, *School Psychology for the 21st Century: Foundations and Practices*, invokes the temporal element of change and references the previous and current development of the field. Early in the first decade of this new century, we as authors began a discussion that led to the conception and creation of the first edition of this volume. As we discussed the feasibility of writing an introduction to school psychology, we quickly found that we shared a viewpoint and vision for our professional field and that we were all enthusiastic about the possibilities that exist at this important juncture. We embarked on this work not only to provide a solid introduction to school psychology but also to help shape the further development and progress of the field.

This volume is designed to provide an introduction and orientation to the field of school psychology. We especially intend for it to be of interest and use to graduate students who are beginning to prepare for careers in the field. Almost all of the hundreds of graduate programs in school psychology in the United States and Canada offer an introductory class on the field and its professional issues. Students typically take this class during their first year of graduate study, often during their first semester or term. We believe that it is ideally suited for use in such introductory graduate classes, where we hope that it will help to shape the views and practices of the emerging generation of school psychologists. We believe that it will also be of interest to undergraduate students in psychology and education who are considering graduate studies and careers in these fields and who desire to learn more about the possibilities that school psychology may hold for them. We also intend this book to be of use to individuals who are considering a career change into school psychology and need a resource to help them explore the field. Individuals who currently work as school psychology practitioners, trainers, administrators, and researchers will find this volume to be a fresh introduction and guide to our dynamic and exciting field.

The first two chapters present a foundation and context for understanding school psychology. Chapter 1 provides an introduction to the field, and Chapter 2 gives an overview of the history of school psychology as well as the historical context of its place in psychology and American education. Chapter 3 provides a foundation for effective school psychology practices in an increasingly diverse cultural context. Chapters 4 through 6 provide a foundation for the professional practice of school psychology, focusing on training and credentialing, employment trends and issues, and legal and ethical aspects of practice in this field. Chapters 7 through 12 provide the details of our vision of best practice in school psychology and focus on the wide range of roles that we believe school psychologists should pursue, including a data-oriented problem-solving approach to practice; assessment; prevention and intervention; facilitating systems-level change via implementing a public health perspective on school psychology services; and being involved as a consumer and producer of research and evaluation. Chapter 13 provides some concluding comments regarding moving the field of school psychology forward and mapping our own future as professionals. Together, the 13 chapters in this book provide a comprehensive and, in our view, state-of-the-art introduction to the field of school psychology.

This volume was written deliberately to reflect our shared points of view as well as a shared vision of what school psychology can become. As we began to discuss the possibility of writing an introductory volume to school psychology, none of us was interested in simply providing another overview of the history, current status, and issues of the field. Rather, we wrote this book because we were interested in promoting a forward-thinking vision of the exciting and dynamic possibilities within the field of school psychology. We believe that school psychology has much to offer and that its potential is just beginning to emerge. The possibilities for this field to make a strong positive impact in schools and other settings and in the lives of children, adolescents, and their families are simply enormous. We also believe that there are still several barriers to achieving this vision, foremost of which are the low expectations of many professionals and institutions for school psychology, some of which have unfortunately been perpetuated by the narrow vision of school psychology that is held by some of its own practitioners and trainers. We are not naive about the challenges, obstacles, and barriers that many school psychologists face in using their professional skills and interests to achieve the maximum good. Rather, we believe that, through a concerted effort over time, school psychologists can individually and collectively advance the field at all levels, and that in doing so, school psychology will make an enormous positive impact.

Although each chapter within this book is unique, these chapters were developed through a collective vision for the book. Some of the "big ideas" on which this book and our vision for the field of school psychology are based include the following:

• North American society has become increasingly diverse and pluralistic with respect to the cultural background, race, ethnicity, and language of its citizens, and it will continue to become increasingly diverse during the 21st century. School psychologists should develop cultural competence so that they can work appropriately and effectively with individuals and groups from a variety of backgrounds (see Chapter 3).

• School psychology practice has been and should continue to be primarily focused in school or other educational settings. The educational setting is a primary focus of our vision and of this book. However, school psychologists have much to offer outside of the context of school settings, and we encourage the practice of school psychology in a variety of settings and contexts (see Chapter 5).

• School psychology practice should be outcome focused and data driven. School psychologists should base their decisions on valid data and use effective data collection techniques to inform, monitor, and modify intervention activities (see Chapter 7).

• Assessment of children and adolescents has been and will continue to be a mainstay activity of school psychologists. However, the types of assessment methods and the process of assessment have evolved over time. Assessment activities should do more than simply describe or diagnose problems. Rather, the most useful assessment strategies are those that provide a foundation for implementing and monitoring effective interventions (see Chapter 8).

• School psychologists have historically worked with a limited segment of student populations, primarily those who have or are suspected of having disabilities and those who are otherwise at high risk for negative outcomes in life. We believe that there will always be a need for school psychologists to focus some of their efforts on the small percentage of students who have serious learning, behavioral, and social–emotional problems. We also recognize that longitudinal research points to the chronic nature of such problems and the critical need for *early* intervention if negative long-term outcomes are to be curtailed. Thus, we strongly contend that school psychologists should use their unique expertise to positively affect *all students in school settings*, not just those who currently exhibit serious learning, behavioral, or social–emotional problems.

• Effective prevention and intervention activities should occupy a significant percentage of school psychologists' time. Such activities should occur within the context of a problem-solving, evidence-based practice model (see Chapters 9 and 10).

• Prevention and intervention activities can occur with individuals, within small groups, within classrooms, within entire schools, and within school district- or community-based contexts. School psychologists should engage in prevention and intervention activities at each of these levels, so that a larger number of individuals may be positively influenced (see Chapters 9 and 10).

• School psychologists do not typically function in isolation but work as part of a system. School psychologists should strive to use their expertise to develop a solid understanding of the systems in which they work and to help facilitate systems-level change as needed (see Chapter 11).

• School psychologists should be savvy consumers of research and should have the skills to engage in research and evaluation activities within their respective settings that will help to advance practice (see Chapter 12).

• School psychology is a field with incredible potential for helping to solve the "big" problems facing education. And yet this potential is still not fully realized. We believe that school psychologists should play an active and important role in this regard. This book is built on the foundation of a progressive, forward-thinking vision of school psychology, and we are optimistic that collectively individual school psychologists can continue to move the field forward through their efforts (see Chapter 13).

We hope that this book will receive a broad audience and that it will meet the needs of those who use it, perhaps even inspire them to think about and practice school psychology in a new way. In sum, school psychology is a dynamic and exciting field that has incredible and still unrealized potential for positively affecting education, psychology, and the lives of children, adolescents, and their families. It is our hope that this book will provide a useful and engaging guide to the field of school psychology and will help the field continue to move forward.

Comments on the Second Edition

The second edition of this volume maintains the same vision, unifying themes, and chapter/organizational structures as the first edition. What is different in the current edition of this volume is a number of updates and improvements that reflect developments in the fields of school psychology and education since 2006, new legal issues impacting the field, new research findings, and recent social and demographic trends in the field and in society in general. Some of the specific changes from the first edition include:

• Hundreds of new references that reflect updates to the critical literature in the field, new research findings in education and psychology, and the latest legal, ethical, and social developments.

- Enhanced discussion and coverage of response-to-intervention (RTI) methods of assessing and supporting students, which have become a major development in the field in a remarkably short period of time, since the implementation of the 2004 Individuals with Disabilities Education Improvement Act (IDEIA).
- Expanded coverage of issues related to supporting the increasing number of culturally and linguistically diverse students in schools, including enhanced and updated content in Chapter 3 as well as updated content infused across other chapters.
- Up-to-date coverage of the changes in school psychology training programs, professional standards, and demographic trends in the field that have emerged since the publication of the first edition of this volume.
- Updates on some of the latest trends, programs, and tools for assessment and intervention with children and adolescents in educational and related settings.
- Analysis of some of the recent economic, demographic, and social changes that have occurred in the United States and Canada (and worldwide, in some cases) since the first edition of this volume, particularly those changes and trends that impact education, children and adolescents, and families.
- Expanded coverage of the evidence-based practice model in addressing mental health concerns as well as expanded coverage of empirically supported mental health interventions.

Acknowledgments

We have enjoyed the support of many colleagues as we have developed the first and second editions of this volume, and we wish to acknowledge their contributions. In particular, we would like to acknowledge Randy Floyd for his supportive consultation and expertise. We are indebted to Chris Jennison, former Publisher, Education, at The Guilford Press, who provided the persistent encouragement (and occasional nudging) to one of us (KWM) over a period of 2 years to write an introductory book on the field of school psychology that led to this book becoming a reality in its first edition in 2006. At Guilford, Craig Thomas, Senior Editor; Natalie Graham, Editor; and Anna Nelson, Senior Production Editor, have all provided invaluable assistance to us in moving forward the second edition of this volume as well as other volumes we have published with Guilford both individually and collectively. We are indebted to our colleagues and students at our respective institutions (University of Oregon, University of British Columbia, and Utah State University) for helping to create intellectual environments in which we could conceptualize and articulate what we think is a progressive view of school psychology. We are also grateful to our own mentors and past colleagues in the field. Finally, we are indebted to the many scholars, practitioners, and leaders in the field of school psychology over the past several decades who, through their life's work, have helped bring the field to the critical and promising point where it is at the present time.

Contents

Introduction to the Field of School Psychology

I t is fitting for the first chapter of this introductory volume about school psychology to provide a general exploration of this exciting field. If you are investigating this field or are new to it, you probably have some basic questions, and this chapter is an attempt to answer some of them and to provide a useful orientation to this book. The chapter begins with a discussion of the various definitions of school psychology and how these definitions inform and shape the field. General characteristics of school psychologists are described, including such aspects as the number and location of individuals who work in the field, demographic characteristics of school psychologists, professional organizations, and level of training. To help provide a more direct introduction to the field, we present four composite vignettes of individuals who work in school psychology. These vignettes show the diversity, strength, creativity, and challenges within the profession. Some aspects of entry into the field are described, including graduate training and credentialing. School psychology is differentiated from some of the more closely related fields in psychology and education. Finally, we include a guide to using this book and an overview of some of the "big ideas" on which the book was developed.

Defining School Psychology

At the beginning of a book introducing readers to the field of school psychology, it is reasonable to consider the questions "What is school psychology?" and "What is a school psychologist?" Individuals who have worked in this field for several years might assume that the meaning and definition of school psychology are self-evident. However, a closer look at the development of the field, the evolution of a professional identity, and some of the controversies regarding issues that to outsiders appear to be straightforward show us that in order to define school psychology we must examine it closely and consider the importance of "what's in a definition."

1

Previous Definitions

It is interesting to look through the literature from a few decades ago to see how the defining characteristics of school psychology have evolved over time. In their 1961 book *The School Psychologist*, White and Harris stated, "In our view school psychology is that branch of psychology which concerns itself with the personality of the pupil in interaction with the educational process," and argued that the field "encompasses not only the learning process, as part of education, but also the personality of the learner as a member of school society, as a member of a family unit, and as a member of the community" (p. 1). In her landmark book *The Psychologist in the Schools*, the original treatise on problem solving as the professional aspiration of school psychologists, Susan Gray (1963) posited that school psychologists had two primary roles: one as *data-oriented problem solvers* in schools and the other as *transmitters of psychological knowledge and skills.* Bardon and Bennett, in their book *School Psychology* (1974), wrote, "The specialty in psychology concerned with how schooling affects children in general and with the pupil in interaction with a specific school is called school psychology. The specialty includes knowledge about research and theory dealing with what happens between children and others when they are together in schools; more than that, school psychology deals with how school for a child in Jackson Junior High is different than school for a child in Wilson Junior High" (p. x).

Current Definitions

In contrast to these notable statements from the 1960s and 1970s, which tended to define the field by focusing on what school psychologists do or should do rather than on what the specialty is, the most current definitions of school psychology tend to be more direct in defining the essential characteristics of school psychology. In the About School Psychology section of the National Association of School Psychologists (NASP) website, the answer to "What is a school psychologist?" is provided:

> School psychologists help children and youth succeed academically, socially, behaviorally, and emotionally. They collaborate with educators, parents, and other professionals to create safe, healthy, and supportive learning environments that strengthen connections between home, school, and the community for all students.
>
> School psychologists are highly trained in both psychology and education, completing a minimum of a specialist-level degree program (at least 60 graduate semester hours) that includes a year-long supervised internship. This training emphasizes preparation in mental health and educational interventions, child development, learning, behavior, motivation, curriculum and instruction, assessment, consultation, collaboration, school law, and systems. School psychologists must be certified and/or licensed by the state in which they work. They also may be nationally certified by the National School Psychology Certification Board (NSPCB). The National Association of School Psychologists sets ethical and training standards for practice and service delivery. (NASP, 2010d, paragraphs 1 and 2)

Another definition or description of school psychology is provided by the Division of School Psychology (Division 16) of the American Psychological Association (APA). In the Goals & Objectives section of their website, the archival description of the specialty of school psychology reads:

> School Psychology is a general practice and health service provider specialty of professional psychology that is concerned with the science and practice of psychology with

children, youth, families; learners of all ages; and the schooling process. The basic education and training of school psychologists prepares them to provide a range of psychological assessment, intervention, prevention, health promotion, and program development and evaluation services with a special focus on the developmental processes of children and youth within the context of schools, families, and other systems.

School psychologists are prepared to intervene at the individual and system level, and develop, implement, and evaluate preventive programs. In these efforts, they conduct ecologically valid assessments and intervene to promote positive learning environments within which children and youth from diverse backgrounds have equal access to effective educational and psychological services to promote healthy development. (APA Division of School Psychology, 2010, paragraphs 1 and 2)

Because these definitions are from the two most influential entities representing the field of school psychology in the United States, they have particular importance. What do these definitions have in common? They indicate that school psychology is a profession concerned with the development, mental health, and education of children and youth. They indicate that school psychologists provide services to children, youth, and their families within the context of educational settings but are not limited to those settings. They indicate that school psychologists are concerned with supporting children, youth, their families, and other professionals who work with them in educational and other settings. Importantly, these definitions tell us that school psychology is part of the broader field of psychology and that it also is connected to the field of education and to other professional fields as well. Formulating definitions of school psychology and subsequent efforts to refine these definitions have been exceedingly difficult at times. These issues are not trivial. Professional identity and activities are shaped in great measure by how a specialty is defined. The short answer to "What's in a definition?" is "more than you might think."

Characteristics of School Psychologists

Definitions aside, another way to obtain a snapshot of the field of school psychology is to look at the characteristics of school psychologists. Like a good working definition of the field, it is surprisingly complex to provide a simple description of those who call themselves school psychologists. Because the practice of school psychology is governed by various credentialing bodies within the individual states and provinces, and because membership in professional organizations is voluntary, there is no unitary list or registry of school psychologists. This section provides some basic data regarding school psychologists, particularly the number of individuals who are estimated to work in the field, and some of their basic demographic characteristics, including gender and ethnicity. In Chapter 5, we provide more details regarding the characteristics of school psychologists, specifically in the context of employment.

Perhaps the most direct way to make inferences regarding basic characteristics of school psychologists is to look at available data from national organizations. However, even this method is fraught with challenges because the actual percentage of school psychologists who join professional organizations is unknown and many school psychologists (like ourselves) belong to two or more professional organizations that represent the field.

Data provided to the authors by the NASP's Membership Department indicated that as of March 18, 2010, there were 26,085 members of the association. The majority of these NASP members resided in the United States, but 300 lived in Canada and 133 were from other nations. On the basis of our own experiences and conversations with school psychologists, we estimate that 60 to 65% of school psychologists in the United States are members of NASP, and the figure for school psychologists in Canada is somewhat less. If we are correct, then a reasonable estimate of the number of school psychologists in the two nations ranges from 39,000 to 43,000. Of course, this number is nothing more than an educated guess. Not only do we not know the actual percentage of school psychologists who belong to NASP, but we must also recognize that there are some individuals who are NASP members who are not specifically trained as school psychologists or who are working in related fields. That said, our estimate is very consistent with data from a Charvat (2005) survey of state departments of education educational licensing agencies, which indicated there were nearly 38,000 certified or licensed school psychologists in the United States alone. This estimate is also in line with other recent estimates taking into account U.S. school psychologists only. For example, Fagan (2008) noted that a "reasonable figure" for school psychologists within the United States is in the 30,000–35,000 range, and Charvat (2008) estimated that there were approximately 35,400 credentialed school psychologists in the United States in 2008, with 28,500 of these individuals being practicing school psychologists.

Using APA Division 16 data is less informative in terms of estimating the number of school psychologists. On March 18, 2010, we were informed by the division's vice president of membership that at the end of 2009 there were approximately 2,200 members of Division 16. This figure is obviously not a proxy figure in any respect for the total number of school psychologists in the United States, because it is widely understood that far fewer school psychologists join APA than NASP, and it is unknown how many individuals are members of both organizations. One reason that APA Division 16 has far fewer members than NASP is that a doctoral degree is required for full APA membership, but a large majority of practicing school psychologists do not have doctoral degrees.

Internationally, the number of school psychologists is also something of a puzzle, and it is even more difficult to ascertain than the number within the United States. Several years ago, Oakland and Cunningham (1992) conducted an international survey and estimated the number of individuals globally in the field of school psychology to be 87,000. More recently, Jimerson, Stewart, Skokut, Cardenas, and Malone (2009) estimated that there were 76,122 school psychologists in 48 countries, including 32,300 in the United States and 3,500 in Canada. After the United States, Turkey had the next largest estimated number of school psychologists (11,327), followed by Spain (3,600), and then both Canada and Japan (3,500 each). Jimerson et al. noted that estimates for school psychologists for the three countries with the largest number of children (India, China, and Indonesia) could not be obtained, and in Indonesia there was no evidence of school psychology practice. It does seem likely that the 76,122 figure somewhat underestimates the number of school psychologists internationally and that Oakland's (2007) estimate of 100,000 may be a better reflection of the number of school psychologists worldwide.

Although we are using the term *school psychologists* very generally to make these worldwide comparisons, it is worth noting that the role of school psychologists outside of the United States and Canada (who are also referred to in some nations as "educational psychologists") may differ considerably from the role of school psychologists in the United States and Canada. Particularly in the United States, the role of the school psychologist has been strongly linked to public law for education of students with disabilities. In most other nations, this is not the case. That being said, many of the basic core functions of school psychologists in terms of consultation, intervention, and assessment are likely similar across many countries (Oakland, 2007; Oakland & Jimerson, 2008). (More information on the practice of school psychology worldwide is available at the International School Psychology Association website: *www.ispaweb.org.*)

With respect to gender of school psychologists, there is considerable evidence that the field has become a female-dominated profession in the past two or three decades, and the percentage of women in the field continues to increase slightly. The most recent membership survey data available from NASP (from 2004 to 2005) indicated that approximately 74% of NASP members are women, reflecting increases from the November 1999 estimate of 72% reported by Fagan and Wise (2000) and from their 1994 estimate of 67%. In commenting on the fairly recent shift in gender composition of school psychologists since about the 1970s, Reschly (2000) stated that the increased proportion of women in the field during this time period constituted "the clearest changes in school psychology during the past two decades" (p. 508).

Future trends regarding the characteristics of school psychologists are difficult to predict. Because the field does not exist in isolation, future trends will inevitably be shaped by external forces, such as economic conditions, the development of public education, new federal laws and mandates, advocacy by national and state organizations, and national and worldwide social trends. However, it appears that in the immediate future several trends are very likely. The field of school psychology should continue to grow at least modestly, and school psychologists will continue to enjoy adequate to good employment prospects in most regions, even during times of economic downturn. Public school settings will almost certainly continue to be the primary place of employment for school psychologists, although expansion into nontraditional settings will continue. The large majority of school psychology practitioners will hold master's or specialist degrees as their highest academic degrees, although the percentage of school psychologists with doctoral degrees may increase slightly, as it has in recent years. For the foreseeable future, the large majority of school psychologists will be women, and it is likely that the percentage of women in the field may even continue to increase.

It is important to recognize that the clear evidence of professional gender imbalance is not limited to school psychology alone, but seems to be evident in most areas of specialization within graduate training programs in psychology, at the doctoral, master's, and specialist levels. For example, a 2007 APA survey (APA, 2007a) of recent doctoral recipients in the field of psychology found that 76% of all respondents were women, which reflected an increase of 7 percentage points over 10 years and 24 percentage points in 21 years since previous surveys had been completed. Fagan (2008) asserted that "the proportion of women in school psychology may rise to as high as 80%" (p. 2070). Although Fagan stated that "effects of the increasing female representation have not been studied" (p. 2071), he did note that the increase in women in the psychology field has helped the profession maintain its ability to meet the needs of its clientele and has likely led to the increase in certain research/service areas (e.g., women's issues, bullying).

Being There: Four Stories from the Field

Although the general professional definitions and descriptions of school psychology are extremely important and have broad impact on how the field is perceived both internally and externally, they give us only a small glimpse of what school psychologists do in their day-to-day work. Definitions cannot capture the diversity of roles that school psychologists fill, nor can they adequately convey how each practicing school psychologist is in a unique situation and setting and has a unique perspective on the field. In addition, general definitions cannot possibly convey the wealth of experience, passion, and personal commitment that individual school psychologists bring to their work. Perhaps a better way to illustrate what school psychology looks like at the point of actual practice is to present a glimpse into the professional lives of several school psychologists. The following four composite vignettes contain elements of the professional lives of several school psychologists whom we know and have spoken to extensively about their work. Although these vignettes are composite scenarios of more than one person and do not contain identifying information, all are based on actual persons.

Alexa: "A Tough but Rewarding Field"

Alexa is currently in her second year working as a school psychologist in a large county school district in the southwestern United States, comprising a large urban area, its immediate suburbs, and an outlying rural region that is sparsely populated. Alexa has responsibility for three schools (two elementary schools and a middle school), and she also provides training and consultation across the district to help teachers adapt to the system's new response-to-intervention model (RTI) for identifying and supporting students who have learning problems. Alexa arrived here after completing her doctoral program and internship from a nationally recognized training program. Prior to her doctoral studies, she received a bachelor's degree in psychology in her home state in the Midwest, and then earned a specialist degree in school psychology at an institution in the Mountain West region. Alexa did not fall into the field happenstance or after a late discovery: She has been focused on her goal of a career in school psychology since her senior year in high school.

Alexa's days are full. Her three schools all have pressing needs and problems. Not only are there the usual array of student concerns, but the area has been hit hard by the severe economic recession that began in 2008, and a large military base nearby means that many of the children at her schools have a parent who is deployed overseas in Iraq, Afghanistan, or elsewhere. The population in her school district has historically been transient, which creates a revolving door of incoming and outgoing students with special needs. In addition, the district has a significant and growing population of English language learners, most of whom speak Spanish at home. As a result of these factors, many of the students in her schools have notable stressors in their lives, and it manifests in a variety of academic, behavioral, and social–emotional problems. In addition, the district's adoption of an RTI model the year she arrived has created a strong need for Alexa to consult and train with specialists and teachers. Not only is assisting with RTI implementation a part of her job description, but RTI was an integral component of her doctoral training program, and Alexa carved out a strong area of interest and specialization in RTI during her training.

Although her initial goal in accepting her current position was to work 2 to 3 years and then pursue an academic position at a research institution with a doctoral program, Alexa has been rethinking that idea. "I'm finding the district's move to an RTI model to be very rewarding and exciting, and I like working as a practitioner more than I thought I would. I also really enjoy the relationships and friendships I have formed with my colleagues. And I'm probably making more money now than I would if I moved to a university trainer position. I'm getting a good start to paying off my student loans and I finally was able to buy a decent car!"

But Alexa's enthusiasm for her professional role is tempered by the realities of some of its challenges. "The move to RTI happened more quickly than most of the staff expected, and I don't think it was carefully enough planned and orchestrated in the beginning," she says. As a result, she has encountered significant resistance to the idea from staff at two of her three schools. "In my specialist program internship, I mostly gave standardized cognitive assessments, participated in team meetings, and did some consultation with parents and teachers. I liked it, but I often questioned how it was helping kids. What I am doing now is so much more satisfying and useful than what I was doing then. But it is not easy, and the kinds of changes we need to put in place are moving slowly."

Despite those sometimes hard realities and challenges in her professional role, Alexa is convinced she made a good choice by going into school psychology: "This is important work. When we get it right, I can see the results in the lives of our students and their families, not to mention our teachers. And what I really like about it is being able to follow through with kids over time, to see them progress when we are able to put together the right combination of programming for them. This field can be tough, but it's so rewarding."

Roger: "Like Putting Water on a Dying Plant"

Unlike Alexa, Roger got a later start to his career in school psychology. Currently in his late 30s, Roger is in his seventh year of a second career as a school psychologist. A native of California, he graduated with honors from a small liberal arts college in the Pacific Northwest and then went through a master's program in business administration at a large, prestigious university in California. "I wanted to move up the corporate ladder in management and sales, and I wanted to make lots of money. At least that's what I thought and what my family seemed to expect." After receiving his MBA, he joined a large company and began the climb upward in the sales division. He stayed with the company 5 years, earning two promotions and a very healthy salary. But after about 3 years he began questioning his pursuit and found it increasingly a poor match for his idealism and sense of social justice. He also became interested in exploring other options. "I was becoming more and more frustrated, and although it was a good job and there was nothing wrong with that industry, I wanted to do something that I felt was making more of a difference in people's lives day to day." His introduction to school psychology came in the unlikeliest of places. "I would work out at a gym three or four nights a week, and got to know a group of five or six other regulars there. One of them was a school psychologist, and I found myself wanting to ask her lots of questions about her work, then I started researching the field." He was soon convinced that this was a good direction for him, and the next year he applied for and received admission into a specialist-level master's program in his home state. "I loved my school psychology training—It was hard, but so much different and more satisfying to me than my MBA program."

Roger completed his internship with a school district in the San Francisco Bay area, accepted a regular position there, and has been there ever since. The district is large, mostly urban, and very diverse. About 40% of the students are Asian and about 25% are Latino; white and African American students each constitute about 10% of the district's population. There are also many immigrants from the Middle East and quite a few students for whom English is not their first language. Roger feels that his own Asian ethnicity helps him with initial cultural acceptance issues when dealing with Asian students and families, but he does not see it as an advantage with students from other groups, stating that after the initial work has started "what really matters is connecting with people and coming up with plans that can help students and make a noticeable difference in their education." He is assigned to an alternative middle school/high school program for at-risk students, including many students with disabilities, and also provides services to an elementary school one day a week. Roger likes the elementary school and says "it gives me a sense of perspective," but his clear passion is the alternative middle-secondary program: "These kids come to our school basically having failed or been thrown out or seen as the bad kid, but for most of them, they come here and it's like a new start. We get the right things into place for them and it's like putting water on a dying plant. I love it." The alternative school is relatively small, and one of Roger's assignments is to serve as the special services coordinator and assistant principal. He oversees the coordination of referrals for special education eligibility and mental health services. He also works individually with students and co-leads social and emotional learning classes with three to four teachers per week. "It's incredible how quickly some of these kids make gains. We still have lots of challenges, but we see on a weekly basis major positive changes happening in their lives."

In the past 4 years, Roger has sought out additional training in positive behavior support and has helped to introduce it schoolwide. "It's cut down our office discipline referrals by 45% since we started, and now that it's part of the routine, it really doesn't take that much time." His expertise in applied behavior analysis and functional assessment from graduate school provide a natural springboard for him to use in developing plans for the students who continue to act out even with positive behavior support in place, and he is integrally involved in writing behavioral goals and objectives for students who are on individualized education plans (IEPs).

Roger clearly loves his work and does not regret his decision to leave the corporate world, but he wishes there were greater resources available: "We need a full-time mental health specialist, and we could use two more teachers. And the supplies and materials and facilities are really pathetic. The corporate world wouldn't put up with these conditions for a minute." Despite the challenges, Roger would absolutely recommend a career in school psychology. "For someone who is not afraid to work hard and be flexible, it's a great way to make a definitive impact for good. If you have the right training and tools, you can measure what you are doing, and sometimes it amazes me how well we are able to get things turned around."

Dana: "A Great Time to Be a School Psychologist"

Dana works as a school psychologist in a large suburban school district in the midwestern United States, adjacent to one of the nation's largest cities. She serves one middle school (1,600 students) and one large elementary school (900 students). In addition, she serves on the district's crisis intervention response team and on a steering committee charged with guiding the district's practices and policies for at-risk and underserved students. In her mid-40s, Dana is a veteran school psychologist with 16 years of professional experience, including 3 years with a large urban school district in another state immediately after completion of her EdS degree.

Dana has worked in the field long enough to have seen some significant changes. Her graduate training emphasized individual cognitive and academic assessment as well as individual and small-group counseling. For her first few years in the field, much of her time was devoted to conducting individual psychoeducational assessments and participating in decision-making processes to determine which students would receive special education services because of a specific learning disability, guided by the traditional ability–achievement discrepancy model. She also carried a small caseload of students from her schools' programs for youth with emotional disturbances who required individual counseling.

Much has changed for Dana in recent years. "As soon as the 2004 Individuals with Disabilities Education Improvement Act was in place, we were positioned to begin moving to an RTI model for assessing students with learning problems, because some of our psychologists and our special education director had been moving in this direction. Now I give far fewer individual intelligence and achievement tests, and I spend more time helping teachers and the student support teams gather data and develop and monitor interventions. At first it was a hard transition, because I didn't have much training in those kind of tasks, but I got up to speed fairly soon. I really find that this is a better use of my skills—we're helping students earlier, and we spend much less time doing assessment just for the purpose of eligibility decisions."

Another major shift for Dana has been in how she supports students who have behavioral and emotional problems. She has always had a strong interest in this area, and has specifically stayed in her current assignment for so long because both of her schools have strong programs for supporting students who are eligible for special services under the behaviorally disabled (BD) category (her state's name for the federal "emotionally disturbed" [ED] category). Initially, most of her intervention work with BD/ED students was in individual counseling and small-group social skills training interventions. "These were good to an extent, but we were only serving a very small number of kids, out of necessity. But we moved to schoolwide positive behavior support about 10 years ago, and for the past 4 years both of my schools have been emphasizing social and emotional learning schoolwide and classwide, not just in small groups. We're now seeing much better results and I'm helping a lot more kids as a result." With regard to her interest in the BD/ED area, Dana states: "I'm not only involved in assessment, service eligibility, and providing services to students with BD, but I'm actively involved in helping the district focus on ethnic overrepresentation issues in the BD program. As an African American myself, I've been really aware and frustrated that our BD programs are identifying African American kids—particularly boys—at a rate so much higher than their presence in the school system in general. Some of these identifications are appropriate, but way too many have been questionable, and I tend to advocate very actively for not only making data-based decisions, but looking at cultural issues too. We've made some progress here, but have a long way to go."

Dana admits her work can be stressful and has had 1 or 2 years that were particularly challenging (she played a key role in responding to the aftermath of a school shooting a few years ago). Overall, however, she finds her profession and career to be very satisfying and rewarding. "Now is a really great time to be a school psychologist. Even with all the economic and budget and social issues we are facing, we have some really exciting possibilities. I wish the field was at the point it is now when I went through grad school and started my first job—I could have helped so many more kids."

Mariana: "One of the Most Rewarding Things I Can Imagine"

Mariana is a school psychology program faculty member at a regional state college in a small eastern U.S college town, a position she has held for 7 years. She was awarded tenure and promotion to the rank of associate professor 1 year ago. She mostly teaches graduate-level classes in her department's certificate of advanced graduate study (specialist-level) school psychology program, but also teaches two undergraduate courses in psychology each year, and she supervises her advisees' graduate thesis research. Prior to the start of her career as a university educator and school psychology trainer, Mariana completed her predoctoral internship and 1 additional year of work as a school psychologist in an urban school district in the northeastern United States. Her doctoral training was at a prominent program that had a strong orientation toward behavioral theory and school psychologists as problem solvers.

Mariana enjoyed her 2 years working as a full-time practitioner but was focused on the goal of becoming a faculty member from the start: "I've always loved the university setting, and the opportunity to be around new ideas and innovations that come with it. At first, I thought I wanted to focus a lot on research and work as a faculty member in a PhD program, but I found that I really loved the teaching and mentoring of students, and was less enthusiastic about teaching less but being expected to publish a lot more." Her greatest surprise in making the transition from practitioner to trainer was how much work was involved. "I knew that my mentor and the other faculty from grad school worked hard, but I really had no idea. The first 2 years I was constantly struggling just to be prepared for my classes and meetings the next day, and got almost no scholarship done. There are a lot of complex demands, and the job doesn't have as clear a starting and stopping point every day as I had in my work as a practitioner." After that initial transition, Mariana found her footing, improved her time management, and began to carve out an area of scholarship related to multicultural educational issues as well as mental health service delivery in schools. "These are really important areas, and there is so much to be done." Mariana loves working in her present role, and rates her mentorship of students as the single most satisfying part of the job. "To see these students progress from knowing very little about the field to becoming highly effective and respected school psychologists is one of the most rewarding things I can imagine. My work is impacting so many students indirectly, through the work of the students I trained. I honestly have no interest in doing anything else at this point in my career."

Tying It Together

The variety, personal investment, challenges, and impact reflected in the professional lives of the four composite school psychologists featured in these vignettes could easily be duplicated by conducting similar interviews with any four randomly selected school psychologists. It is also noteworthy that professional lives evolve over time. Those school psychologists profiled in this section have seen their career paths develop and change, sometimes in ways they never anticipated. The same could be said for any school psychologist who is committed to making in impact in the field. Although tied together by a collective professional identity and associations, every school psychologist has a unique story, makes unique contributions, and follows a unique path. And yet there is a commonality among them that ties them together and reflects the shared vision and unique identity that defines school psychology. We believe that this vision and identity stem from a focus on affecting the academic, behavioral, and social–emotional problems of children and youth in educational settings through the effective use of psychological principles and procedures and through the medium of "school psychology." This vision is also clearly tied to the personal commitment and idealism of those individuals who choose to join the field of school psychology. Although school psychologists have differing backgrounds, job descriptions, expectations, and professional ambitions, as a group they share a collective desire to positively influence the lives of children, adolescents, and their families. It is the incredible power of this collective individual idealism that fuels the impact and potential of the field.

How Does One Become a School Psychologist?

Having established a definition of school psychology and some of the characteristics of school psychologists, the next question that might be asked by someone exploring the field is "How does one become a school psychologist?" This question is dealt with in extensive detail in Chapter 4, which covers training and credentialing issues. To help us establish our basic introduction to school psychology, a few of the more elemental details regarding the paths that must be traveled to become a school psychologist are covered in this section.

To become a school psychologist, one must have completed a graduate-level program in school psychology and have received a credential (i.e., a certificate or license) to practice in the field. The specialist-degree level of training has become the minimum standard of preparation for entering the field. This level of training typically (but not always) requires approximately 2 years of full-time graduate study beyond the bachelor's degree and includes a field experience component (practicum and internship). NASP has advocated for a specialist standard of preparation requiring a minimum of 60 semester credits of graduate study and including a full-time academic-year internship. Because these standards are integrated into NASP's Nationally Certified School Psychologist credential (the NCSP, which is promoted and offered by NASP's National School Psychology Certification Board), the 60-credit/1,200-internship-hour specialist level of training has become the *de facto* standard in the field. It is worth noting that many graduate programs do not offer a specialist degree by that name but provide an equivalent level of training through a master's degree (MS, MA, or MEd) or certificate of advanced graduate study program.

Although the efforts of NASP to advocate for minimum training at the 60/1,200 specialist level have created a general standard, it is important to recognize that neither NASP nor any other professional organization actually credentials school psychologists for work in the field. There is no national-level licensing body that provides clearance to work as a school psychologist anywhere. Rather, credentialing of school psychologists is the responsibility of individual states and provinces. For school psychologists to work in public school settings, they must usually obtain a credential, which may be called a certificate or a license, from the educational licensing agency of the particular state or province where they intend to work. Usually, these agencies are part of the state or provincial department of education. Each state sets its own standards for entry into the field in that state, and some states have lower entry-level requirements than others. However, the NASP-advocated specialist level of training is almost always sufficient for credentialing in any state or province.

As if the differentiation between NASP professional standards and various state education department standards was not confusing enough, newcomers to the field are frequently surprised to find that there is another level of credentialing that is usually necessary to practice as a school psychologist outside of school settings. To become licensed as a psychologist to practice independently or to practice in settings such as hospitals, clinics, and community mental health agencies with the use of the title "psychologist," one must hold a doctoral degree in psychology (school psychology, counseling psychology, or clinical psychology) and be licensed by the professional psychology licensing board of a particular state or province. The doctoral level of professional psychology training, which usually requires 1 year of supervised predoctoral internship and 1 year of supervised postdoctoral residency (although, as noted in Chapters 4 and 5, several states no longer require supervised postdoctoral hours) as well as passing written and oral competency examinations that are required by many states, is what is advocated by APA and its various state affiliates. However, the APA position, as well as most state psychology licensing laws, includes provisions for the use of the title "school psychologist" (as opposed to "psychologist" or "licensed professional psychologist") with less than the doctoral level of training and without a psychology license, providing that the work is limited to school settings and is conducted under the banner of a school psychology credential from a state department of education.

There are currently close to 250 institutions of higher education in the United States and Canada that provide graduate training in school psychology at some level, and more than 300 different training programs exist at these institutions (Miller, 2008). Although the specialist level of graduate training has become the standard and typical mode of entry into the field for most school psychologists, a substantial percentage of school psychologists have earned doctoral degrees. Recent estimates of the percentage of school psychologists who have doctoral degrees have been around 32% for all school psychologists, although the percentage is lower (24.4%) for practitioners (Curtis, Lopez, et al., 2008). For about the past 30 years, the trend has been in the direction of steady but small increases in the proportion of school psychologists with doctoral degrees.

Individuals who enroll in school psychology graduate training programs have a variety of undergraduate backgrounds, the most common of which are psychology and education. A generation ago, it was not uncommon for individuals entering the field of school psychology to have had backgrounds in education, perhaps some experience as teachers, and in many cases to be midcareer (i.e., in their 30s or 40s), but these background characteristics appear to be less common now. We are not aware of any studies or data that have tracked the age, undergraduate preparation, and background of students entering school psychology programs over the years, but it has been our experience that the trend has been toward students entering graduate school in their early to mid-20s, more often than not with an undergraduate degree in psychology and often with limited volunteer or professional experience in psychology or education. We anticipate that as education and mental health fields become increasingly professionalized and that as higher levels of educational attainment become more common, these trends in school psychology training will continue and become even more noticeable.

Differentiating School Psychology from Related Professions

In addition to understanding what school psychology is all about and how one becomes a school psychologist, prospective graduate students who are beginning to explore the possibility of a career in this field must also decide whether to pursue school psychology or some closely related field. As school psychology faculty members, we visit with prospective graduate students on an ongoing basis. Although many prospective school psychologists have a very clear idea what being a school psychologist involves and how school psychology differs from some of its sister fields, many do not. Most trainers have likely sat through meetings with prospective students who assumed that they were considering entering a school counseling training program, for example. Because there are important differences not only in the entry-level requirements but also in the typical role and function of various fields, it is very important for prospective graduate students to get a clear picture of how school psychology is both similar to and different from its sister fields in psychology and education.

Related Fields in Psychology

At the doctoral level of training, there are other areas of professional psychology that overlap considerably with school psychology and that may prepare professional psychologists to work with children, adolescents, and their families. Historically, school psychology has been included with two other fields, *clinical psychology* and *counseling psychology*, as one of the three applied areas of professional psychology. Completing a doctoral program in any one of these three fields will, in part, prepare one to become a board-licensed professional psychologist and to work in a variety of clinic, private practice, community, and medical settings. Clinical and counseling psychology programs have not traditionally focused on schools and educational issues as school psychology has, and they do not typically prepare students to work primarily in school settings. However, many clinical and counseling psychology programs focus on working with children, adolescents, and their families and provide a path toward a predoctoral internship and postdoctoral residency year in a child-focused setting, providing assessment, intervention, and consultation services. Historically, there have been some important differences between clinical and counseling psychology, with the former field focusing more on abnormal behavior and psychopathology and the latter on normal developmental and adjustment issues of life. However, these distinctions have become increasingly blurred in recent years, and today it is not uncommon to find clinical psychologists working in college counseling centers and counseling psychologists working in hospitals and community mental health clinics.

Within clinical, counseling, and school psychology, some subspecialties focusing on children, youth, and their families have emerged in recent years, and these subspecialties are usually not specific to one field of psychology. For example, just as APA has a division devoted to school psychology (Division 16), it has separate divisions devoted to child, family, and youth services (Division 37), clinical child and adolescent psychology (Division 53), and pediatric psychology (Division 54). Child and adolescent neuropsychology has also emerged as a strong subspecialty within the division of neuropsychology (Division 40). These specialty areas include doctoral-level psychologists who are graduates of school, clinical, or counseling psychology programs, who have received specific specialty training, and who have developed particular expertise and interests in the respective specialty area.

With these related psychology fields and specialty areas, school psychology shares a focus on children, youth, and their families. What makes school psychology unique among these related areas within psychology is the specific focus on schools as practice settings and on educational and learning issues as primary concerns. Although some overlap exists among these areas, they all have a unique identity.

Related Fields in Education

Because school psychology is rooted in education as well as psychology, there are professions specific to education with which we share common concerns and professional overlap. *School counseling* is perhaps the best known of these related educational professions. This field grew out of the mental hygiene and child guidance movements of the

early 20th century, and its focus has evolved from vocational guidance and college placement to the promotion of a comprehensive model of student development, adjustment,
and growth at all grade levels. The American School Counselor Association has been
in existence since 1952 and currently has more than 27,000 members internationally.
Many more school counselors than school psychologists are employed in schools. Within
the United States, the national average ratio of school counselors to students is slightly
less than 1:500 (American School Counselor Association, 2010), whereas the national
average for school psychologists is estimated at about 1:1,500 (Fagan & Wise, 2007). In
terms of differences in training and job focus between the two fields, school psychologists tend to receive more training in individual assessment methods and intervention
techniques than do school counselors and have historically focused more on students
with disabilities. School counselors are more likely to be assigned to work at a single
school, whereas school psychologists are often itinerant and may have responsibility for
two to four schools or may work on a districtwide basis. Much of this difference in site-
based versus itinerant service models is related to the large differences in professional to
student ratios, which are much smaller for school counselors.

In addition to school psychologists and school counselors, *school social workers* are also
employed in public and private schools. This profession is part of the larger field of social
work, and it began in the early 1900s in the large urban areas of the northeast United
States out of a concern for underprivileged youth and their families. The first school
social workers often were part of psychological clinics in the schools and had the title
of "visiting teachers." Their role was often focused on home visits and advocacy for children and their families who were living in tenements in industrial areas. Today, school
social workers maintain some of the same historical emphasis on advocacy and working
with at-risk students, but they tend to work on multidisciplinary teams with psychologists,
counselors, teachers, and nurses and to focus on a broad array of mental health and
social–behavioral adjustment issues. It is difficult to estimate the number of school social
workers nationwide. It is widely understood that there are far fewer school social workers
than school psychologists, although an exact professional-to-student ratio is not known.

Although school counseling and school social work are the two best known professions within education that are closely related to school psychology, there are other
professional roles in schools that have much in common with our field. These other roles
are not necessarily defined as separate professions but have evolved as specialty positions
in education in many school systems. Special education consultants, service coordina-
tors, behavioral specialists, or consulting teachers are often employed in larger school
districts and have the responsibility of working with teachers, other educators, and parents in developing appropriate educational programs for students, especially those who
are at risk for negative outcomes or who are otherwise having difficulty in school. Such
consultant or coordinator positions are often filled from the ranks of experienced and
talented teachers, but sometimes they are filled by individuals with school psychology
backgrounds. These roles usually involve extensive indirect intervention through consultation, and they may have a problem-solving or training focus as well. In addition, some
schools hire teachers or counselors to serve as educational diagnosticians or educational
assessment specialists. These types of positions include an exclusive focus on individual
assessment of students with learning and behavior problems, and on the surface they
seem quite similar to the role of school psychologists who are in very traditional "test-
and-place" assessment roles.

Although most school psychologists remain employed with that title, those who have
the aptitude and interest to pursue other roles within schools often find that there are

opportunities for career shifts within school systems. Some school psychologists move into educational leadership positions, such as pupil personnel directors, special education administrators, and school principals. Typically, career moves of this type require the individual to obtain additional graduate-level education in order to receive an administrative credential. School psychologists who have particular expertise in research methods, statistics, and psychometrics sometimes move into district-level positions as directors of research services, directors of testing/assessment and analysis, and so forth.

Using This Book: A Vision for School Psychology

As stated in the preface, this book is designed to provide an introduction and orientation to the field of school psychology. We especially intend for this book to be of interest to graduate students who are beginning to prepare for careers in the field of school psychology. This book is also designed to be an exploratory resource for individuals who are considering careers in school psychology as well as those who are currently working as school psychologists and who are interested in a guide to this dynamic and exciting field.

Chapter 2 of this text provides brief overviews of the historical context of the field as well as of history and trends in American education. Chapters 3 through 6 provide a foundation for the professional practice of school psychology, focusing on cultural and linguistic diversity, training and credentialing issues, employment trends and challenges, and legal and ethical aspects of practice in this field. Chapters 7 through 12 detail our vision of best practice in school psychology and focus on the wide range of goals that we believe school psychologists should pursue, including a data-oriented problem-solving approach to practice; assessment; prevention and intervention; facilitation of systems-level change; and involvement as a consumer and producer of research and evaluation. Chapter 13 provides some concluding comments regarding moving the field of school psychology forward and mapping our own future as professionals. Together, the 13 chapters in this book provide a comprehensive and, in our view, state-of-the-art introduction to the field of school psychology.

You may have noted that we use the phrase "school psychology for the 21st century" in the title of this book. Our focus on the 21st century was a very deliberate choice. In deciding to write this book, we were not interested in simply providing an overview of the history and current status of the field, which have been well documented in other sources. Rather, we were interested in promoting a forward-thinking vision of the exciting and dynamic possibilities within the field of school psychology. We believe that the field of school psychology has much to offer and that its potential is just beginning to emerge. The possibilities of this field making a strong positive impact in schools and other settings and in the lives of children, adolescents, and their families are simply enormous. We also believe that there are still several barriers to achieving this vision, foremost of which are the low expectations of other professionals for school psychology, which have unfortunately often been perpetuated by the narrow vision of some school psychologists and school psychology trainers. We are not naive about the institutional challenges, obstacles, and barriers that many school psychologists face in using their professional skills and interests to achieve the maximum good. Rather, we believe that through a concerted effort over time school psychologists can individually and collectively advance the field at all levels and that, in doing so, school psychology will make an enormous positive impact.

Although each chapter within this book is unique, they were developed through a collective vision. Some of the "big ideas" on which this book and our vision for the field of school psychology are based include the following:

• The general fields of psychology and education, as well as the specific field of school psychology, have given us rich and sometimes challenging historical precedents for the present practice of school psychology. Although it is important to have a strong understanding of these historical elements and how they have shaped the present, we agree with the premise that *the past is not necessarily the future*, and we advocate that the time has come for the field of school psychology to move forward from some of the historical challenges that have limited it in realizing its full potential.

• American society has become increasingly diverse and pluralistic with respect to cultural background, race, ethnicity, and language of its citizens, and it will continue to become increasingly diverse during the 21st century. School psychologists should develop cultural competence so that they can work appropriately and effectively with individuals and groups from a variety of backgrounds (see Chapter 3).

• School psychology has been and should continue to be primarily focused in school or other educational settings. The educational setting is a main focus of our vision and of this book. However, school psychologists have much to offer outside the context of school settings, and we encourage the practice of school psychology in a variety of settings and contexts (see Chapters 4 and 5).

• Individual psychoeducational assessment of children and adolescents has been and will continue to be an important activity of school psychologists. However, individual assessment activities should do more than simply describe or diagnose problems. Rather, the most useful assessment strategies are those that are part of the problem-solving process and provide a foundation for effective interventions (see Chapter 8).

• School psychology practice should be data oriented or data driven. School psychologists should base their decisions on valid data and use effective data collection techniques to inform, monitor, and modify intervention activities (see Chapter 7).

• School psychologists should be savvy consumers of research and should have the skills to engage in research and evaluation activities within their respective settings that will help to advance practice (see Chapter 12).

• School psychologists have historically worked with a limited segment of student populations, primarily those who have or are suspected of having disabilities and those who are otherwise at high risk for negative outcomes in life. We believe that there will always be a need for school psychologists to focus some of their effort on the small percentage of students who have serious learning, behavioral, and social–emotional problems. We also recognize that longitudinal research points to the chronic nature of such problems and the critical need for *early* intervention/prevention if negative long-term outcomes are to be curtailed. Thus, we strongly contend that school psychologists should use their unique expertise to positively affect *all students in school settings*, not just those who have severe needs.

• Although assessment activities have had and will continue to have an important place among the school psychologist's varied responsibilities, effective prevention and intervention activities should occupy a significant percentage of his or her time (see Chapters 9 and 10).

- Prevention and intervention activities can occur with individuals, within small groups, within classrooms, within entire schools, and within school district or community-based contexts. School psychologists should engage in prevention and intervention activities, including consultation, at each of these levels, so that a larger number of individuals may be positively influenced (see Chapters 9 and 10).

- School psychologists do not typically function in isolation but instead work in consultation and collaboration with others and as part of a system. School psychologists should strive to use their expertise to develop a solid understanding of the systems in which they work and to help facilitate systems-level change as needed (see Chapter 11).

- School psychology is a field with incredible potential for helping to solve the "big" problems facing education. And yet this potential is still largely unrealized. We believe that school psychologists should play an active, important, and essential role in this regard. This book is built on the foundation of a progressive, forward-thinking vision of school psychology, and we are optimistic that collectively individual school psychologists can continue to move the field forward through their efforts (see Chapter 13).

In sum, school psychology is a dynamic and exciting field that has incredible and still unrealized potential for positively affecting education, psychology, and the lives of children, adolescents, and their families. It is our hope that this book will provide a useful and engaging guide to the field of school psychology and will help to continue to move the field forward.

DISCUSSION QUESTIONS AND ACTIVITIES

1. Individuals who are being introduced to the field of school psychology are often surprised to find that the definition of school psychology is not necessarily clear-cut and has, at times, been a point of controversy. Discuss the power of definitions and how they can shape the field of school psychology and how it is perceived.

2. During the past several decades, the characteristics of school psychologists have changed somewhat. Characterize some of these changes, and describe the current characteristics of those who work in the field of school psychology.

3. Interview one or more school psychologists in your area. Find out how they entered the field, what their career trajectory has been, what their responsibilities and roles are, and how they spend a typical day, week, and month in their workplace. Ask what they like most or find most rewarding about their work as school psychologists and what they find to be most frustrating or difficult.

4. One of the first decisions that new graduate students in school psychology make is whether to pursue a master's/specialist degree or a doctoral degree. How do the two levels of training differ, and what are the costs and benefits, pros and cons, to each?

5. Differentiate the training and roles of school psychologists at the doctoral level from that of the two other primary areas of professional psychology: clinical psychology and counseling psychology. Differentiate the training and roles of school psychologists at the specialist or master's level from that in the fields of school counseling and school social work.

CHAPTER 2

The Historical Context of School Psychology

In comparison to many other established scientific and academic fields, school psychology is relatively young. It has been in existence for barely a century and has been a formidable organized professional entity for only a few decades. To fully understand the field of school psychology in the 21st century, it is essential to understand its roots. As can be inferred from Chapter 1, we agree with Reschly and Ysseldyke's (2002) observation that the past is not necessarily the future with respect to the field of school psychology, but we also believe that a basic understanding of the past is essential if we are to continue to move the field forward. This chapter provides a brief excursion into the historical context of school psychology. First, we explore its philosophical and intellectual foundations, ranging from classical Greek to modern European influences. Some of the major events, movements, and individuals in the emergence of the field of psychology in general, and the field of school psychology in particular, are examined. We then detail aspects of the historical context of American education as they relate to the development of school psychology. We provide an overview of major events and issues in the development and professionalization of the field of school psychology and link them to the recent history of the field, with a particular emphasis on legal developments and training and credentialing issues that have had a strong impact on the recent history of school psychology. Ongoing tensions or "culture wars" that have surrounded school psychology's rise to prominence are examined, including values conflicts within various dimensions of the field and the historical and current differences between the two primary organizations representing the field. The chapter ends with some discussion of what lessons and trends have been apparent in the history of the field and what these issues may portend for the future.

Philosophical, Intellectual, and Social–Cultural Foundations

The most influential historian in the field of school psychology, Thomas Fagan, has stated that "no significant aspect of contemporary school psychology, including its practitioners, training programs, or credentialing, existed before the 1890s" (Fagan & Wise, 2007, p. 25). Thus, at first glance, it appears that there may not be any point to tracing the historical context of the field prior to the late 19th century. However, it is important to recognize that school psychology did not develop in a social or cultural vacuum. Rather, its emergence was the product of a confluence of forces and timing. Therefore, it is useful to look at some of the more notable historical forces that contributed not only to the birth of school psychology but also to the larger fields of psychology and education in general.

Classical Greek Influences

Psychology is considered to be a Western discipline, given that its philosophical, intellectual, and cultural foundations stem from ancient and modern forces flowing from the classical world of ancient Greece to modern Europe. It has been said that there is no distinctive aspect of psychology that cannot be traced to the philosophical world of the Greeks (Leahey, 1987). Specifically, most modern psychological thought can be traced to the various philosophies espoused and shaped in succession by three prominent Greek philosophers: Socrates (470–399 B.C.), his student Plato (428–348 B.C.), and particularly Plato's student Aristotle (384–322 B.C.), a founder of the philosophy of science who was known as the "first professor."

Socrates was an itinerant teacher whose work focused on the meaning of general ideas or constructs, especially truth, justice, and beauty. Socrates was antagonistic toward the Sophists, a group of Athenian teachers who espoused a worldview that we might today term *humanistic relativism* or *postmodernism*. The Sophists proposed that "man is the measure of all things," meaning that all experience is subjective and that it is not possible to derive an ultimate reality because of individual differences in the way that reality is perceived. Socrates believed that the ideas of the Sophists were dangerous and could lead to moral anarchy. By posing provocative questions that contrasted sharply with the views of the Sophists, he promoted the notion that ultimate general truths existed and that there were enduring laws or principles that could lead to such truth. However, Socrates did not provide answers to most of his own questions. Rather, it was his famous student Plato who provided answers through written dialogues based on Socrates's questions.

Plato extended Socrates's quest for general universal truths to encompass a quest for all forms of knowledge. Thus, *epistemology*, or the study of theories of knowledge or various *ways of knowing*, was born. Although Plato was concerned with ways of deriving knowledge, his focus and methods did not lend themselves very well to the scientific study of human behavior. It was Aristotle who first promoted the philosophy of empiricism, which ultimately became a foundation of modern psychology. Aristotle's views were in many ways antithetical to those of his teacher, Plato. Aristotle moved away from the somewhat mystical ideas of Plato and firmly established a foundation for scientific thought that was based on observation. It is worth noting that Aristotle was the first to conduct a systematic "literature review" of the works of earlier thinkers (Leahey, 1987), a technique for laying the groundwork for particular problems that later became a bedrock practice of psychological science and a practice that is certainly familiar to any graduate student in school psychology.

The cultural, artistic, and philosophical activity of the Greek and Roman worlds began to decline noticeably around 300 A.D. By the fall of Rome in the late fifth century, the intellectual energy characterized by the work of the Greek philosophers had largely dissipated, and it was centuries before there was a revival of significant cultural and intellectual life in the Western world. The Dark Ages marked a long period of retrench-ment in these areas, and it affected every level of society. However, despite the ending of the incredible accomplishments of the classical era, an important legacy was left to influence future generations. In particular, one of the hallmark intellectual tensions that emerged in the Greek period—the conflict between rationalism and empiricism—carried into greater European culture and became one of the primary foundational influences that led to the emergence of psychology.

Modern European Influences

By the time the new discipline of psychology emerged in the late 19th century, and public education was becoming an increasingly important aspect of American society, the West-ern world had emerged from centuries of intellectual and artistic retrenchment. During the church–state-controlled medieval period, virtually the only persons who could read and write in most of Europe were clerics, and rigid rules were imposed regarding the development and dissemination of written literature. In addition, questions regarding the structure, function, and meaning of human behavior, which had flowed with great energy during the classical period, became the nearly exclusive province of the religious orthodoxy. Individuals who dared challenge the status quo often put their liberty and even their lives at risk. A couple of famous examples illustrate very well the rigid and oppressive hierarchical intellectual climate of those times. Italian scientist-philosopher Galileo Galilei (1564–1642) spent the latter part of his life under house arrest because his Copernicanistic views of the universe (i.e., that the earth and other planets revolved around the sun) were found to be heretical. Protestant scholar and Englishman Wil-liam Tyndale (c. 1494–1536) was brutally killed and his body burned for the offense of secretly translating much of the Bible from Greek into English and making it available to nonclerics.

Despite the restrictive and oppressive intellectual tone of the times, the new energy and ideas that began to flow during the Renaissance period did stem from some roots that were established during the middle ages. It is interesting to consider that the com-mingling of Christianity, Islam, and Judaism in the Near East produced and preserved some important written works and that Tyndale's unauthorized translation of the Bible into vernacular language was an important intellectual development, not just a religious issue.

By the 17th century, the modern scientific revolution had begun. Prominent figures such as René Descartes (1596–1650) and John Locke (1632–1704) emerged and revital-ized the philosophy of science and its empirical and epistemological roots. Descartes wrote and taught regarding the process of seeking truth in a skeptical manner, of the native physical or material structure of the world, and, importantly, of the *dualism* of the body and mind of humans, which he saw as distinct elements. Descartes's identi-fication of thought as a central component of human experience led him to coin his famous axiom "I think, therefore I am." Locke, on the other hand, dismissed the notion of innate moral and metaphysical truths and advocated discovering truth through per-sonal experience. An important aspect of Locke's work for the formation of psychology and the advancement of education was his focus on the mind and on the process of using reflection or introspection to gain knowledge. In many ways, Locke's work was a pre-cursor to the science of the mind, paving the way for theories of intelligence, learning, and cognitive processing. Other 17th-century thinkers also provided important founda-tions for the emergence of psychology and the refinement of educational pedagogy. For example, Thomas Hobbes (1588–1679) was the first intellectual who explored the connection between the development of speech and the development of reasoning. He also introduced the concept of *natural law*, the notion that there were regulations inherent in nature, whether or not humans recognized them. This concept was a precursor to the psychological principle that behavior is lawful and is governed by basic principles, a concept that became especially important in behavioral psychology.

The 18th century is considered a period of enlightenment in the Western world, with major developments (and revolutions) in science, philosophy, art, and politics. Many of the developments of this period provided a further foundation for the emergence of psychology during the next century. David Hume (1711–1776) was a moderate skeptic who wrote extensively on the notion of *habit* or *custom*, the propensity to behave, think, and feel in customary and predictable ways. Hume desired to apply Newtonian-like laws to predict human behavior, using the technique of introspection to generate his ideas. One particularly psychological contribution of Hume was his development of a classification of the contents of the human mind, which focused on perceptions and distinguished between impressions and ideas.

In opposition to the notions espoused by Hume and various other skeptics, a school of thought emerged out of Scotland by the mid-18th century that espoused "common sense" in analyzing and understanding human behavior. This assertion of common sense, typified by the writing of Thomas Reid (1710–1796) and his student Dugald Stewart (1753–1828), ridiculed the claims of philosophy and posited that everyday experience provides a better foundation for understanding human thought and behavior than the theories of skeptics, which they considered to be absurd. The writings of both these men dissected the mind into component faculties and advocated the practical value of the study of human behavior and thought. One of the foremost thinkers of the century was German philosopher Immanuel Kant (1724–1804). Kant developed a science of understanding humanity, which he called anthropology but which actually bears more similarity to psychology. He studied human intelligence, moral character, the notion of self, and other constructs that would become important within psychology. Kant's work greatly influenced fellow German Wilhelm Wundt, who later developed the first psychology laboratory. Another Enlightenment-era figure whose writings proved to be highly influential in psychology (and in education and politics) was Genevois philosopher Jean-Jacques Rousseau (1712–1778). Rousseau became known for many things, including his influence on political revolutionaries Marx and Engel, who were intrigued with his notions of free will and of the innate freedom of humans and with his criticism of Enlightenment-era scientific and technological advances, which Rousseau viewed as chaining or enslaving people. He advocated for education as the means of overcoming the corrupt state of civilization. Rousseau was one of the first intellectuals to discuss in detail the *nature versus nurture* dichotomy of the influence on human behavior, and he weighed in on the side of nurture, believing that external conditions and influences, rather than innate drives, shaped the individual. Interestingly and somewhat paradoxically, his belief in human malleability foreshadowed B. F. Skinner's advocacy of using a carefully controlled society to enhance human potential (as espoused in his book *Walden II*, in which he admitted to shouting at his animal research subjects *"Behave damn you! Behave as you ought!"* when his predictions went awry) and also served as inspiration for "whole child" education advocates, who rejected highly structured and sequenced teaching of basic skills as advocated by Skinner.

In sum, 17th- and 18th-century intellectual developments, which are often referred to as the Age of Reason and the Age of Enlightenment, helped move Western thinking out of the Dark Ages and the medieval period and provided the intellectual foundation for the birth of psychology, as well as developments in education, that would provide an impetus for school psychology. And unlike the classic Greek philosophers, whose work was foundational for psychology, many of the prominent intellectuals of the 17th and 18th centuries overtly concerned themselves with issues and constructs that were distinctly psychological, regardless of the fact that the field had not yet emerged.

The Emergence of Psychology

Although the foundation of psychology had been laid in the preceding centuries, the discipline formally emerged in the mid- to late 19th century, first in Europe, and then in America. Certain 19th-century influences made a strong impression on the emerging field. One of the foremost influences was the work of English naturalist Charles Darwin (1809–1882), whose elucidation of a scientific theory of natural selection in evolution revolutionized science. His 1859 seminal work *On the Origin of Species* broadly influenced Western intellectual circles, and his later works on the descent of humans and the expression of emotions in humans and animals became cornerstone literature in the fledgling field of psychology. German physiologist Franz Joseph Gall (1758–1828) developed the science of phrenology, or the description and prediction of human traits from bumps on the head and the shape of the cranium. Although phrenology is now relegated to a status only slightly higher than an amusing footnote, it must be understood that it was an enormously influential enterprise. More important, phrenology focused the seat of human behavior clearly on the brain, correlating specific regions of the brain with specific behavioral functions. In a sense, Gall's phrenology was the first formal expression of physiological psychology, especially the study of brain–behavior relationships.

By late in the 19th century, the discipline of psychology became formally established and legitimized, and three forms of psychology had emerged: the psychology of consciousness, the psychology of the unconscious, and the psychology of adaptation. German scientist and philosopher Wilhelm Wundt (1832–1920) is credited with establishing the first psychology laboratory in 1879 and establishing psychology as an independent experimental science. Wundt's work focused on the experimental study of individual consciousness. On the other hand, Viennese physician Sigmund Freud (1856–1939), who is credited as being the father of psychiatry, introduced ideas as radical as Darwin's by suggesting that unconscious desires and motives shape much of human behavior. Freud's deterministic views of human behavior and the unconscious were truly revolutionary. Although many of his theories have now been rejected even by proponents of the psychodynamic approach he pioneered, one must not overlook the enormity of his contributions and influence. Even today, his metaphor of the conscious mind as being the "tip of the iceberg" of human experience is widely used, the notion of the "subconscious" mind is part of the popular vernacular, and the influence of his work in Western cultures cannot be minimized. In addition, the psychology of adaptation, with roots in Darwin's theory of natural selection, focused on how the individual adjusts to the environment and, ultimately, how the environment shapes behavior. This psychology later developed into behaviorism, which became perhaps the most influential force of the 20th century in academic psychology.

By the end of the 19th century, psychology had moved from an emerging to an established field. American and European universities established psychology curricula and began awarding academic degrees in psychology. The APA was established in 1891.

Seminal texts were published, and scientific journals were established. Although the clinical or practical application of psychology was not yet established, all the pieces were in place for that to happen. Through these events and forces, the conditions that allowed for the development and establishment of school psychology were established.

Developments in American Education

We have tried to make it clear that the field of school psychology was hatched from a confluence of intellectual and social developments in both psychology and education. This section provides additional discussion regarding some of the important historical developments in American education that were important in this confluence.

Colonial Foundations

Although most educational historians have identified the period of about 1825 to 1875 as the era during which the building blocks of American public education were put into place (i.e., Butts, 1978; Calhoun, 1969), there were important historical antecedents during the prior two centuries that led to this series of developments. During the American colonial period in the 17th century, public schools as we now know them did not exist, but the idea of public education began to sprout, particularly in the New England colonies. Although there was generally no public taxation for schools or compulsory education laws during this period, the notion of education for the public good became more prominent, and the idea that formal education of youth would serve a greater civic purpose began to take hold. Most of the formal efforts to educate young people involved a primary component of religious instruction, and the preparation of future clerics was a major emphasis in this regard. By the early to mid-1700s, colonial society was becoming increasingly pluralistic with respect to religious views (albeit within the general Christian worldview, particularly the Protestant version; see Smith, 1967). Tensions were increasing regarding the appropriate place of religious instruction and influence within civic or public life and the legitimacy of public efforts to promote the superiority of one religion over another (Butts, 1978). These tensions ultimately helped lead to the "establishment" clause in the U.S. Constitution and to the weakening of legal bonds between established churches and new states following the revolutionary period.

With the establishment of the first state constitutions in the late 1700s, some states (such as North Carolina, Georgia, and Pennsylvania) adopted specific provisions for public schooling, although it would be many years before these efforts resulted in a strong system of public education. During this same time period, there was considerable national tension between those leaders who favored a strong centralized role for national government (the Federalists) and those who advocated for a weaker federal system and the sovereignty of individual states (the Democratic-Republicans). Interestingly, during this late-18th-century debate regarding the proper role of the federal government, several prominent voices argued in favor of a strong national system of public education, including a national university, goals that never came to fruition. Ultimately, the framers of the U.S. Constitution left somewhat vague the appropriate role of the federal government in public education, with education considered a "creature of the states." As the 19th century emerged, conditions varied greatly from state to state regarding public education efforts, which had not yet risen as a visible, identifiable entity (Butts, 1978; Calhoun, 1969).

19th-Century Steps

During the 1800s, significant steps were taken toward the development of systems of public education. Underlying this development was the growing belief that voluntary and private efforts to formally educate America's young citizens were insufficient and that the new democracy could not flourish under such conditions. As many of the cities in the northeastern United States grew rapidly with industrialization, so did the number of poor and uneducated youth. This, along with deteriorating social conditions, led to a public outcry to reverse the trend and improve the situation. As a result, "common schools," the precursor to today's public schools, began to be established (Butts, 1978; Ravitch, 1974), primarily in the mid-Atlantic and New England states but also in Virginia and the Carolinas. The growth of the abolition movement and the relative lack of common schools in the southern states set the stage further for the development of public systems of education.

Following the horrors of the Civil War and the end of the institution of slavery, the nation was in massive debt, many of the southern cities were in shambles from the war, and the industrialization that had swept the northern cities slowly began to move to the urban areas southward. Thus, the Reconstruction period saw further expansion of the common schools, increasing efforts to ensure that African American youth received a public education, and an expansion of compulsory schooling laws, particularly in urban centers (Best & Sidwell, 1967; Tyack, 1967). This period of expansion was aided by the increasingly centralized power of governments at both the state and national levels. As governmental authority became more centralized, typically a concurrent increase occurred in efforts to promote common schools and to provide a financial base from which to support them (Berlin, 1974).

20th-Century Developments, Persistent Issues

By the early 1900s, the combination of (1) systems of public and compulsory education in the United States, (2) social conditions following industrialization and reconstruction, and (3) the emergence of new educational tools and scientific technologies was becoming extremely complex. The field of public education began to grow rapidly at the same time that the budding discipline of psychology was emerging in the United States. Thus, the conditions were in place that allowed, or perhaps required, the incipient field of school psychology to begin its toehold during what has come to be known as the Progressive Era in American social history (Tyack, 1967). One of the greatest impacts of the Progressive Era on education was the combination of more far-reaching child labor laws and compulsory education laws. By the end of the first decade of the 20th century, all states had compulsory education laws of some type in place, and by 1920 almost all American children attended schools, at least through the elementary school level (History of American Education Web Project, 2010; Tyack, 1967).

Before we move into the beginnings of the field of school psychology, it is worth considering that by the first quarter of the 20th century two persistent and significant issues in American education had developed that would have long-lasting implications (even to the present day) for school psychology: the development of the IQ or mental ability testing movement and the common state of racial segregation and inequality in schools. We consider these two issues in more detail, because they both have had a major impact on school psychology. The movers in the mental ability testing arena had, by the end of World War I, developed great confidence in the potential of IQ tests to measure the human mind, and this confidence spread throughout much of public education. Most of the individuals who were influential in this movement, such as Lewis Terman and Henry Goddard, held a *nativist* view of intelligence, interpreting it as inherited, essentially fixed, and difficult if not impossible to modify in any meaningful way through education. The power of the IQ testing movement became enormous and led to what distinguished educational historian Diane Ravitch (2000) termed "a brutal pessimism" regarding educational programming, tracking, and opportunities. In essence, the results of IQ tests were used—initially with little criticism—to determine in great measure individuals' opportunities and future. "The intelligence testers promoted fatalism, a rueful acceptance that achievement in school is the result of innate ability, not sustained effort by teachers and students. The cult of the IQ became an all purpose rationale for students' lack of effort and for poor teaching: Why study hard in school if IQ predicts outcomes? Why work hard to teach slow learners if their IQs predict they cannot do well in school?" (Ravitch, 2000, p. 161). As anyone familiar with school psychology knows, the development of the field ultimately became inextricably linked to the IQ testing movement, a connection that, we argue, plagues the field to this day despite the recent influence of the RTI approach, and that is still commonly cited as a barrier to moving the role of school psychologists to a greater focus on prevention, intervention, and consultation. This issue is discussed in greater detail in several other chapters of this volume. It is also worth considering that the IQ movement influenced American education well beyond the practice of school psychology. The practices and notions that came from this movement were often used as a basis for excluding children with disabilities from public schools (an issue discussed in more detail in Chapter 6), for routing students into vocational versus academic tracks, and for reducing the focus on alterable variables (such as student and teacher effort, curriculum delivery, school structure) within schools (Ravitch, 2000).

With respect to racial segregation, tension, and inequalities in American public education, the struggle has been long and divisive, and it has taken legal precedents from the nation's highest courts to steer improvements and standards that are still evolving and trying to fulfill their promise. During the colonial period and the early years of the nation, public education efforts were aimed almost exclusively at white children: Native Americans were essentially left out, Asians and individuals of Hispanic descent did not yet exist in large enough numbers to develop a critical mass for advocacy, and laws throughout the southern states prohibited educating African American slaves, who existed in large numbers. There were relatively few exceptions to this state of affairs. By the advent of the Reconstruction era in the late 1800s, African American children began to be offered formal opportunities for public schooling in increasingly greater numbers, but for the most part and for many years these opportunities existed in separate systems that were operated at a severe disadvantage, with far fewer resources than other public schools. As educational opportunities for African Americans increased, serious debates took place among the community of black leaders regarding what direction was best, as typified by the debates between Booker T. Washington (who advocated for a practical, industrial education for blacks) and W. E. B. Du Bois (who advocated for an intellectually rigorous education for blacks and derided practical education efforts as second class).

As the 20th century evolved, two forces began to merge that gradually began to chip away at these historical antecedents. First, American society was becoming increasingly diverse and pluralistic as a result of patterns of immigration dating to the late 1800s. Second, legal advocacy and public discourse regarding the education of children from minority group backgrounds increased. The 1954 landmark ruling of the U.S. Supreme Court in *Brown v. Board of Education* was the culmination of many years of advocacy to change inequity. This ruling held that segregated educational environments were bad for children and that the notion of "separate but equal" treatment in America (which became the law of the land in the court's 1892 *Plessy v. Ferguson* decision) was a cruel myth. With the passing of the 50th anniversary of *Brown*, it is now apparent that, notwithstanding the substantial gains made following this and other court decisions, the full promise of equality has yet to be fulfilled. School psychologists are currently dealing with two major issues related to race, ethnicity, and social class: (1) The "achievement gap" (between white/Asian and black/Hispanic/Native American students) in educational attainment is becoming an increasingly serious issue for educators and policymakers, and (2) minority misrepresentation in special education programs (particularly overrepresentation among African American youth) continues to present significant challenges. In addition, the past two to three decades have witnessed increased emphasis on developing and using culturally and linguistically appropriate assessment and intervention techniques. Issues related to ethnic and cultural issues in public schools are addressed in more detail in other chapters of this volume, particularly Chapter 3.

Beginnings of School Psychology

Although Fagan's assertion that no significant aspect of school psychology existed before the 1890s (Fagan & Wise, 2007) is indeed accurate, it is important to understand that the seeds from which the field would spring were already planted by that time. In addition to the establishment of psychology as a unique discipline by the late 1800s, other forces paved the way for the emergence of school psychology. As we have noted, the industrialization and urbanization of America, increased support for public education, the beginnings of the compulsory schooling movement, and post-Civil War social changes all contributed to a need for professionals to focus on education, child development, mental health, and other aspects of support, training, and supervision for children in an increasingly complex society.

One of the seminal events in the beginnings of school psychology was the 1896 establishment of a psychological clinic by Lightner Witmer at the University of Pennsylvania in Philadelphia. This clinic has been referred to as the first child guidance clinic. Witmer's goal was to prepare psychologists to help educators solve children's learning problems (Bardon & Bennett, 1974). With this contribution, Witmer has been credited as the founder of both school psychology and clinical psychology. This clinic was clearly the first effort of its kind in North America. However, a somewhat similar laboratory clinic had been established by Sir Francis Galton at University College in London in 1884, predating Witmer's American clinic by 12 years. Although the primary purpose of Galton's laboratory was the measurement of individual human differences rather than direct service, one of its first endeavors was to assist local schools in selecting and classifying pupils. Thus, some writers have argued that the birth of school psychology may be more appropriately credited to Galton's laboratory in England (White & Harris, 1961).

One of the events almost always mentioned in the same breath as the beginning of school psychology is the publication of the Binet–Simon scales in 1905. We have previously addressed the impact of the IQ testing movement on American education and school psychology, but it is worthwhile to consider the beginnings of this movement in more detail. Psychologist Alfred Binet and psychiatrist Theophile Simon were commissioned by the Minister of Public Education in Paris to develop a methodology for classifying and sorting children who were not successful in the general education settings and who could not profit from the regular curriculum for the purpose of providing them specially designed training in other settings. Together, they developed the Binet–Simon scales, the first modern intelligence test, which was not only used in France but also later adapted by Lewis Terman of Stanford University into an English language version for use in the United States. Thus, the early history of school psychology became inextricably linked to intelligence testing and individual assessment and classification. These efforts proved to be instrumental in expanding the field of school psychology in later years and also served to entrench many school psychologists in a psychometric-driven role of sorter or gatekeeper. Of course, part of the early entrenchment of school psychologists in the psychometric gatekeeper role could also be attributed to the fact that the field of psychology had not yet developed a technology for effective intervention selection and implementation.

In the United States, the 1890s and early 1900s marked an increasing emphasis on providing educational and mental health services for youth whom we would today consider as being "at risk." Many urban public school districts in the larger cities of the eastern United States had established special educational programs and classes by this time, aimed at assisting students with significant learning problems. In 1899, William Healey established a clinic in Chicago for a juvenile court in the public school system, perhaps the precursor to today's special programs for students with emotional and behavioral disorders. The mental health field became formally established by 1910, with the founding of the "mental hygiene" movement that year. A primary focus of the incipient mental health field was the founding of child guidance clinics to help prevent and treat juvenile delinquency. Although these efforts were not necessarily specific to the field of school psychology nor conducted by individuals who were known as school psychologists, they nevertheless were early manifestations of activity in the field.

By the 1920s, the terms *school psychology* and *school psychologist* had emerged, indicating that the field was becoming increasingly established, with the signs of a distinct profession. Arnold Gesell became the first person to be appointed to the position of school psychologist, and he served in that role in Connecticut between 1915 and 1919. The term *school psychologist* also had appeared in the literature by this time. Thus, the field of school psychology, although barely in its infancy and without any formal structure or specific professional organization, had arrived.

Development and Professionalization of the Field

The late 1920s witnessed the first efforts to establish training programs and credentialing for school psychologists. During the 1930s, these efforts were expanded. The young field was beginning to grapple with increasing regulation and recognition, a sign that it had arrived. However, the practice of psychology in the schools was still largely unregulated, and individuals who fulfilled psychological service roles in schools had a wide range of professional training and went by a plethora of titles, such as psychological examiner, psychoclinician, and clinical or consulting psychologist. The first book on school psychology, *Psychological Service for School Problems*, authored by pioneering school psychologist Gertrude Hildreth, was published in 1930. Interestingly, one of the features of this book was the illustration of a typical day for a school psychologist and of the division of different activities within a work day. Hildreth's view on school psychology service delivery was fairly broad. Although individual testing and diagnosis played a prominent role in her breakdown of a professional day, consulting with teachers, administrators, parents, and other individuals through conferences appeared to be the single activity that consumed the most time.

During the 1940s and 1950s, the field of school psychology continued to expand. During this era, two important professional conferences with strong implications for the future of school psychology were held. The Boulder Conference on Clinical Psychology was held in 1949, shortly after the end of World War II and during the time when the practice of psychology was expanding greatly as a result of the development of the Veterans Administration hospitals and clinics to provide medical services to personnel who had served in the military during the war effort. The Boulder Conference resulted in the articulation of the scientist-practitioner model of psychology training and models for credentialing of psychologists. The impact of the Boulder Conference was to further legitimize the applied professional practice of psychology, which had previously taken a back seat in status to the academic or scientific aspect of the field. The Thayer Conference of 1954 was held for the purpose of advancing and shaping training, credentialing, and practice in school psychology. The proceedings of the Thayer Conference provided the first comprehensive picture of the field of school psychology and its circumstances. During this era, a division of the APA emerged (Division 16) that was specifically focused on school psychology, and the first few state school psychology associations were started. However, there was no strong link between national and state organizations and efforts similar to those increasingly enjoyed by the field of clinical psychology during this time. Part of the reason for the lack of a cohesive school psychology organizing body stemmed from the huge disparity in procedures for credentialing of school psychologists across the various states. Many states still did not have any formal recognition or training standards for psychologists to practice in schools. In addition, the doctoral versus nondoctoral conflict in psychology had begun to surface, and it clearly affected the status and organization of school psychologists. Unlike clinical psychologists, who were increasingly trained at the doctoral level and followed similar routes to credentialing and practice across states, school psychologists were primarily nondoctoral practitioners, and there was little consistency from state to state with regard to credentialing.

During the 1950s and 1960s, a social or demographic development occurred that had a major impact on American education and culture and ultimately on the development of school psychology: the post-World War II "baby boom" (children born between 1946 and 1964). Because such a large percentage of young American men were involved in military service, and because of the war effort in general (with a large percentage of young American women working in civilian-military roles and war-related industries), marriages and birthrates declined substantially during this time. As the war ended, an enormous number of young men and women, whose lives had been "on hold" during the war, resumed normal life. Most married, many pursued higher education with the assistance of the new G.I. bill, and almost all members of this generation began to raise their own families. Thus, a period of extensive growth in the numbers of children and youth in the United States began. By the mid-1950s, this growth spilled into the public schools, which began to expand at an unprecedented rate, continuing into the 1970s. At the same time, federally funded efforts were made to improve mathematics and science education, which in part led to the expansion of school guidance services.

As the number of schoolchildren expanded greatly, so did the numbers of students who had disabilities or who otherwise struggled with respect to their academic and behavioral adjustment in the school setting. These rapidly expanding numbers of "exceptional" students spurred the growth of school psychology, as parents, teachers, and administrators looked for solutions to learning and behavioral problems. Although no federal law for the education of students with disabilities was passed until 1975, many states and larger school districts expanded and refined their programs for meeting the needs of exceptional children, and school psychologists were usually a part of these efforts. The passage of new laws for the education of students with disabilities ultimately proved to be a watershed set of events for the field of school psychology.

The era of increasing emphasis on awareness and laws for education of students with disabilities corresponds to a great extent with the emergence of a new era of growth in school psychology. According to school psychology historian Thomas Fagan, the field's historical development can be divided into two distinct eras: the hybrid years of 1890 to 1969, when school psychology was emerging and beginning to develop an identity; and the thoroughbred years of 1970 to 2000 and beyond, when school psychology had clearly emerged as a unique field with a stable professional identity. Without question, the culminating symbol of the bridge between the two eras was the establishment of NASP, which held its first convention in St. Louis in 1969. The founding of NASP was significant not only because it signaled that the field had achieved a strong professional identity and professional structure but also because it represented the beginnings of a shift in the voice of the field (Fagan & Wise, 2007).

Division 16 of APA had previously served as the only national-level voice of the field of school psychology and was the first national organization within the field (Fagan, 2002). However, after NASP was established, its membership numbers quickly surpassed those of APA's Division 16, giving it increased credibility and visibility. Division 16, through its connection with APA and its advocacy of the doctoral degree as a necessity for independent practice, positioned itself as the voice of psychology within the greater body of American psychology. NASP, on the other hand, was a free-standing organization representing what was viewed as a unique field and as a mission to advocate for the interests of master's- and specialist-level school psychologists. These differences between APA and NASP had enormous implications for some of the later tensions and dynamics that would shape the field and that continue today.

Recent History of School Psychology

History is constantly being written and rewritten. The history of school psychology includes not only the foundations and early period but also recent events and issues. The beginning of Fagan's thoroughbred years in 1970 can be considered a starting point for a brief overview of some of the recent history of the field, two aspects of which are discussed in this section: the impact of the public law for education of students with disabilities and the impact of the development of training and credentialing standards for school psychology training programs and practitioners.

Public Law 94-142/Individuals with Disabilities Education Act

Some of the most important recent historical developments in the field of school psychology have been attributable to the impact of new laws and court decisions. These legal issues and related ethical issues are covered in more detail in Chapter 6, but they are briefly introduced here with an emphasis on how they have been critical in shaping the field. Specifically, the passage by the U.S. Congress of Public Law 94-142 in 1975, originally referred to as the Education for All Handicapped Children Act, proved to be incredibly important in the development of school psychology; its impact cannot be overstated. For the first time, there was a unified federal law rather than a patchwork of state laws and policies mandating a free and appropriate public education for students with disabilities. Three areas show the immediate and continuing impact of this law on the recent history of the field of school psychology.

First, because of the mandates for appropriate special education eligibility assessment of students, greater numbers of school psychologists were needed. This need resulted in a significant expansion of school psychology training programs and in the numbers of practicing school psychologists from the 1970s through the 1990s. For example, it has been estimated that the number of training programs doubled from about 100 to more than 200 during this period and that the number of NASP members likewise more than doubled. In short, the significant expansion of school psychology can be attributed in large measure to the impact of the federal law.

Second, the legal mandate for eligibility assessment not only expanded the field but also served to further entrench school psychologists in a gatekeeper or sorter role, a legacy that, while changing as more schools are adopting a problem-solving/RTI model, has been highly resistant to change. Many of the generation of school psychologists who entered the field within the few years immediately after the enactment of Public Law 94-142 were trained with the expectation of functioning primarily as psychometricians, and their expectations were in many cases further shaped in this direction by school administrators. The historical entrenchment in the gatekeeper/sorter role was (and continues to be in many schools) a source of frustration to many in the field who desired to engage in a broader range of services and to play an intervention-focused role.

Third, some of the specific mandates of Public Law 94-142 and its successors (the Individuals with Disabilities Education Act [IDEA], 1990, 1997, and 2004) have shaped professional practice. Perhaps the singular most important example is the original definition of learning disabilities (LDs) in the public law, which defined LDs primarily on the basis of a significant discrepancy between a student's intellectual ability and academic achievement. This definition not only further entrenched the field in the psychometric gatekeeper model but also actually resulted in day-to-day practice constraints. Two generations of school psychologists learned to live with a standardized intelligence test kit in one hand and a standardized academic achievement test in the other, much to the chagrin of many who believe that this type of assessment activity not only is questionable in terms of the premises on which it is based and the results it produces but also does little or nothing to help children and, in fact, may lead to harm if services provided following the evaluation do not effectively address a child's difficulties (Reschly, 2008). The most recent (2004) reauthorization of IDEA (which allowed the use of RTI procedures as an alternative to the ability–achievement discrepancy model for LD eligibility assessments) has reduced dependency on the ability–achievement assessment paradigm and has generally been received in the field in a positive manner. Although it is too early to tell whether this change will result in a significant broadening of roles for school psychologists, as discussed in later chapters, it does appear that RTI procedures are increasingly being adopted by schools and that the role of the school psychologist is expanding to incorporate some of the prevention/intervention work that is part of the RTI model. A larger unknown is how the RTI processes will fit in and be used for classification/diagnostic purposes. Will some states adopt rigid, formulaic RTI processes that simply shift the reliance on cognitive test kits to another set of practices that don't particularly inform interventions, or will the promotion of RTI prove to be a watershed event? Stay tuned: We are hopeful that the latter case will be true, and we've made sure that this edition discusses RTI in many places where it is relevant. But we've been disappointed before. Without question, IDEA and other public laws will continue to evolve, and as they do, they will likely affect the role of school psychologists.

Training Standards and Credentialing

Chapter 4 discusses training and credentialing of school psychologists in detail. As a precursor to that chapter, it is worth noting that the recent history of the field has seen some important developments in this arena. This section details some of the important historical developments related to training standards and credentialing of individual school psychologists and training programs.

APA Accreditation of Doctoral Programs

Although Division 16 of APA began to pursue efforts for the accreditation of doctoral programs in school psychology in the 1960s, it was not until 1971 that the first program was accredited (Fagan & Wells, 2000). Before then, no nationally accredited training programs in school psychology existed at any level. In the decade following the first accreditation of a school psychology program, interest and activity in this area moved slowly, and most doctoral programs in the field either did not meet the minimum criteria for accreditation or were not interested in pursuing accreditation. By 1980, there were 20 accredited doctoral programs. However, the perceived importance of APA accreditation gradually built steam. By 1990, 38 programs had received accreditation; by 2000, this number had increased to 52. By 2010, there were 60 APA-accredited doctoral programs in school psychology and an additional eight APA-accredited doctoral programs in the combined professional–scientific psychology category, which list school psychology as one of their focus areas. Although only one of these programs is in Canada, APA is phasing out of accrediting Canadian programs and will cease to accredit them as of September 2015. Instead, these programs will be eligible for accreditation through the Canadian Psychological Association.

NASP Approval of Specialist Programs

With respect to master's and specialist programs (i.e., 60-semester-credit graduate programs in school psychology), Fagan and Wells (2000) noted that the use of standards specifically for school psychology training did not occur within the relationship of NASP and the National Council for Accreditation of Teacher Education (NCATE) until the 1980s and that the NASP folio review for program accreditation was implemented in 1988. By the end of that decade, NASP program approval could be gained by adherence to the training standards developed by NASP, either through an institution's NCATE review process for all education credentialing programs or separately through the NASP training program review board. Like APA accreditation for doctoral programs, NASP approval for specialist programs increasingly became perceived as important. By 2010, 156 specialist-level programs and 63 doctoral-level programs were approved by NASP. Currently, an agreement exists between NASP and APA that allows for doctoral programs to receive joint APA accreditation and NASP approval within the same accreditation process. Thus, when a doctoral program receives APA accreditation in school psychology, it may also be awarded doctoral-level program approval by NASP.

The NCSP Credential

Credentialing of individual practitioners is another area in which recent history has witnessed significant developments that have affected both training and practice. Because individual states dictate their own standards and procedures for both psychological board licensing for independent practice and department of education certification to practice in the schools, there has been much variation among the states, which has sometimes created difficulties for practitioners who train in one state and then want to work in another. One important development in this area was NASP's establishment in 1988 of the National School Psychology Certification System. This system leads to the granting of the Nationally Certified School Psychologist (NCSP) credential to those individuals who are ascertained to have completed minimum standards of training and competence. Obtaining this credential requires practitioners to have completed an NASP-approved training program or its equivalent (consisting of at least 60 semester credits of graduate-level coursework in an identified school psychology program plus a 1,200-clock-hour internship under the supervision of a credentialed school psychologist) and passing a standardized national examination. The purpose in enacting this system was to promote the NASP training standard for quality assurance and to make it easier for holders of the NCSP credential to receive state department of education certification to practice as school psychologists as they move from one state to another.

Initially, the national certification program took off slowly, and few states signed agreements allowing certification or license reciprocity for holders of the NCSP credential. However, after more than two decades of existence, it has gradually increased in visibility and influence. By 2010 the majority of U.S. states—31 in all—recognized the NCSP credential as a complete or partial basis for awarding their own state practice licenses or certificates. It is also worth noting that the number of practitioners holding the NCSP credential has continued to rise steadily, with more than 11,500 individuals listed as of 2010. This figure represents nearly one-third of the membership of NASP and a reasonably large percentage of all school psychologists. The trend is clearly moving toward all or most U.S. states accepting the NCSP as a basis for licensure or certification and for a significant percentage of school psychologists striving to hold this credential.

Growth through Tension and Opposition

Are stress, tension, and opposition natural prerequisites to growth and development? We think they are, both personally and professionally. If this notion is true, then the field of school psychology has had ample opportunities for growth! Perhaps more so than the other areas of professional psychology (clinical and counseling), school psychology has experienced not only the general tensions inherent in all of psychology but some unique turmoil as well. This section explores some of these tensions, including some ongoing "culture wars."

Two Cultures of Psychology

In a 1984 study published in *American Psychologist*, Gregory Kimble articulated a "scientist–humanist" dimension in belief systems and values among psychologists that has created an underlying tension in the field for many years. The scientist–humanist dimension was his label for the dichotomy that he found through a survey of psychologists that utilized sophisticated sampling and survey techniques. The implication is that psychologists can be roughly divided into two distinct cultures: one representing the scientist end of the dimension, and the other representing the humanist end. Because school psychology is part of the larger field of psychology and is certainly included in this dichotomy, it is worth reviewing the six major areas in which this cultural division is said to be manifest.

Scientific versus Human Values

This conflict involves the tension between the principles of objective science and the values of some practitioners who might be consumers of the science. A good illustration in the field of school psychology involves the application of behavioral theory to promote the use of positive reinforcement within a classroom to increase appropriate behavior and decrease inappropriate behavior. Although there is a virtual mountain of evidence that increasing reinforcement for positive behaviors of students will lead to positive results, doing so goes against the value systems of many teachers and some school psychology practitioners, who might be opposed to the notion of "bribing" or otherwise hold the belief that external reinforcement systems are mechanistic and inappropriate, an idea popularized by journalist Alfie Kohn (1993) in the influential book *Punished by Rewards*.

Determinism versus Indeterminism

This second area of conflict has been in existence for centuries or longer. It is reflected in the tension between the notion that behavioral or personal outcomes are the result of fixed laws or determinants and the notion that outcomes are malleable and that individuals can alter their personal destinies. A good example of the unfolding of this conflict in our field is the hoopla that surrounded the publication of *The Bell Curve* by Herrnstein and Murray (1994). The conclusion of these authors was that intelligence was, for the most part, hereditary or native and that educational achievement and related outcomes of individuals low in ability cannot be meaningfully affected through well-meaning intervention programs. Strong advocates of this view argue that early intervention programs such as Head Start are a poor use of resources. However, there is an impressive array of evidence to the contrary, as detailed in Hart and Risley's (1995) *Meaningful Differences in the Everyday Experience of Young American Children*, which documents in painstaking detail that intellectual skills of young children are significantly affected by their early environments and that early life experiences set the stage for later accomplishments.

Objectivism versus Intuitionism

Those who value objectivism may use the axiom "in evidence we trust," whereas those who value intuitionism may reject data-driven approaches and instead make evaluations based on subjective feelings. A good example of this conflict within school psychology involves the selection and use of projective-expression assessment techniques for evaluating children's social–emotional status. Although objective data in this area overwhelmingly raise caution regarding the questionable technical properties of many tools, such as drawing and sentence completion tests, many practitioners continue to have a strong allegiance to such methods and view their intuitive value as compensating for their technical flaws, no matter how damning those flaws may be (Merrell, 2008).

Laboratory versus Field

This dimension of conflict is between results and methods refined in laboratory settings and those applied in naturalistic field settings. Because school psychology, as opposed to some branches of psychology, is an extraordinarily applied field, this conflict does not rear its head to a significant extent in our world. However, instances do exist. When functional behavioral assessment (FBA) became a mandated assessment practice through the 1997 reauthorization of the IDEA, many practitioners were frustrated with and perhaps resented the necessity of implementing in school settings a technology that had been developed primarily in laboratory or clinic settings with individuals who had low-incidence disabilities. Conversely, a number of FBA adherents who had honed their research in laboratory settings were not happy that FBA had been mandated in school settings prior to it being sufficiently refined and evaluated for those settings.

Nomothetic versus Idiographic

This interesting conflict will require some background for most readers to fully understand it. These two terms were first proposed in 1894 by Wilhelm Windelband, a German philosopher of science, as the two primary and somewhat opposing methods of scientific inquiry. Nomothetic inquiry involves procedures and methods designed to cover *general laws* and is concerned with *similarities among phenomena* such as population averages, aggregate statistical methods, and psychometrics. Idiographic inquiry involves attempts to understand a particular event or individual or the *uniqueness of a phenomenon*. Idiographic inquiry would support the use of qualitative analysis and single-case designs. The reality in school psychology is that both methods of inquiry are used by most practitioners and researchers, and for most it does not pose a significant conflict. For example, a school psychologist might assess a student's reading ability using curriculum-based assessment methods (an idiographic approach) but place the results in context for intervention planning by comparing the results with averages from the classroom or group (a nomothetic approach).

Elementism versus Holism

Elementism is reflected in the notion of looking at very small parts or elements of human behavior and in isolation, whereas holism involves looking at the "whole" person and not considering any particular aspect of their characteristics or behavior in isolation. Like the conflict between laboratory and field, this particular conflict has not been as much of a controversy in school psychology as it has been in some other branches of psychology. However, there are clear precedents for this conflict in our field. A good example is the use of individual subtest or item-level analysis of assessment data versus relying on total scores. Some practitioners may find a great deal of intuitive value in the former, whereas psychometric fundamentalists will likely decry such practices as being fraught with unreliability.

In sum, school psychology is not immune to the tensions that have existed within the field of psychology in general. The two cultures of psychology identified by Kimble (1984) still appear to be distinctive enough to warrant this discussion, and they appear to have some very specific manifestations within school psychology. Again, it is important to recognize that the stress produced by this tension is not a bad thing for school psychology. Not only can it help the field to grow but it can also work like a system of checks and balances: Advocates at each end of the dimension help to curb possible excesses of the opposite end.

NASP and APA

No discussion of tensions within the field of school psychology could be complete without an examination of the historic and ongoing tensions between NASP and APA that has waxed and waned over the years but has never fully gone away. This discussion is provided not to inflame any wounds or to promote a particular point of view. Rather, it is considered to be an essential part of the recent history and ongoing development of this dynamic field.

Although there are several historical issues that characterize the conflict, in many ways the tension that has existed between NASP and APA comes down to one overriding issue: disagreement and debate regarding the doctoral versus specialist level of training, both for use of the term *school psychologist* and for independent practice outside of school settings. NASP was founded in 1969 for the purpose of providing an organized voice to practicing school psychologists, the vast majority of whom did not have doctoral degrees in psychology. Although the percentage of school psychologists who have earned the doctoral degree has increased slightly over the years, it is still true that the vast majority of school psychologists (currently about 70% of all school psychologists and 75% of practitioners) do not have doctoral degrees. APA is the oldest and largest organization of psychologists, and it has attempted to be the advocate and voice of the broad field of psychology in America. NASP, on the other hand, was specifically founded to represent the interests of practicing school psychologists. Because the founding of NASP was brought about in great part by perceptions among many school psychologists that APA was either an ineffective voice for them or was actively ignoring or excluding them, it did not take long for tensions to arise.

The position of APA in the mid- to late 20th century was always either implicit or explicit in contending that the doctoral degree should be the minimum level for the use of the title "psychologist" or "professional psychologist." Within only 6 years following the founding of NASP, this position was formally codified by APA's 1977 stance that the doctoral degree in psychology is the minimum level of training needed for engagement in independent practice, state board licensing, and use of the title "psychologist." However, the APA position statement, APA's Model Licensure Act (MLA), and the language of most state psychology licensing boards (which are usually informed greatly by the MLA) included a provision for individuals who were trained at the master's or specialist level and were appropriately credentialed by their state department of education to use the title "school psychologist" within the scope of their school-based practice. In other words, the stance of APA and general professional psychology was that one must be a doctoral-level psychologist to receive a board license and to practice independently and call oneself a psychologist, but one could use the title "school psychologist" with less than doctoral-level training providing the work was specifically limited to school settings and conducted under the authority of a state department of education certificate. This statement represents the current APA position, although as discussed in greater detail later, there were recent discussions of the MLA within APA that almost led to the removal of this exemption.

APA's position on independent practice restrictions has never been accepted by NASP, and it has always been a point of some tension between the two organizations. In fact, NASP has supported the efforts of its state affiliates to promote legislation allowing specialist-level school psychologists to become licensed for independent practice, whereas APA and its state affiliates have continued to actively oppose such efforts. Although it has waxed and waned over the years, this conflict has always been present and is enormously complicated, especially given that many school psychologists are members of both APA and NASP and support both organizations.

This conflict has been complicated by several developments and issues over the years. Fagan and Wells (2000) noted that the U.S. Department of Education resurrected the jurisdictional conflict between APA and NASP by questioning the designation of two separate accrediting bodies for the same profession. In response, APA and NASP established a joint task force in 1978 (the Inter-Organization Committee, or IOC) to work cooperatively to resolve the conflict. This body established a collaborative pilot effort in 1983 for joint APA and NASP/NCATE accreditation of doctoral programs. However, whereas APA supported this effort, NCATE did not, and joint site visits were discontinued. Even with these tensions, doctoral programs accredited by APA have still been able to automatically qualify for NASP program approval, although the future of this historical cooperative process is still uncertain. One of the interesting questions of the doctoral versus nondoctoral conflict is whether there is any evidence that supports one position over the other. In general, there has not been any such evidence, although a review by Reschly and Wilson (1997) opined that the specialist level of training was not sufficient for the independent practice of school psychology in non-school settings. In 1988, at the NASP convention in Chicago, one of us (KWM) attended a town hall-type meeting on the doctoral versus nondoctoral issue, moderated by then-NASP president Thomas Fagan. What was striking about this meeting was the large number of participants who attended, whose impassioned arguments at the open microphones appeared to surprise even the moderator, who stated that he was under the impression that concern about this issue had diminished over time. Clearly, this issue will not simply go away anytime soon, and some leaders in the field have even acknowledged that it appears to be intractable (Short, 2002).

It is probably simplistic to view the historical and continuing rift between APA and NASP as being exclusively the result of the entry-level-training disagreement. Rather, the tension seems to include differences in the broader culture and worldviews of the two organizations. According to Short (2002), there are distinct cultural differences in how the two organizations perceive school psychology within the broader context of professional psychology, with APA representing a culture of school psychology as part of professional psychology and NASP representing a culture of school psychology as a separate profession. Thus, "APA views school psychology as a specialty within American psychology, sharing significant commonalities with other specialties in terms of skills, knowledge, and competencies," whereas NASP asserts "that school psychology is a separate profession from professional psychology" (Short, 2002, p. 111). To an outsider or someone newly initiated to the field, these differences may seem to be trite, even pointless, yet they persist and continue to have ramifications for the development of the field, siphoning off tremendous energy that might otherwise be used to move the practice and science of school psychology forward. In 2002, APA's board of directors voted to withdraw their participation from the APA–NASP IOC, based on the conclusion "that the IOC had failed in its mission to gain consensus on important issues" (Clark, 2002, p. 40). It is evident that history is continuing to be written in this arena and that the APA–NASP tension has not yet subsided.

Despite the lack of evidence that interorganizational tensions between APA and NASP are diminishing, there have recently been some encouraging signs, sort of a "silver lining" in the dark clouds if you will. From 2007 through early 2010, it was very clear that the process of revising the APA's MLA was going in the direction of taking the unprecedented step of advising state psychology licensing boards to work toward not allowing the use of the title "school psychologist" by anyone who was not a board-licensed, doctoral-level psychologist trained in school psychology, even if they were working in school settings and credentialed by that state's department of education. Not surprisingly, this issue inflamed tensions between APA and NASP to a level that many observers (us included) considered to be unprecedented. NASP actively opposed the effort and urged its members to do the same. Early in the process, it was unclear whether or not APA's Division 16 leadership would ultimately take a stand for or against the proposed MLA language, which further escalated tensions as the issue was studied and its membership provided input. Ultimately, the Division 16 leadership took a strong stand in alignment with NASP, arguing for retaining the exemption for the title "school psychologist" in the MLA (although not advocating for independent practice recognition for nondoctoral practitioners). Through the hard work and advocacy of some very influential Division 16 leaders during 2009 and early 2010, the APA Council of Representatives was convinced to abandon the course that had been charted, and the exemption was retained in a vote of the council on February 20, 2010. Although many school psychologists were only vaguely aware of the behind-the-scenes activity, the eventual result was an extraordinary achievement, an impressive sign of collaboration between NASP and APA's Division 16. It remains unclear whether this achievement represents a denouement to the historical drama or is merely an interlude. We would not be surprised to see the issue revived by APA in the future, and it's clear that the independent practice issue is going to continue to be one of détente or stalemate. Despite the possibility that the current goodwill won't last forever, the successful 2009–2010 efforts of APA Division 16 leadership to amicably resolve the issue will certainly be remembered as a milestone in the history of the field.

Leaving Adolescence: Toward the Maturation of the Field

Some of the most important dates and landmark events in the history of school psychology that have been described in this chapter are detailed in Table 2.1. It is clear that school psychology is a relatively young field. It has a brief but rich history that is inseparable from the fields of both psychology and American education. If we accept that school psychology is a young field, just how young is it in developmental terms? School psychology is clearly out of the infancy state, having emerged as a distinctive profession with strong voices, major influences, and extensive numbers of professionals. One can also easily make the case that the field has left its childhood, given that we have moved from Fagan's hybrid years to the thoroughbred years. If identity confusion and turmoil are essential components of adolescence, as some influential developmental psychologists have proposed, then it would be hard to argue that school psychology has totally left adolescence. Rather, like the 20- or 30-something emerging adult "twixter" who continues to live in his or her parents' basement and is not quite ready to take on the full responsibilities of adult life, our field appears to be in a delayed or extended period of adolescence. Adulthood and full maturity appear to be just around the corner and even in sight, but the field still seems hesitant or unsure regarding making the next steps to get there.

The Spanish philosopher and poet George Santayana is credited with making the statement "Those who forget the past are doomed to repeat it." Our foray into school psychology's brief history in this chapter might well be concluded by considering the

TABLE 2.1. Some Important Dates and Landmark Events in the History of School Psychology

1892	American Psychological Association is founded.
1896	Lightner Witmer establishes first psychological/child guidance clinic at University of Pennsylvania.
1899	First school-based psychological clinic is established in Chicago public schools.
1905	Binet–Simon intelligence scales are published in Paris, France.
1915	Arnold Gesell of Connecticut becomes first person hired as "school psychologist."
1916	American/English language revision of Binet–Simon scales is published by Lewis Terman at Stanford University ("Stanford–Binet").
1928	First school psychology training program is established at New York University.
1930	First book on school psychology, *Psychological Service for School Problems*, is published by Gertrude Hildreth of Columbia University.
1943	Ohio School Psychologists Association is founded, becomes first state school psychology organization.
1945	APA is reorganized into divisions, and first national organization for school psychology (APA Division 16) is established.
1954	Thayer conference, first national school psychology conference, is held in West Point, New York.
1962	*Journal of School Psychology* is founded, becomes first school psychology journal.
1969	National Association of School Psychologists is founded at organizational meeting in St. Louis, Missouri.
1971	PhD program in school psychology at University of Texas at Austin becomes first APA-accredited doctoral program in school psychology.
1975	Public Law 94-142, Education of All Handicapped Children Act, is enacted by U.S. Congress and takes effect in 1977.
1977	APA council resolution declares that doctoral degree is required for use of "professional psychologist" title and increases tension with NASP.
1978	Joint APA–NASP Inter-Organizational Committee is established to work out differences between two organizations.
1988	NASP begins training program approval process with folio review system and approves first training programs.
1988	NASP institutes Nationally School Psychology Certification Board and administers first national certification exam; first NCSP certificates are granted in 1989.
1997	APA grants specialty recognition to school psychology.
2002	Future of School Psychology Invitational Conference is held in Indianapolis, Indiana.
2002	APA board of directors votes to withdraw from joint APA–NASP Inter-Organizational Committee.
2004	Individuals with Disabilities Education Improvement Act reauthorization removes requirement for IQ–achievement discrepancy and allows for use of RTI procedures in LD classifications.

accomplishments and disappointments of the field to date and pondering when it will take leave of the basement of postadolescence and move into maturity. We believe that a "paradigm shift" is taking place in the field (Reschly & Ysseldyke, 2002; Reschly, 2008) and that the past is not necessarily the future. However, the past is important, even critical, to our current understanding of the field. We have provided a background in this chapter that we hope the reader will not forget within the context of the road map that subsequent chapters present regarding moving the field forward.

DISCUSSION QUESTIONS AND ACTIVITIES

1. Go to the "Today in the History of Psychology" website at *www.cwu.edu/~warren/today.html* and use the search engine to locate important historical events in the chronology of psychology that occurred on your birthday (day and month). Are any of the events you identified specifically relevant to the history of school psychology?

2. Select an individual who played a prominent role in the history of school psychology and write or present a brief overview of his or her life and accomplishments. We particularly encourage you to consider researching someone who is a lesser known or overlooked "pioneer" from the field.

3. For those who have recently entered a graduate program in school psychology, what were the features of this field that attracted your interest? Why did you choose to train for a career in school psychology rather than other professional fields of psychology (clinical or counseling psychology) or related educational or mental health fields (such as school counseling, social work, or teaching)?

4. The history of school psychology has clearly been tied to the role of gatekeeper or sorter and to the work of psychoeducational assessment. What are your views regarding the opportunities, risks, and barriers to moving school psychologists into broader roles that reduce substantially the amount of time spent conducting individual psychoeducational assessments?

5. The ongoing conflict between the sometimes opposing views and values represented by APA and NASP has clearly taken up a tremendous amount of time, talent, and energy that might otherwise be used to move the field forward in other ways. How do you view this cultural tension, and what do you think it will take for the field to settle these concerns and rise above them?

CHAPTER 3

The Changing Face
of School Psychology

Responding Effectively to Cultural and Linguistic Diversity

with Elsa Arroyos

The title of this chapter recognizes the importance of including a discussion of issues related to cultural and linguistic diversity. As the field of school psychology continues to establish its professional identity, it does so in the face of an ever-changing population of children, adolescents, and their families. The United States continues to experience rapid and unprecedented changes in the demographic makeup of its population. Ethnic groups that have historically been in the minority of the population are quickly becoming a majority. In addition, although the United States has historically been a linguistically diverse society, it is also experiencing a new and powerful influx of persons whose native language is not English. This is exemplified by the 140% increase across the last three decades in the population speaking a language other than English at home (U.S. Bureau of the Census, 2010a). These demographic shifts are being reflected in our school systems, and this diversification of the student body clearly affects the delivery of school psychological services.

In this chapter, we provide an introductory discussion of the relevant issues and concepts related to cultural and linguistic diversity and associated implications for school psychology practice. The chapter begins with a brief overview of the demographic shifts and changes that are occurring in the United States, highlighting the implications of these changes for the field of school psychology. With this change in the population, it is inevitable that "differences" will become more pronounced. However, in order to avoid

Elsa Arroyos, PhD, is Associate Professor and Director of Training, School Psychology Program, Department of Counseling and Educational Psychology, New Mexico State University, Las Cruces, New Mexico.

the pitfall of equating differences with stereotypes, a discussion of within-group and between-group differences is included. The need to recruit and retain school psychologists from diverse backgrounds is highlighted as a significant challenge facing the field, given the ever-changing student population and the need to provide culturally responsive school psychological services. In addition, some key concepts and issues related to cultural and linguistic diversity in general are provided to highlight the important variables that school psychologists need to consider in their work with diverse groups and/ or individuals. This chapter includes a brief overview of the components of culturally competent or culturally effective school psychology practice, including an overview of culturally responsive RTI that is emphasized in this volume, as well as a discussion of the issue of minority misrepresentation in special education programs. Finally, the chapter concludes with a discussion of why the data-driven problem-solving model (discussed more extensively in Chapter 7) may be particularly beneficial in helping school psychologists to reduce bias in their practice and to better aid children and their families from all cultural and linguistic backgrounds.

Demographic Trends:
The Changing Linguistic, Ethnic, and Cultural Landscape

Although the United States has been a multicultural and multilingual nation since its inception, recent trends indicate substantial diversification of its demographic makeup. In 1992, it was estimated that by 2050 the Latino population would become the largest minority group in the United States (Pratt & Rittenhouse, 1998; U.S. Bureau of the Census, 1992). This prediction has been realized even earlier than anticipated. Data from the U. S Census Bureau for 2009 confirm that Latinos currently make up the largest non-European ethnic group in the United States, exceeding the population that identifies as African American or black (U.S. Bureau of the Census, 2010b). Currently, Latinos make up approximately 15.8% of the population, with African Americans/blacks constituting 12.9%, Asian American/Pacific Islanders 4.8%, and American Indian/Native Alaskans 1.0%, indicating slight increases across all groups reported for the 2000 census. Furthermore, 17.9% of the U.S. population speaks a language other than English, and 11% of individuals in the United States are foreign born (U.S. Bureau of the Census, 2010b).

These demographic trends are also being paralleled in our school systems, where more students and more diverse populations are being served than ever before (National Center for Education Statistics [NCES], 2010a). Thus, there is a tremendous and unprecedented need for school psychologists to develop more culturally competent and responsive practices. In general, our schools are even more diverse than the U.S. population as a whole, largely because of demographic characteristics previously discussed and birthrates across ethnic groups. For example, recent immigrants to the United States are more likely to be younger than the U.S. population in general, and some of the ethnic minority groups in the United States have higher birthrates than the U.S. population in general. As reported for fall 2010, 55.2 million students are entering public and private elementary and secondary schools in the United States (NCES, 2010a). Of the approximately 49 million children in the public PreK–12 educational system, the percentage of Caucasian students declined from 68% (28 million) in 1988 to 55% (26.7 million) in 2008. Increases in Latino/a enrollments were seen over this time period, with a 2008 population of 10.4 million (22% of school enrollees) compared with a 1998 population of 4.5 million (11% of school enrollees). Although the total number of African American/black students increased from 1988 to 2008 (from 6.8 to 7.5 million), the percentage decreased slightly (from 17% to 16%). All other ethnic groups comprised less than 5% of the population individually in 2008: Asians, 3.7%; Pacific Islanders, 0.2%; American Indian/Alaska Natives, 0.9%; and students of two or more races, 2.6% (NCES, 2010b).

The field of school psychology has not been blind to these expansive demographic shifts. Many writers in our field have clearly recognized the need to employ more culturally responsive practices in an increasingly diverse society (e.g., Gopaul-McNicol, 1997; Gollnick & Chinn, 2009; Halsell, 2002; Ortiz & Flanagan, 2002; Ortiz, Flanagan, & Dynda, 2008; Ysseldyke et al., 1997). With these changes in demographics comes a range of experiences from the increasingly diverse groups and the individuals within the population. These individuals bring with them a multitude of cultural and linguistic experiences that add richness to our population and that need to be recognized and valued in our schools and by society as a whole.

Beyond Stereotypes: Within-Group and Between-Group Differences

The rapid changes occurring in the linguistic, cultural, and ethnic makeup of the U.S. population accentuate the differences that make these groups diverse in the first place. Although we need to recognize these differences in our work as school psychologists, we also must be careful not to equate these differences with stereotypical descriptions and/ or expectations for individuals from diverse groups. That is, there is a fine line between acknowledging differences and interpreting them in stereotypical fashion. It is critical to understand the role that within-group and between-group differences play in working with culturally and linguistically diverse individuals.

Stereotypes

Humans have a natural inclination to socially categorize individuals based on some salient feature such as age, gender, race, ethnicity, socioeconomic status, and so forth. There is a purpose to socially categorizing, or stereotyping, individuals, as the case may be, in that it serves as a means of simplifying a complex social world. However, in doing so, we run the risk of minimizing or even erasing the individuality of people, including what makes them different, if we stereotype their identity and behavior based solely on their group membership.

By way of definition, the action of stereotyping is to have "rigid preconceptions we hold about *all* people who are members of a particular group" (p. 154) that is designed to define that group, erasing individuality and difference (Sue & Sue, 2008). By engaging in stereotyping, we are, in essence, engaging in a form of prejudicial behavior. Although stereotyping may sometimes be benign, it may also lead to discrimination against groups to which one does not belong in favor of one's own group. Furthermore, one runs the risk of overstating differences between groups or highlighting the similarities between self and other members of one's own group. Finally, stereotypes can serve as a means to "justify" the behavior of individuals from a particular group, which can further eradicate individuality by reinforcing a "they're all alike" attitude or perception. Stereotypes may also lead to the development of certain expectations about an individual's abilities, behaviors, and so forth that can lead to interpreting subsequent behavior(s) in a manner that "fits" expectation for a person from "that" group. As practitioners working with the general public (i.e., schools and their associated members), it becomes our responsibility to acknowledge differences but in a manner that does not alienate or harm individuals. This is a challenging responsibility. It requires a conscious effort to overcome one's own stereotypic expectations and not to rely on general stereotypes as professional judgments are formed.

Within- and between-Group Differences

To move beyond stereotypic representations of individuals from various cultural and linguistic groups, we must understand the implications or relevance of within- and between-group differences. Individual differences obviously refer to how individuals differ from one another in some aspect, whereas group differences refer to how individuals from one group typically differ from those of another group. In understanding individual and group differences, there are two important considerations: (1) There is significant variability *within* any one group and (2) there is always significant overlap *between* groups (Merrell, 2008). Given these facts, it becomes essential for professionals to be careful not to draw undue inferences about students' characteristics, abilities, behaviors, and so forth simply on the basis of their group membership (e.g., gender, ethnic background, cultural background). Furthermore, in understanding the overlap between groups, it is crucial to consider that the typical differences between groups do not necessarily apply to individual members of those groups. In other words, although there may be characteristics that describe a group as a whole (e.g., whether a group is individualistic or collectivistic), the characteristic does not automatically get ascribed to *all* individuals within the group (e.g., not all Latino/a people are collectivistic).

By understanding that individuals from the same group are not necessarily alike in every respect and that there may be similarities across different groups, we become less prone to making stereotypical interpretation of individuals. It comes down to understanding our clientele on an individual, case-by-case basis. We are not suggesting that school psychologists need not take into account individuals' group memberships; on the contrary, it is still crucial to understand group memberships and the role these play in personal development. However, at the same time, school psychologists still need to acknowledge clients' individuality by taking into account factors other than their group membership. For example, many school psychologists may be prone to automatically using nonverbal assessment methods for students whose native language is not English and/or who are considered bilingual. However, it is also important to consider variables such as generational status, level of acculturation, and so forth. It may be appropriate to use traditional tests such as standardized ability and achievement tests that have been normed primarily on individuals from the dominant (Anglo) culture with a Latino student, for example, who was born and raised in the United States, is highly acculturated, and is fluent in English and Spanish (and prefers English). It is especially important to understand the individual as a part of both his or her own ethnic/cultural group and family group as well as society at large and to understand what the intermingling has been or continues to be between them. There are many factors that may distinguish individuals from their cultural groups and from mainstream culture as well as other factors that make them similar to those from their cultural group and mainstream society. It is the responsibility of multiculturally competent and effective school psychologists to evaluate these factors in the most culturally sensitive manner possible.

Ethnic Minority Underrepresentation among the Ranks of School Psychologists: A Major Challenge for the Field

Professionals in our field have long recognized the disparity in numbers of culturally and linguistically diverse (CLD) school psychologists to serve the needs of students in ever-changing school settings. Reschly (2000) noted that CLD school psychologists have historically been vastly underrepresented in the field, and more recent surveys continue to validate this. In a survey of school psychologists during the 2004–2005 school year (Curtis, Lopez, et al., 2008), it was found that school psychologists of color represented only 7.4% of the field (1.9% African American, 3.0% Hispanic, 0.9% Asian/Pacific Islander, and 0.8% Native American/Native Alaskan, and 0.8% other). There continues to be very little gender diversity, with 74% of all school psychologists and 77% of practitioners being female (Curtis, Lopez, et al., 2008). Only 9.7% (one of 10) previously reported fluency in a language other than English (Curtis, Hunley, Walker, & Baker, 1999; Curtis, Grier, & Hunley, 2004). Furthermore, if we consider other characteristics that "match" the clientele we serve, only 2.6% reported having a disability (Curtis et al., 1999). Clearly, these figures indicate that the demographic makeup of professionals in school psychology is much different from that of the population that is served by school psychologists (Fagan, 2002, 2008). In addition, when considering that more than 70% of school psychologists are women, yet males are disproportionately more likely to be recipients of special education and other remedial educational services, the demographic disparity between school psychologists and the youth they serve is even more striking.

According to Reschly (2000), some studies indicate that minority representation in graduate programs and faculty has increased; however, because this increase in minority representation has not kept pace with the demographic changes of the U.S. population in general, the makeup of the field will still remain overwhelmingly European American for the next decade. There is no denying that many of these white, middle-class females are committed to working with issues of diversity and becoming more informed about best practices with a diverse student population, but there is still the possibility of a cultural mismatch between them and individuals from CLD backgrounds (Reschly, 2000).

At the start of the 21st century, Reschly (2000) summed up the then current (and future) status of the field with the following statement, which we think is still true more than a decade later:

> There is reason to believe that school psychology is becoming more ethnically diverse; however, the pace of change is not sufficient to improve markedly the current imbalance in the characteristics of school psychologists and the populations they serve.... School psychologists can expect to be challenged in the next decade and beyond by issues relating to disproportionate minority representation, valid and culturally sensitive assessment and interventions, and improved outcomes for all children. (p. 519)

Other professionals in the field also refer to the importance of a paradigm shift in order to meet the new demands of a changing population. For example, Sheridan and Gutkin (2000), also commenting on the state of the field at the dawn of the 21st century, reiterated the importance of making necessary changes to the field, via a paradigm shift, to meet the needs of the populations we serve. Their words still ring true:

> School psychology must be reflective of, responsive to, and proactive toward the multiple and changing systems within which we operate (e.g., school, family, societal, legislative

systems) including the increasingly diverse populations whom we serve (e.g., children, families, educators, administrators, community leaders) and the settings in which they function (e.g., homes, schools, agencies, hospital). (p. 489)

One way in which the field of school psychology can be "reflective of, responsive to, and proactive toward" the changing systems in which we work is through the recruitment and retention of culturally and linguistically diverse school psychologists at all levels—from practitioners to administrators to trainers. These individuals not only would become valuable new assets to the field but would also facilitate and reinforce work already being done regarding culturally responsive service delivery (Curtis et al., 1999; Zhou et al., 2004).

To better serve our youth and meet their mental health and educational needs, NASP has recognized the need to "actively increase" the number of culturally and linguistically diverse school psychologists to work with these students. Furthermore, the organization also sees the need to recruit and retain culturally and linguistically diverse trainers in school psychology programs. In its current position statement regarding this issue, NASP delineates its recruitment and retention efforts that are being put into place to meet to meet their goal of remedying the "disproportionately few culturally and linguistically diverse school psychologists to serve the greater number of diverse students in both regular and special education" (NASP, 2009). Other efforts include the NASP minority scholarship program as well as the Multicultural Affairs Committee and the presidential initiative of the Minority Recruitment and Retention Task Force, the latter two of which have the goal of increasing the number of CLD school psychologists at all levels in the field.

These efforts are similar to those put forth by other governing bodies, such as the APA and its Division 16. As a major organization in the field of psychology, APA has committed itself through many efforts to increase the number of culturally and linguistically diverse trainers and practitioners in the field of psychology as well as to enhance services to diverse populations. For example, APA has issued its *Guidelines on Multicultural Education, Training, Research, Practice, and Organizational Change for Psychologists* (APA, 2002) and *Guidelines for Providers of Psychological Services to Ethnic, Linguistic, and Culturally Diverse Populations* (APA, 1990). It also established the Office of Ethnic Minority Affairs in 1979, which, among its many efforts, seeks to promote recruitment, retention, and training opportunities for ethnically diverse individuals in psychology. Other APA organizational initiatives in this area include the Committee on Ethnic Minority Affairs; the Commission on Ethnic Minority Recruitment, Retention, and Training in Psychology Task Force; and the Council of National Psychological Associations for the Advancement of Ethnic Minority Interests. Finally, Division 16 also supports recruitment and retention efforts, as is indicated in its stated objective to "encourage opportunities for the ethnic minority participation in the specialty [of school psychology]" (*www.indiana.edu/~div16/G&O. htm*). More recently, NASP and Division 16 of APA have joined forces to develop a joint position article that addresses the overall shortage of school psychologists in the field by drafting guidelines for professional psychologists trained with a clinical or counseling psychology focus to "respecialize" in school psychology (Tharinger & Palomares, 2004). It is unclear whether this effort will result in more diversity within school psychology, but it may help somewhat in alleviating overall personnel shortages. It is important to appreciate that these efforts to diversify the ranks of professionals in the field require a shift in thinking about diversity and approaches to working in diverse school and learning environments.

Key Concepts and Issues in Cultural and Linguistic Diversity

Although there is currently a call to increase the number of culturally and linguistically diverse school psychologists in the field to help serve an even more diverse student population, it may take many, many years for the field to meet this goal. However, it must also be acknowledged that increasing the number of CLD school psychologists in the field is only one means of increasing cultural responsiveness of practitioners in the field. We must recognize that *all* school psychologists need to be aware of key issues in working with culturally and linguistically diverse clientele. Stated simply, we cannot assume that the challenge of responding effectively to increasing cultural and linguistic diversity of students and families in our schools will be met by enhanced recruitment and retention of diverse professionals within the field. Rather, it is incumbent on all school psychologists to enhance their own multicultural competence or effectiveness.

One starting point is in how we define *culture*. We agree with other professionals in the field who call for consideration of diversity from a broad perspective as part of the need for school psychologists to change their role to meet the demands of the new millennium (Bradley-Johnson & Dean, 2000). For example, Bradley-Johnson and Dean (2000) concur with other professionals in the field (e.g., Nastasi, Varjas, Sarkar, & Jayasena, 1998) that "culture" should be more broadly defined to include place of residence (urban vs. rural), geographic location (native vs. international), age, gender, socioeconomic status, sexual orientation, and specific family traditions, along with the more limited definition of culture as race and ethnicity. A broader definition of culture would compel practitioners to take account of many more factors that could be potential contributors to current functioning that would not have otherwise been considered if the focus had simply been on race or ethnicity. The drawback on focusing exclusively on the latter could be an overinterpretation of characteristics based on race or ethnicity alone to the exclusion of other important factors.

Second, there is also a need to consider other moderating variables in working with culturally and linguistically diverse individuals. Moderator variables such as *acculturation, worldview,* and *identity* (Dana, 1993) differentiate and help to deepen understanding of within-group and between-group differences and similarities in theory and research (Vázquez, 1997). By taking moderator variables into account when working with culturally and linguistically diverse individuals, school psychologists will be better able to obtain a more reliable estimate of the potential contribution of cultural variance in their evaluation procedures (Dana, 1993). Acculturation, worldview, and identity are discussed briefly next.

Acculturation

Acculturation is the process of psychological change in values, beliefs, and behaviors when adapting to a new culture (Takushi & Uomoto, 2001). With school populations increasing in diversity, this process is an important issue that warrants consideration. School psychologists need to be aware of this process and to interpret students' behavior in light of it so as not to assume that a particular response is necessarily associated with a learning disability, emotional disability, or other form of within-person pathology. It may be the case that the students' behavioral responses may be associated with the process of acculturation or adaptation to a new cultural environment such as the school. It may also be true that individuals who are less acculturated into the dominant culture—those who have more of a traditional cultural orientation—are more likely to function in ways that are more consistent with some of the known generalizations regarding their particular ethnic or cultural minority group. Competent evaluation of culturally and linguistically diverse individuals needs to account for the contribution of culture; therefore, it is necessary to know to what level the person has acculturated to an environment. Many acculturation instruments have been developed to assist school psychologists in evaluating this construct with their clientele.

However, as with many constructs in psychology, there is no single measurement model of acculturation. These acculturation measurement models consist of conceptualizing acculturation along a single unilinear continuum (e.g., Berry & Annis, 1974) or using a bilinear model (e.g., Szapocznik, Kurtines, & Fernandez, 1980a, 1980b) and can further be classified as based on a single or on multiple cultures (i.e., monocultural or dual-cultural; Kim & Abreu, 2001). Kim and Abreu (2001) conducted a search of acculturation instruments and found 33 tools for use with either African Americans, Asian Americans, Hispanic Americans, Native Americans, or Native Hawaiians and one instrument for all ethnic minority groups. More recently, Taras (2008) conducted a similar search and identified 59 acculturation assessment tools. Acculturation scales for Hispanic populations are by far the most developed, which is not surprising given the rapid growth of this segment of the population. In addition, many acculturation scales had initially been developed on the adult population, but more recently a focus on children and, in particular, adolescents has been noted.

Rhodes, Ochoa, and Ortiz (2005) suggest using interviews and observations in addition to the questionnaire/survey method of assessment to measure level of acculturation. Using an interview helps one to determine or judge the level of acculturation (i.e., distance between individual's own acculturation and that of the mainstream culture). In addition, observation as a tool for assessing acculturation allows one to observe patterns of preference, identification, participation, and affiliation with mainstream culture, as well as language preference, manner/style of dress, celebration of holidays, and explicit expressions of cultural knowledge. Although some methods may be better (i.e., interviews and surveys) than others (observations) for assessing acculturation, what is most important is that acculturation level is assessed in the first place. Another variable to consider besides level of acculturation is the stress that can be directly associated with it.

The process of acculturation itself can be a stressful encounter for individuals. The effect of experiencing what has been termed *acculturative stress* may lead to certain problems, such as anxiety, depression, marginality and alienation, or identity confusion (e.g., Williams & Berry, 1991). Therefore, it is critical as part of our work with culturally diverse individuals that we take into account the process of acculturation and possible associated stressors in order to best meet the needs of these individuals.

Worldview

The concept of worldview has been defined as *people's insight regarding their culture and individuality* (Sue & Sue, 2008), or how they perceive the world given their own experiences, culture, and so forth. People's beliefs and assumptions are rooted in their worldview (Takushi & Uomoto, 2001). Furthermore, worldview encompasses group identity, individual identity, beliefs, values, and language. It influences all perceptions, including what and how we learn. Thus, culture and worldview can have an impact on how individuals perform on evaluative procedures and on their communication style (e.g., verbal and nonverbal behaviors). It is also critical for school psychologists to be aware of their own worldviews and subsequent beliefs and assumptions, because they may differ significantly from those of their clientele. Many times school psychologists acknowledge the importance of taking cultural diversity into account in their work but do little to put aside or even examine their own cultural assumptions, values, and beliefs to consider how their clients might view the world differently than they do (e.g., Savage, Prout, & Chard, 2004).

Many of the practices in school psychology, as well as the systems in which school psychologists work, adhere to a Western worldview. The Western worldview can be described as being influenced by Judeo-Christianity and "concerned with individualism, autonomy, and the need to control and survive" (Ibraham, Roysircar-Sodowsky, & Ohnishi, 2001, p. 441). Because of the pervasive influence of this worldview in American society, there is often a general expectation that all students need to adhere to it in order to function and/or succeed in a society that also adheres to a Western worldview. But are we doing more harm than good by expecting certain groups of students to put aside their beliefs and assumptions in order to stay within the status quo? This is a difficult question.

Because worldview encompasses an individual's group and individual identities, beliefs, values, and even language(s) used, it directly influences his or her perceptions, including what and how he or she learns. Thus, it follows that it is important to take an individual's worldview into account because it can have a significant impact on his or her performance in a classroom. Expecting students to adopt a Western worldview is in some ways an unfortunate practice given that their worldviews are directly related to their cultural and ethnic identities (i.e., a shared cultural heritage, social relatedness, and cultural ties; Sodowsky, Kwan, & Pannu, 1995); ethnic identity has also been identified as an important moderator variable. What message are we sending to these students about the value of their own culture or ethnicity? Unfortunately, perhaps the message that is being received by many students is that they are not valued. If so, then this may lead to a self-fulfilling prophecy related to poor academic and social performance at school.

To become culturally responsive, competent, and effective, all practitioners need to start with an exploration of their own cultural beliefs and assumptions and to understand how their worldviews may differ from those of their clients to ensure that this "difference" will not interfere with meeting the needs of students. It is also critical that practitioners be aware of their own ethnic identity development to best serve their diverse clientele.

Identity

Being aware of where students are regarding their identity development will give the school psychologist a better indication of these students' cultural background and characteristics as well as their perspective on how they will approach the world. It is through acknowledgment of a student's identity that a school psychologist can avoid stereotyping them or approaching them in a stereotypical manner. It is through understanding identity development that the school psychologist can learn about and appreciate the experience of culturally and ethnically diverse clientele. As a result of much research, several models of racial and ethnic identity development have been developed. This section highlights some of the prominent models and/or experts in this area.

Cross (1971, as cited in Atkinson, Morten, & Sue, 1998) was one of the first individuals to develop the idea of the racial identity model (Negro-to-Black Convergence Experience) that dealt with the issues of racial oppression and African Americans' identity development in relation to it. Cross's models addressed the notion that individuals have varying racial and cultural levels of identity, which allowed service providers to clearly identify clients' level of racial identity and encouraged them to be culturally competent in order to provide effective services. Because of this positive influence (i.e., service providers' consideration of racial/cultural variables), Cross's models had a profound impact on the profession of psychology. Many identity development models designed for various ethnic groups were patterned after Cross's original models (e.g., Atkinson et al., 1998; Sue & Sue, 1981, 1999, 2008).

Cross's model (1971, 1972; Hall, Cross, & Freedle, 1972, 1995, as cited in Sue & Sue, 2008) outlined four stages of black identity development: *preencounter, encounter, immersion–emersion,* and *internalization.* In this process, individuals move from a white frame of reference to a positive black frame of reference, from the preencounter stage, in which a person is not aware of the implications of his or her race or ethnicity) to processes that involve consciously or unconsciously diminishing one's "blackness," to achievement of a sense of inner security as conflicts between "old" and "new" identities are resolved during *internalization* (which involves reaching a balance and developing a level of comfort regarding their race/ethnicity; Sue & Sue, 1999). In sum, "global anti-White feelings subside as the person becomes more flexible, more tolerant, and more bicultural/multicultural" (Sue & Sue, 2008, p. 237).

Atkinson et al. (1998) developed a five-stage minority identity development model, which, unlike Cross's model, is based on the assumption that all minority groups experience the common force of oppression and that, as a result, all will generate attitudes and behaviors consistent with a natural internal struggle to develop a strong sense of self- and group identity. These authors conceptualized their model as a continuous process in which the stages blend into one another without clear or abrupt separation: *conformity, dissonance, resistance and immersion, introspection,* and *synergetic articulation and awareness.* A person's development follows from a preference for dominant cultural values (conformity) to a sense of self-fulfillment regarding his or her ethnic identity (synergetic articulation and awareness). This model again has implications for the school psychologist in understanding the impact of cultural experiences on a person's behavior.

D. W. Sue and D. Sue (1990, 1999, as cited in Sue & Sue, 2008) elaborated on this model and developed the racial/cultural identity development model. Like the previous model, it includes five stages of development that "oppressed people experience as they struggle to understand themselves in terms of their own culture, the dominant culture, and the oppressive relationship between the two cultures: conformity, dissonance, resistance and immersion, introspection, and integrative awareness" (Sue & Sue, 2008, p. 242). The authors further delineate attitudes and beliefs at each stage of development that help service providers understand their clients more thoroughly. These attitudes and beliefs relate to how the clients view themselves, others of the same ethnicity, others of differing minority ethnicity, and those from the majority culture.

In summary, the commonality across these ethnic identity development models is the importance of outlining the cultural experience of individuals from minority backgrounds. That is, in order to provide proper services to individuals from culturally diverse backgrounds, school psychologists need to understand their clients' and their own ethnic identities.

Models for Best Practice in School Psychology Service Delivery

Assessment

As noted throughout this book, the role of the school psychologist appears to be chang-ing, with less emphasis on traditional assessment activities and a greater emphasis on assessment as part of the problem-solving process, but assessment will continue to be an important part of the school psychologist's role even in this new paradigm. As assessment experts, school psychologists are required to make informed decisions regarding evalu-ation procedures with all students. In particular, school psychologists need to attend to the various cultural, ethnic, and linguistic variables that influence the evaluations that we complete. Not only is it best practice to consider cultural, ethnic, and linguistic vari-ables in assessment, but it is also mandated by the Individuals with Disabilities Education Improvement Act (IDEIA) as well as by NASP and APA, all of which make reference to the need to assess these factors. Yet many school psychologists do not receive adequate training in this area (Ochoa, Rivera, & Ford, 1997; Padilla, 2001; Rogers & Lopez, 2002). Padilla and Borsato (2008) corroborate this conclusion by stating that "although the situation is improving, many psychologists are not trained in nonbiased assessment, and as a result, they know little about procedures for evaluating students from diverse back-grounds" (p. 16). Given these observations, the following sections highlight the critical considerations in evaluating students from culturally and linguistically diverse back-grounds.

Nondiscriminatory Assessment

Although there are relatively few hard data to demonstrate this notion conclusively, writ-ers in the fields of psychology and educational assessment have long contended that many tests that are used in educational settings are biased against individuals from minority (racial and ethnic) backgrounds. As such, there has been a significant push to develop assessment procedures and tests that, in particular, are "culturally sensitive," "culture reduced," and/or "culture free." However, it has been argued that it is impos-sible to eliminate the influence of culture (Ortiz, 2008), because it is a multifaceted, multidimensional construct that is too complex to be able to completely account for in evaluations. Thus, many researchers in the field argue not only for the development of assessment instruments that take into account issues of culture and diversity but also that evaluation is a process that we strive to make as "nondiscriminatory" as possible (Ortiz, 2008). Ortiz (2008) suggests that nondiscriminatory assessment is a process that guaran-tees that every individual is evaluated in the least discriminatory manner possible rather than just the search for "the" best unbiased test. He further contends that this process is applicable to all individuals, not just those who are "different" in some way or are from a minority cultural background.

Padilla and Borsato (2008) also argue that assessment of psychological variables is made culturally sensitive through a "continuing and open-ended series of substan-tive and methodological insertions and adaptations [e.g., development of instruments, administration, to interpretation] designed to mesh the process of assessment and evalu-ation with the cultural characteristics of the group being studied" (p. 6). So it is not suf-ficient solely to incorporate instruments that have been designed by considering cultural variables; we must also engage in a "process" that leads to evaluations being culturally responsive to our clients. Padilla and Borsato (2008) advocate for a paradigm shift in which evaluations take into account the unique values of specific ethnic groups, which do not necessitate comparison with other groups, especially if the comparison is likely to be biased. Further, they argue that there is a need to increase the cross-cultural competencies of those individuals administering assessments. That is, these individuals need to become more knowledgeable and comfortable with the customs and communicative styles of the diversity of persons who are not representative of the prototypical individual on whom most assessments are based (e.g., white, middle-class persons). Last, given the bias inherent in many tests, it is also critical that test examiners be knowledgeable about psychometric theory and test construction as well as administration and interpretation.

When it comes to nondiscriminatory assessment of culturally and linguistically diverse students, there are no clear-cut formulas for what to do (i.e., a "use this test with this student"-type approach). Rather, one has to consider each case individually, while keeping cultural, ethnic, and linguistic factors in mind, to develop a hypothesis regarding that individual's functioning. Therefore, the goal is to develop and follow strategies that can be implemented with any student; as such, general guidelines have been developed to help accomplish just this. For example, Ortiz (2008, pp. 668–674) offered a comprehensive framework for nondiscriminatory assessment that includes the following components: assess for the purpose of intervention (i.e., intervention-driven evaluation); assess initially with authentic and alternative procedures (e.g., curriculum-based materials); assess and evaluate the learning ecology (i.e., extrinsic cause of learning difficulties); assess and evaluate language proficiency and opportunity for learning; assess and evaluate educationally relevant cultural and linguistic factors (e.g., exposure to different cultures and languages); evaluate, revise, and retest hypotheses (i.e., to reduce making incorrect inferences about assessment data based on preconceived notions); determine the need for and language(s) of assessment; reduce bias in traditional testing practices (i.e., either administering tests in a standardized way and attempting to evaluate results in a nondiscriminatory manner or modifying testing in way that is less discriminatory initially); and support conclusions via data convergence and multiple indicators. Although this model provides a very thorough assessment of cultural factors, one must still consider the application of this model on a case-by-case basis. For further study, Martines (2008) also provides a compilation of critical factors (e.g., determining ethnicity and decision-making guidelines), models (e.g., multicultural assessment procedure and bicultural model), and assessment practices (alternative methods, preschool assessment) necessary for evaluating students who are CLD. Lau and Blatchley (2009) also provide a multidimensional, multi-task evaluation model for students who are CLD that, like Lopez's model, emphasizes the importance of cultural and linguistic variables for inter- and intrapersonal comparisons, the former comparison to those of similar cultural, educational, and socioeconomic backgrounds.

Assessing Language

Aside from the assessment of cultural variables such as acculturation, worldview, and ethnic identity, a school psychologist also must be competent in assessing language and language proficiency. However, before the actual assessment process begins, a school psychologist needs to have fundamental knowledge regarding language proficiency and development. Often, what is deemed abnormal or a language deficit is actually a natural consequence of developing two languages simultaneously or acquiring a second language. During second-language acquisition, children may go through some learning processes such as *code switching* (i.e., mixing languages), *interference* (i.e., having one language interfere with the other, such as when a child has to translate from one language to the other cognitively), and *silent periods* that could be perceived as deficits (Rhodes et al., 2005). These are normal processes and should not be taken as signs of language delays or disorders. Frequently, some behaviors of bilingual students or second-language learners are interpreted as being similar to those of children with learning disabilities: being withdrawn, distractible, moving more during English class; hesitating to speak; making mistakes in verbal or written English because of the use of the L1 (first-language) phonetic system; difficulty in math because of limited vocabulary in English; and making similar mistakes in reading, such as losing his or her place in the text, making substitutions, repeating words, and so forth. However, it is critical to assess where a student is with regard to language development and proficiency.

Cummins's (1984) work is central to understanding development of language proficiency. He has suggested that it takes 2 to 3 years to develop basic interpersonal communication skills (BICS), or what is equated with "social" language, whereas it may take 5 to 7 years for acquirement of cognitive academic language proficiency (CALP), or the language of "school" (i.e., that which facilitates academic success). BICS and CALP help us understand why a student learning a second language is able to converse in the second language much sooner than he or she succeeds with written and oral language related to schoolwork and learning in academic areas. Thus, oral language proficiency can be deceiving, because a student may appear to be very fluent in a social context (Yansen & Shulman, 1996) but may be challenged in other facets.

Language proficiency has typically been measured on a continuum from nonspeaker of a language to fluent speaker (Yansen & Shulman, 1996). According to Yansen and Shulman (1996), language proficiency can be classified under five levels of proficiency: level 1, nonspeaker; level 2, very limited speaker; level 3, limited speaker; level 4, functional speaker, and level 5, fluent speaker. In addition to assessing language development and proficiency, it is equally important to assess language dominance. A school psychologist can use a home language survey (Ortiz, 1992, as cited in Yansen & Shulman, 1996) to assess information regarding language use patterns, language first learned, and language preference. Yansen and Shulman (1996) recommend an additional method: using story narration stemming from picture or book prompts, which helps give an indication of a student's capacity for self-expression in both languages. More formal methods of assessments that have been used include the Language Assessment Scales (DeAvila & Duncan, 2005), the Bilingual Syntax Measure (Burt, Dulay, & Hernandez Chavez, 1980), the Bilingual Verbal Abilities Tests (Muñoz-Sandoval, Cummins, Alvarado, & Ruef, 2000), and La Bateria III Woodcock-Muñoz (Bateria III; Muñoz-Sandoval, Woodcock, McGrew, & Mather, 2005). Again, the method of choice will depend on several factors, including the referral question and other sources of information related to language development and proficiency.

Use of an Interpreter

Another consideration for school psychologists is whether to use an interpreter during evaluation procedures or for other facets of school psychological services. However, using an interpreter takes serious consideration, given the complexity inherent in bringing in an additional person to serve as an intermediary. Not only must the interpreter be competent in interpretation, but also the school psychologist must be competent in working with interpreters and both must possess essential skills and competencies in order to meet with successful outcomes for the students served through this process. For example, interpreters need to possess knowledge regarding the cultural backgrounds of the students with whom they work in addition to skills in translation and understanding the education and psychological issues faced by the school psychologist with whom they are collaborating (Lopez, 2008). In turn, the school psychologist needs to be able to work collaboratively with the interpreter and have skills in obtaining and reporting data obtained through an interpreter to understand the issues involved in working through an interpreter (Lopez, 2008). In addition, school psychologists must be able to establish rapport with students and families to interview, to conduct meetings, and so forth through an interpreter (see Lopez, 2008, for a more thorough description of these individual competencies as well as the shared competencies of interpreter and school psychologist). Lopez provides many recommendations for each phase of working with interpreters that cut across the various functions of the school psychologist: briefing session (addressing seating arrangements, providing context to the interpreter, discussing ethics, deciding what type of oral translation to use, discussion of technical terms, providing an opportunity to translator to review documents, addressing cross-cultural communication and behaviors, and providing the interpreter an opportunity to ask questions); active phase (establishing rapport with client, using audiotapes, allowing time for translation, note taking, assessing the comprehension of the client, and observation of verbal and nonverbal interactions); and debriefing session (discussing outcomes of session and cross-cultural issues, encouraging the interpreter to ask questions, revisiting issues or concerns during the session, and learning from the experience as a means to improve subsequent sessions). It is also important for a school psychologist to evaluate the translation process by taking a critical look at the data collected and consider what he or she will do differently in subsequent sessions that will improve outcomes for the students and families. In using an interpreter, various potential problems can arise, and one must be able to anticipate issues such as the interpreter's lack of "psychological" knowledge or his or her attitudes and beliefs that may interfere with the process (Vázquez, 2003). In sum, the use of interpreters in school psychology practice, particularly in assessment, is an extremely complex matter that has only recently begun to receive the detailed attention it requires.

Consultation

Another area of focus for service provision by school psychologists is consultation. Consultation is an indirect service delivery model emphasizing prevention and problem solving of student issues. School consultation is a critical component of school psychology work and is likely to increase in prominence with the current emphasis on RTI. In schools, consultation involves interaction between school personnel (including school psychologists) and families in conferring and collaborating as a team to identify the needs of students (Dettmer, Thurston, & Dyck, 2005). Furthermore, school consultants aid in the implementation, evaluation, and revision of educational programs that have been designed to serve the learning and behavioral needs of the students they serve.

Culturally competent educators should work toward reducing stereotyping and preventing prejudice of culturally diverse groups, but just as important is the goal of promoting contributions from culturally diverse groups (Dettmer et al., 2005). Dettmer and colleagues see the role of the consultant as being facilitative and supportive in this endeavor, particularly in the area of assessing the instructional environment and designing effective instruction for culturally diverse groups. Dettmer and colleagues reiterate the multicultural competencies of collaborative consultants to include assessing one's own cultural awareness and sensitivity as a means to develop and strengthen skills in working with diverse groups. They also highlight the importance of being aware of one's own cultural background so as to enhance abilities for acknowledging cultural differences that may arise through the consultative process.

Furthermore, Booker (2009) provides a rationale for considering culture in school consultation. Namely, she discusses two primary viewpoints: the need to be an ethical practitioner and the need to effectively understand culture-related dynamics in the classroom. Booker states, "To be capable of working in schools and to practice in an ethical manner require becoming adept at understanding individual and cultural differences" (p. 174). As such, she argues that we have professional ethical obligations in relation to the increase in diversity of our school's populations to integrate culture in to consultative practices. She further discusses the differential school practices (e.g., educational placements) that have occurred historically and presently that underscore why culture is important to consider and, therefore, an important first step in being an agent of change. She concludes, "More than just individual differences will likely impinge upon the effectiveness of consultation in schools. Working on understanding culture will create only a more competent consultant" (p. 187).

Significant attention has been given to further understanding and explicitly outlining the need to incorporate multicultural variables into the consultation framework (e.g., Ingraham, 2000; Rogers, 2000; Sheridan, 2000). Ingraham (2000, p. 323) stated that there is a need for a conceptual framework for multicultural school consultation that "considers diversity issues in the structures, processes, context, and their interactions for practice." Ingraham suggested that a multicultural framework for consultation is needed that incorporates diversity in its broadest form, that focuses on all individuals involved in consultation (and their interrelationships), that takes into account the cultural context of consultation, that considers issues and constructs resulting from consultation across and within cultures, that clearly articulates competencies of consultants and consultees alike, and that increases attention to areas of much-needed research. A multicultural school consultant regards culture as influencing the "thoughts, expectations, and behaviors for each party in the consultation and makes adjustments to develop and maintain rapport and understanding with the consultee(s) and client(s)" (Ingraham, 2000, p. 326). Ingraham offered five components of a multicultural school consultation (MSC) framework that underlie the theory and practice of MSC. These domains are related to consultant learning and development, consultee learning and development, cultural variations in the consultation constellation, contextual and power influences, and hypothesized methods for supporting consultee and client success. In addition, Sheridan (2000) considered the impact of multiculturalism and diversity in behavioral consultation with parents and teachers and noted that much empirical support exists for the use of behavioral or conjoint behavioral consultation in the schools but that much less research exists on the use of this model when the individuals involved in the consultation process represent different areas of diversity.

Rogers (2000) summarized the themes related to cross-cultural competencies in consultation that have been identified as "important and necessary for effective consultation" (p. 415). These competencies refer to understanding one's own and other's cultures. It is necessary to be aware of one's own beliefs, assumptions, and prejudices as well as to understand the cultural and sociopolitical backgrounds of clients and to understand and respect their perspectives, values, and histories. Another competency identified is that of developing cross-cultural communication and interpersonal skills. A school consultant must be effective in bridging diverse perspectives and building relationships with those involved (i.e., stakeholders). Additionally, it is necessary to examine the "cultural embeddedness" of consultation. Just as in the assessment role, school psychologists must consider the context, which may necessarily involve using one's cultural lens or perspective throughout the process of consultation. School consultants also need to be skilled in using qualitative and quantitative methodologies for the purpose of data gathering, which is a central component of the consultation process. School consultants are also competent in acquiring culture-specific knowledge (e.g., acculturation, second-language acquisition or bilingualism, bilingual education, emigration, culture-specific issues in assessment, education, and mental health). Finally, school consultants understand and are skilled in working with interpreters (i.e., from finding an interpreter to training and working with him or her).

It has been recognized that consultation frameworks themselves need to incorporate multicultural and diversity issues, and this recognition also needs to be translated into systematic training in graduate training programs. Martines (2003) outlined specific suggestions related to training cross-cultural consultant school psychologists. Martines reiterated the importance of integrating Sue's (1981) cross-cultural competencies (i.e., attitude, knowledge, and skill competencies related to culture and ethnicity) into the course objectives as well as incorporating instructional strategies and assignments related to further understanding and applying these issues. According to Martines (2003), it is not sufficient just to provide "on-the-job training"; students must also be provided with a framework to be able to continue to develop their multicultural competency in their profession (p. 13).

Response to Intervention

As noted throughout this book, there has been a fairly dramatic increase in the use and discussion of the RTI model in school psychology since the first edition of this book was published. While RTI models have been developed to meet the academic and behavioral needs of all students, special consideration has been given to the use of RTI models with culturally and linguistically diverse students or implementing culturally responsive RTI.

For example, Klinger and Edwards (2006) noted that culturally responsive, quality instruction is important to evaluate within an RTI model. Success at Tier 1 would require that teachers have the knowledge and experience with appropriate evidence-based instructional approaches that have been validated with CLD populations. According to Klinger and Edwards, it is unknown what the intensive support at Tier 2 needs to look like for students who are CLD. At Tier 3, a child study team should be diverse and composed of individuals with expertise in culturally responsive pedagogy, nonbiased assessment, and language acquisition. Klinger and Edwards conclude that we need to address the critical issues surrounding providing services to CLD populations so as to avoid reinforcing a "deficit-based approach to sorting children" (p. 115).

Harris-Murri, King, and Rostenberg (2006) argue the need for a culturally responsive RTI model as an approach for reducing disproportionate minority representation of students with emotional disturbance (ED) in special education. They describe several dimensions of a culturally responsive RTI model for students who are at risk for ED. The first dimension refers to the importance of assessing the perceptions and ideologies across the home, school, and community as a means to implement interventions through the recognition of cultural differences this process brings about. The second dimension emphasizes the importance of professional development of educators to include the examination of biases. The emphasis on culturally responsive curriculum and instructional practices is the third dimension. A culturally responsive RTI approach would ensure that students receive appropriate instruction that builds on students' prior knowledge, interest, motivation and home language. Instructional practices would include various forms of scaffolds for students and meaningful learning activities that connect to the home culture and emphasizes the student–teacher relationship. The last dimension refers to culturally appropriate assessment procedures in evaluating a student for ED. Harris-Murri and colleagues (2006) assert that "being culturally responsive is more than a set of practices. Rather, cultural responsiveness provides an additional and necessary dimension to the RTI framework that impacts all levels of intervention for all students" (p. 794).

Brown and Doolittle (2008) describe a three-tier cultural, linguistic, and ecological framework for RTI with students who are English language learners (ELL). Tier 1 includes universal screening and research-based instruction as with the previous models; however, these authors emphasize that the instruction at this level must be not only "effective and appropriate" but also linguistically and culturally congruent (p. 6). This means that the classroom teacher must be knowledgeable about language acquisition and be able to apply this knowledge to providing relevant curricula. At Tier 2, more intensive support, the same argument is made for instructional interventions with students who are ELL that are both linguistically and culturally appropriate. Tier 3, intensive individual support, requires the continued consideration of the student's academic, linguistic, and cultural needs as well as consideration of nonbiased evaluation.

Last, Brown-Chidsey and Steege (2005) argue for fair and equitable practices related to assessment, the cornerstone of RTI practices. They reiterate the importance of recognizing the features present that make students unique and diverse, conducting background-specific assessments, and engaging in appropriate goal setting. Regarding how RTI connects to diverse backgrounds, Brown-Chidsey and Steege remind us that the only "rule" that needs to be followed is that of implementing research-based interventions and using data to determine student outcomes. There is nothing in RTI to require that it be bound by specific ability, culture, language, race, or religious ideologies. For this reason, interventions can be "matched to students' backgrounds and experiences" (p. 107). This reiterates the focus of RTI, which is to provide an education for *all* students. There is nothing to stop us from tailoring that education to the needs of students who are CLD.

Overall, the models previously presented all highlight the importance of taking in to account the specific cultural and linguistic needs of CLD students in the RTI process. They encourage us to look beyond the individual student and consider the various other systemic factors (e.g., teachers and staff) that can have an impact on the success of the CLD student. What can be gleaned from these models regarding culturally responsive RTI is the following: (1) Avoid a deficit-based approach; (2) address teacher and school issues in addition to those of the student; and (3) be knowledgeable about culturally responsive pedagogy and language acquisition processes. The first point highlights the significance of avoiding blaming the student for the challenges he or she is having in the classroom. The second point reiterates the importance of implementing research-based practices and interventions within an RTI approach so as to avoid developing another discriminatory process with students who are CLD. Finally, it is critical that teachers and staff are knowledgeable about culturally responsive pedagogy and practices as well as developmental processes in order to avoid a "one shoe fits all" approach.

School Psychology and the Misrepresentation of Minority Students in Special Education Programs

In direct contrast to what is occurring in the field of school psychology related to the underrepresentation of minority individuals practicing in the field, we are continuing to see overrepresentation of minority students in special education. Thus, responding effectively to cultural and linguistic diversity as school psychologists becomes even more salient. For more than three decades, the overrepresentation of ethnic minority students in special education programs has been a prominent and controversial issue. In the most recent annual report to Congress on the implementation of IDEA, proportionally Native Americans (14.09%) and African Americans/blacks (12.61%) had the highest representation of students in special education. This was followed by whites (8.76%), Latino/as (8.38%), and students of Asian/Pacific Islander descent (4.64%). A high proportion of American Indians/Native Alaskans (7.5%) and African American/blacks (5.65%) had learning disabilities compared with Latino/a (4.74%); white (3.86%), and Asian (1.73%) students. Similarly, 1.87% of blacks and 1.04% of Native Americans were classified as having intellectual disabilities compared with 0.69% for whites, 0.59% for Latino/as, and 0.41% for Asians. Within the ED category, Native American (1.13%) and African American/black (1.38%) students again had higher placement rates than white (0.69%), Latino/a (0.43%), and Asian (0.21%) students (U.S. Department of Education, 2009). These findings are still consistent with previously observed trends by Zhang and Katsiyannis (2002), and the National Center for Education Statistics (2010b), that is, the continued historic disproportionate representation of African American students' as having disabilities, especially intellectual disabilities and ED. The data also show a new trend in that American Indians/Native Alaskans have the highest risk index across all disabilities and ethnicities. Guiberson (2009) found, via a comprehensive literature review, that Hispanic children continue to be overrepresented in special education as having specific learning disabilities or speech–language impairments while being underrepresented as having intellectual disabilities and EDs. Further, Rhodes et al. (2005) discussed the variability of minority students in special education across states/regions, and note that Hispanics, African Americans, Asian/Pacific Islanders, and Native Americans in states that had the largest ethnic populations were more likely to be labeled as having intellectual disabilities, illustrating that national data can mask the disproportion that exists within and across states.

Given all of these findings, educators must ensure that minority students who been identified as having a disability have access to appropriate services despite calls to achieve proportionate representation. For example, Klinger et al. (2005) call for addressing these disproportionate trends through the creation of culturally responsive educational systems. They state, "Instead of determining how to 'fix' culturally and linguistically diverse students' 'deficits,' professionals' biases, or society as a whole, we aim to promote the creation of conditions, produce resources and tools, and support multiple stakeholders in the creation of educational systems that are responsive to cultural diversity" (p. 8). This viewpoint resonates with the message of this chapter: the notion that cultural competence is a response to the individual needs of each student.

Rhodes and colleagues (2005) recommend solutions to minority misrepresentation in five areas: teacher training at both the preservice and inservice levels in instructing diverse students; improvement in early intervention/prereferral activities; research to test the "differential susceptibility" versus the systematic bias hypothesis and related to the interaction between a child's ecology and culture; activities that need to be undertaken by the U.S. Office of Civil Rights (e.g., collecting data and writing reports); and factors that should be considered by the profession (e.g., identification procedures).

In sum, the issue of misrepresentation in special education programs is complex. It may take years of systemic changes at the federal, state, and local levels to address adequately this concern. However, in the absence of such far-reaching efforts, school psychologists can ensure that they engage in best practices in service provision to culturally, ethnically, and linguistically diverse groups so as not to become a part of the problem. As a means to aid both practicing and future school psychologists in the effort to become leaders in the field, ensuring that disparities such as those described earlier dissipate, we offer several suggestions for increasing one's own multicultural competency and effectiveness. These suggestions are listed in Table 3.1. To those who have already begun this journey, we commend your efforts in understanding that "diversity is a gift to be cherished and not a fear to be destroyed because of lack of knowledge" (Vázquez, 1997).

Alternative Viewpoint on the Emphasis of Multicultural Competence

Frisby (2009) posited an alternative viewpoint on the emphasis of multicultural competence in school psychology: "Weak empirical support for the CC [cultural competence] construct, and the lack of research-based answers for troubling gaps in the justification for CC advocacy, should temper the urgency with which the CC movement is promoted in school psychology" (Frisby, 2009, p. 873). Frisby offers a critical analysis of the "evidence" for the construct validity of the concept of "cultural competence." He provides a brief

TABLE 3.1. Suggestions for Strengthening the Multicultural Competency of School Psychologists

1. Be aware of your own values, beliefs, and worldview so as to understand how your perceptions may help or hinder your work with others (families, students, colleagues, administration, etc.).

2. Be aware of where you are in your own ethnic identity development so as to understand your comfort level within your own and others' cultures/backgrounds.

3. Be aware of any potential bias(es) (you may have) related to cultural variables (e.g., race, ethnicity, gender, socioeconomic status, disability, etc.) to best meet the needs of your clientele.

4. Understand your limitations and be willing to seek out consultation from others who may have more multicultural knowledge and/or experience.

5. Be willing to learn about others' cultural backgrounds and experiences to avoid stereotyping and to consider within- and between-group differences and similarities.

6. Seek out information regarding your clients' worldviews, values, and beliefs in order to establish and sustain a productive working relationship.

7. Always consider students' and families' cultural contexts when collecting and interpreting evaluation data.

8. Understand how to use and seek out interpreters and/or translators to assist you in your work with linguistically diverse clientele.

9. Understand individual's preferred method of communication (e.g., preferred language) and understand cultural variations in communication (e.g., showing respect for others).

10. Understand the strengths and limitations of traditional assessment techniques such as the use of tests with individuals from culturally and linguistically diverse populations.

historical overview of the evolution of the concept, presents its strengths and problems associated with the CC movement in the field, and describes several unexamined mediating assumptions in the CC movement. He questions the logical tie for the argument that the school psychology CC movement "portrays increasing American diversity (premise) and the need for CC (conclusion) as a short move from Step A to Step B" (pp. 869–870). Frisby provides this analysis as a means to drive home the message that the multicultural competence movement in school psychology is promoted with such haste and intensity that the field cannot keep up with the validation of the construct. Further, he argues that there are "too many intervening factors" (p. 877) that have also been neglected in research validation that does not provide assurance in CC, as a construct or training need. Frisby argues that as a field we are eager to be culturally competent but without the understanding of what it means to be culturally competent and without empirical support for what and who is culturally competent.

Frisby provides a valid argument in that as a field we need to ensure that we are implementing empirically supported practices, especially in light of the regulations required by IDEIA and No Child Left Behind for empirically validated practices. Despite Frisby's perspective, it is important to recognize that there have been many practices that have been deemed as culturally appropriate, which in turn have dictated culturally competent practice. Take, for example, the vast literature related to nonbiased assessment and evaluation with culturally and linguistically diverse populations, a strength of the field that Frisby himself supports. Further, we believe some of Frisby's viewpoints regarding the lack of validity for cultural competence in school psychology are equivalent to notions of "throwing the baby out with the bath water." It would be detrimental to the field to completely dismiss the practical and real-life experiences that school psychologists have gained in working with students and families who hail from diverse backgrounds.

Certainly, school psychology needs to continue to refine its culturally competent practices. Many in the field would not disagree with this notion given the diversification of the school population. At the same time, we should not discount the achievements that have already been gained in culturally competent school psychological practices but, rather, critically reflect on what has been shown to be effective and work toward addressing areas of practice that have not been thoroughly validated.

Data-Driven Problem Solving: An Approach for Supporting All Students

In Chapter 7 we introduce the data-driven problem solving model for school psychology practice. The problem-solving approach is a keystone of this volume, and it permeates the view we seek to promote for advancing the science and practice of school psychology. In this model, school psychologists move from simply being diagnosticians and sorters to using their professional and scientific training to become integral players in determining student needs, selecting appropriate interventions, and evaluating the efficacy of these interventions in an ongoing manner.

So what does data-driven problem-solving have to do with cultural and linguistic diversity? We chose to initially introduce the problem-solving model, albeit briefly, at the conclusion of this chapter on diversity because we believe it has great potential to enhance the ability of school psychologists to respond effectively to the needs of students, families, and school systems, regardless of the cultural and linguistic characteristics of those involved. We recognize that human cultural and language differences will always provide a unique challenge to effective delivery of educational and psychological services and that professionals in our field are under special obligation to enhance their awareness of their clients' unique backgrounds, of their own values and biases, and of models for culturally sensitive service delivery. That said, we propose that many of the current issues we face in this regard (such as bias in our assessment tools, barriers to effective communication, and minority overrepresentation in special education programs) may be reduced when we begin to move away from a focus on within-child pathology and move toward a focus on environments, contexts, desired outcomes, and assets.

The basis for the data-driven problem-solving approach is that problems are not necessarily viewed as forms of pathology or disorder but are considered to be discrepancies between *what is occurring* and *what is expected within a given context* (e.g., a classroom or a family). This model is *outcome focused*, meaning that the emphasis is on a solution or outcome to the problem rather than simply offering an elegant description of the problem. It is *context specific*, meaning that what constitutes a problem or a viable solution to it may differ across settings or contexts, just as expectations and social ecologies differ across settings. Moreover, the problem-solving approach is driven by *ongoing data collection*, which is essential not only to defining the problem and developing potential solutions but also to determining whether the solutions are resulting in the desired effect. In addition, the problem-solving model we advocate is integrally linked to intervention. It includes assessment and description, but only to the extent that it helps clarify what is needed and what is effective. The four basic steps of this model, as outlined in Chapter 7, include identifying and validating the problem (what is the problem?), analyzing the problem (why is it occurring?), determining what should be done about the problem (developing and implementing an intervention), and evaluating the efficacy of the intervention through follow-up and ongoing data collection.

Some recent examples of innovative problem-solving-based service delivery systems in education have been shown to reduce bias and enhance outcomes for students of various backgrounds. Some of these examples include the problem-solving model developed by the Heartland Area Education Agency in Iowa (see Tilly, 2008) and the System to Enhance Educational Performance, a multiple-gating system for defining problems and developing targets for intervention (see *www.isteep.com/login.aspx* for more details) developed by Witt and colleagues. These innovations show that it is possible to increase the success of students in general education environments while reducing the need for placing so many students in already overburdened special services programs. As data-based problem-solving models, including the recently developed RTI approach, have become more widespread, there is increasing evidence that they hold great promise for promoting academic and behavioral success of all students (e.g., VanDerHeyden, Witt, & Barnett, 2005). Some of the promises of problem-solving RTI models include enhancing academic performance of students from minority backgrounds and from low-performing schools and reducing errors stemming from teacher misidentification of learning problems (e.g., Shinn, Collins, & Gallagher, 1998; VanDerHeyden & Witt, 2005). Although our field is still in the formative stages of learning to use innovative data-based problem-solving models to enhance school and student outcomes, the potential is tremendous. As our society becomes increasingly diverse and pluralistic, the field of school psychology must not only honor and embrace diversity but also adopt practices and service delivery models that reduce bias, meet individual needs, and result in better outcomes for all children and their families.

DISCUSSION QUESTIONS AND ACTIVITIES

1. On the basis of the discussion presented in this chapter, list what you consider to be three important things you can do to ensure that culturally or linguistically diverse students and/ or families are comfortable in your office. Provide your rationale for your choices.

2. Observe different school settings and decide whether the school includes a diverse population of students and, if so, what forms of diversity are present. What indicators, if any, are present that show respect for and value of the diversity?

3. Reflect on your own behaviors (e.g., language and dialect) and determine which are consistent with mainstream American culture. Reflect on your own biases and/or assumptions.

4. Seek out an experience that will enable you to get to know an individual or group that is different from you in some way, such as culture, ethnicity, religion, sexual orientation, race, nationality, or socioeconomic class. The experience needs to be a new one and one that you would not normally encounter if not for this specific assignment. Write a reaction paper describing the experience and relating to one or more concepts or issues discussed in this chapter.

5. What do you consider to be the most important personal or professional characteristic for a culturally competent school psychologist? Provide a rationale for your answer.

6. As a way to begin to understand your own cultural experiences, keep a weekly journal documenting what you read, hear, or experience regarding diversity during the week. Some questions to consider may include the following: What impact did it have on you? How did the information fit with your existing knowledge and/or experiences? What, if anything, did you learn about someone else who is different from you?

7. Refer to NASP's website on culturally competent practice (*www.nasponline.org/resources/ culturalcompetence/index.aspx*) and complete the self-assessment questionnaire (*www. nasponline.org/resources/culturalcompetence/checklist.aspx*).

8. Interview a school psychologist, special education director, or director of psychological services to determine what model of RTI is implemented within his or her school district. In particular, focus questions on determining the role of the school psychologist given the model of RTI implemented and how issues of diversity are integrated into the process.

CHAPTER 4

Becoming a School Psychologist
Training and Credentialing Issues

T he previous chapters in this volume have addressed general characteristics and background regarding the field of school psychology: an introduction to the field, the historical context of the fields of psychology and education as they have influenced school
psychology, and an overview of issues pertaining to the cultural and linguistic diversity
in our schools and society. With that background as a foundation, we now move into the
process of *becoming a school psychologist*. This chapter comprehensively addresses a variety
of issues related to the process of professional entry into the field. In this chapter, we
explore how individuals make the decision to become school psychologists. An extensive
discussion of school psychology training programs and of the characteristics of students
and faculty in these programs makes up a substantial portion of the chapter. We also
explore myriad issues related to the training of future psychologists and the regulation
of the programs that provide the training. An important and unique aspect of preparation to enter the field—practicum and internship training—is detailed, along with
an exploration of the considerations involved in selecting and finding an appropriate
internship. The various processes for credentialing school psychologists (certification
and licensure) are also discussed, and the chapter concludes with a brief discussion of
continuing professional development expectations and opportunities within the field.

Becoming a School Psychologist

Collectively, we have interviewed or fielded inquiries from hundreds of individuals—
maybe more than that—who are interested in learning more about the field of school
psychology, are seeking admission to graduate programs in the field, or are trying to
find answers to questions about the roles and functions of school psychologists. Most of
these interactions have been with prospective graduate students who are considering

careers as school psychologists. In some cases, these individuals are well informed about the field and have a fairly good understanding of what a school psychologist is and how one becomes a member of the profession. We also find many misconceptions about both issues. These experiences, as well as our own experiences that led us personally to the field of school psychology, have caused us to reflect on the paths that lead to our field. Although it is true that everyone's path is somewhat unique, we have found many similarities on the road to becoming a school psychologist.

One typical commonality among individuals who seek entry into the field of school psychology is a strong interest in both psychology and education, because the field is a unique hybrid of both disciplines. Our experience has been that, increasingly, individuals who apply for admission to graduate programs in school psychology have earned undergraduate degrees in psychology. We estimate that at least 80% of applicants to our respective training programs in recent years have their undergraduate degrees in psychology, with the remaining 20% in the fields of education, sociology or social work, or a variety of other disciplines. A minority of applicants to our programs in recent years—maybe 15 to 25%—have previously earned graduate degrees (usually master's level) in psychology, education, social work, or counseling. Some individuals who enter the field have had previous professional experience in one of these other fields or in another area. However, prior graduate degrees and extensive professional experience are not necessarily the norm for entering the field, and it is our experience that the percentage of applicants to graduate programs in school psychology who have extensive professional experience and a prior graduate degree has declined in recent years. Although we have no hard evidence to prove this point, our perception is that the "typical" newcomer to the field of school psychology in recent years is one who enters graduate school in his or her early to mid-20s, having earned an undergraduate degree in psychology within the past year or 2.

The motivations of individuals who enter the field of school psychology are varied and diverse, but there are some common threads tying them together. Primarily, most budding school psychologists have a strong desire to provide support to children and their families and to assist them as they struggle with the challenges of the educational experience. With this general motivation almost always comes a particular interest and desire to support and assist children who are struggling academically or behaviorally or who are otherwise at risk for negative educational and life outcomes. In other words, those attracted to school psychology tend to have a strong humanitarian or service orientation, coupled with a strong sense of social responsibility and a commitment to and interest in public education. Beyond these general motivations, there are certainly some differences among those who desire to enter the profession. Some aspiring school psychologists move into the field with a burning desire to make a major impact in improving and changing educational and social systems, whereas others are content to work within systems as they are. Some are attracted to the field because of the continuing strong job market (even in recent difficult economic times), stable employment situations, and their perceptions of reasonable compensation and benefit packages, whereas others appreciate the good employment opportunities and general stability of the profession but settle for what they consider disappointing compensation packages. Almost all school psychologists enjoy the generally regular work hours, which typically are similar to a school day or business day. Those who work in public school settings often have 9- or 10-month employment contracts, with additional vacation and holiday time off during the school year.

Regardless of the varied backgrounds, aspirations, and motivations of individuals who enter the field, the highway to the profession invariably begins with acceptance to a graduate training program in school psychology. The 3- to 5- or 6-year graduate school experience (depending on whether one pursues specialist or doctoral-level training) provides the foundation for working as a school psychologist and is an important socializing factor in developing an initial model of practice and a worldview of the field. Thus, graduate training programs in the field, as well as the faculty who staff them, are of particular interest in the process of becoming a school psychologist and are the focus of the next section.

School Psychology Training Programs, Students, and Faculty

Without successfully completing a graduate training program in school psychology, it is increasingly not possible in most states to become a school psychologist. The training programs not only function as the initial point of entry into the profession but also serve the essential role of professional socialization into the field as well as transmission of values and practices for new professionals. It is the training programs that have responsibility for implementing the training standards of the national professional organizations (NASP and APA) and for endorsing graduates of the programs for licensure and certification from state departments of education and from state psychology licensing boards. Given the critical role that school psychology training programs play in the development and well-being of the field, we cover in detail various aspects of graduate training programs and the faculty and graduate students who are connected to these programs. In addition, some of the emerging issues and trends that affect training programs are addressed.

School Psychology Training Programs

Characteristics

It is quite difficult to obtain a highly accurate picture of school psychology training programs across the United States and Canada because two separate national organizations (NASP and APA) accredit or approve programs in the United States and because many programs are not accredited and thus do not appear on lists of approved programs, nor do they have reporting responsibilities to the national organizations. In addition, there seems to be a moderate but constant flux in training programs, with a few new programs emerging each year and some programs being shut down. Furthermore, it is complicated to generalize what we do know about training programs and to make inferences about the students and faculty within them. That said, with the information currently available, as well as previous detailed efforts to describe the characteristics of school psychology training programs, it is possible at least to make some generalizations about training programs, their host institutions, and the faculty and students who are involved in these programs.

The most comprehensive prior recent published list of school psychology training programs has been compiled by Miller (2008) in an appendix to the first volume of the eight-volume *Best Practices in School Psychology V* collection (Thomas & Grimes, 2008). According to Miller's compilation, there are 244 institutions of higher education in the

United States and Canada that provide graduate-level training in school psychology at some level. This figure of 244 is a bit deceptive. There are actually more training programs than institutions, because many institutions have both doctoral- and specialist-level training programs. These programs are often counted separately in attempts to define and accredit training programs, especially the many cases where doctoral programs receive program accreditation review by APA, and that program also has a connected specialist-level training program that receives program approval review by NASP. For example, Miller's appendix lists eight training institutions but 14 degree programs (ranging from master's to specialist to doctoral) for the state of Illinois.

The majority of the current training programs are at the specialist-level or other nondoctoral levels, such as master's degree or certification/licensure-only programs. Based on our review of the most recent lists of accredited programs from both NASP and APA, a review of Miller's (2008) extensive appendix, and reviews of previous attempts to consolidate the information on training programs (e.g., Thomas, 1998; Thomas & Grimes, 2002), we can infer that there are slightly more than two specialist-level training programs for every doctoral-level training program in existence. Given that numerous unaccredited training programs exist and that these programs are more likely to be specialist than doctoral programs, the ratio of specialist-level to doctoral-level programs most likely ranges from about 2.2:1 to about 2.5:1. The number of graduates produced by these programs each year is likely to be even more skewed in the direction of nondoctoral programs because specialist programs tend to be larger than doctoral programs in terms of the number of new students accepted each year.

A review of the current lists of accredited training programs from NASP and APA indicates that the large majority of school psychology training programs—roughly 60 to 70%—are found at public rather than private institutions of higher education. Within these institutions, about 75% of the training programs are located within colleges of education (often within departments of educational psychology), whereas about 25% are located within colleges of arts and sciences in departments of psychology. With a few exceptions, doctoral programs are more likely to be found at national research universities than at regional universities or liberal arts colleges, where specialist-level programs are the norm. School psychology programs at all levels exist across the United States and Canada, but they are not necessarily distributed evenly by region. For example, the Midwest and Northeast regions of the United States have a large number of training programs, whereas there are fewer training programs in the western United States and only a small number of programs in Canada. Table 4.1 provides a comprehensive listing of the master's- and specialist-level school psychology training programs in the United States and Canada, and Table 4.2 provides a comprehensive listing of doctoral training programs. We developed these tables based on our own 2010 review of NASP- and APA-accredited program listings, by consulting Miller's (2008) compilation, and through Internet searches for additional training programs. On the basis of our own analysis of the status of school psychology training programs as of mid-2010, we have identified nearly 250 training programs, with 60 doctoral programs accredited by APA and 182 total programs (specialist and doctoral) approved by NASP. We recognize that there may be some inaccuracies in our listings in Tables 4.1 and 4.2 because of the continuous flux in program status over time. However, these data were the most recent and complete currently available as we prepared this chapter in mid-2010.

(text resumes on page 75)

TABLE 4.1. Listing of Master's- and Specialist-Level School Psychology Training Programs in the United States and Canada

University	Master's/ Specialist degree	NASP/ NCATE
Alabama		
Auburn University	EdS	
University of Alabama	EdS	Full
Arizona		
Argosy University–Phoenix	MA	
Northern Arizona University	MA	Full
University of Arizona	EdS	
Arkansas		
Arkansas State University	EdS	Full
University of Central Arkansas	MS	Full
California		
Azusa Pacific University	MAEd + PPSC	Conditional
California State University–Chico	MA	Full
California State University–Fresno	MS	Full
California State University–East Bay/Hayward	MS	Conditional
California State University–Long Beach	MA	Full
California State University–Los Angeles	MS	Full
California State University–Northridge	MS	Conditional
California State University–Sacramento	MA	Full
California State University–San Bernardino	MA	
Chapman–Orange University	EdS	Full
Fresno Pacific University	MA	
Humboldt State University	MA	Full
La Sierra University	EdS, MA	
Loyola Marymount University	MA	Full
National University	MS	
Philips Graduate Institute	MA	
San Diego State University	EdS	Full
San Francisco State University	MS	
University of California–Riverside	MA	
University of California–Santa Barbara	MEd	Full
University of the Pacific	EdS	Full
Colorado		
University of Colorado at Denver and Health Sciences Center	EdS	Full
University of Denver	EdS	Full
University of Northern Colorado	EdS	Full
Connecticut		
Fairfield University	CAS, MA	Conditional
Southern Connecticut State University	CAS, MS	Full
University of Connecticut	EdS, MA	Full
University of Hartford	CAS, MS	Conditional
Delaware		
University of Delaware	EdS, MA	Full

(cont.)

TABLE 4.1. *(cont.)*

University	Master's/ Specialist degree	NASP/ NCATE
District of Columbia		
Gallaudet University	PsyS	Full
Howard University	CAGS, MA/MEd	
Florida		
Argosy University/Sarasota	MA	
Barry University	SSP, MA	Full
Florida International University	EdS	
Florida State University	EdS, MS	Conditional
Nova Southeastern University	PsyS	Conditional
University of Central Florida	EdS	Full
University of Florida	EdS	Full
University of South Florida	EdS	Full
Georgia		
Georgia Southern University	EdS, MEd	
Georgia State University	EdS, MEd	
Valdosta State University	EdS	Full
Hawaii		
Argosy University–Hawaii	MA	
Idaho		
Idaho State University	EdS, MEd	Full
University of Idaho	EdS	Conditional
Illinois		
Chicago School of Professional Psychology	EdS	Conditional
Eastern Illinois University	SSP	Conditional
Illinois State University	SSP	Full
Loyola University of Chicago	EdS	Full
National–Louis University	EdS, MEd	Full
Northern Illinois University	MA	Full
Southern Illinois University–Edwardsville	SSP, MS	Full
Western Illinois University	SSP	Full
Indiana		
Ball State University	EdS, MA	Full
Indiana State University	EdS, MEd	Full
Indiana University–Bloomington	EdS	Full
Valparaiso University	EdS	Full
Iowa		
University of Iowa	EdS	
University of Northern Iowa	EdS, MAE	Full
Kansas		
Emporia State University	EdS, MS	Full
Fort Hays University	EdS, MS	
Pittsburg State University	EdS	
University of Kansas	EdS	Full
Wichita State University	EdS, MEd	Full

(cont.)

TABLE 4.1. *(cont.)*

University	Master's/ Specialist degree	NASP/ NCATE
Kentucky		
Eastern Kentucky University	PsyS	Full
Murray State University	EdS	
University of Kentucky	EdS, MSEd	Full
Western Kentucky University	EdS	Full
Louisiana		
Louisiana State University–Shreveport	PsyS	Full
Nicholls State University	SSP	Full
University of Louisiana–Monroe	SSP, MS	Conditional
Maine		
University of Southern Maine	MS	Full
Maryland		
Bowie State University	MA/CAS	Conditional
Towson University	CAS	Full
University of Maryland–College Park	CAGS	Conditional
Massachusetts		
Massachusetts School of Professional Psychology	CAGS	Full
Northeastern University	MS, CAGS	Full
Tufts University	MA	Full
University of Massachusetts–Amherst	CAGS	Full
University of Massachusetts–Boston	CAGS	Full
Michigan		
Andrews University	EdS	Full
Central Michigan University	SPsyS, MA	Full
Michigan State University	EdS	Full
University of Detroit–Mercy	SSP	
Wayne State University	MA	Full
Minnesota		
Capella University	CAS, MA	Conditional
Minnesota State University–Moorhead	PsyS, MA	Full
University of Minnesota	EdS	Full
Mississippi		
Mississippi State University	EdS, MS	Full
Missouri		
University of Missouri–Columbia	EdS	
University of Missouri–St. Louis	EdS	Full
Montana		
University of Montana	EdS	Full
Nebraska		
University of Nebraska–Kearney	EdS	Full
University of Nebraska–Lincoln	EdS	Full
University of Nebraska–Omaha	EdS, MS	Full
New Hampshire		
Plymouth State University	CAGS, MEd	

(cont.)

TABLE 4.1. *(cont.)*

University	Master's/ Specialist degree	NASP/ NCATE
Nevada		
University of Nevada–Las Vegas	EdS	Full
University of Nevada–Reno	EdS	
New Jersey		
Fairleigh Dickinson University	MA	
Georgian Court University	CAGS, MA	Full
Kean University	PD, MA	Conditional
New Jersey City University	PD, MA	Full
Rider University	EdS	Full
Rowan University	EdS, MA	Full
Seton Hall University	EdS, MA	
New Mexico		
New Mexico State University	EdS	Full
New York		
Adelphi University	MA	
Alfred University	CAS	Full
City University of New York, Brooklyn College	CAS, MSEd	Full
City University of New York, Queens College	CAS	Full
College of New Rochelle	MA	
College of Saint Rose	CAS, MS	Full
Columbia University, Teachers College	EdM	Full
Fordham University–Lincoln Center	MSE	Full
Iona College	MA	Conditional
Long Island University–Brooklyn Campus	MSEd	
Long Island University–Westchester Graduate Campus	MSEd	
Marist College	CAS, MA	
Mercy College	MS	
Niagara University	CAS, MS	
Pace University–New York City	MSEd	
Roberts Wesleyan University	CAS, MS	Full
Rochester Institute of Technology	CAS, MS	Full
St. John's University	MS	Full
State University of New York–Oswego	CAS, MA	Full
State University of New York–Plattsburgh	CAS, MA	Full
Touro College	MS	
University at Albany, State University of New York	CAS	Full
University at Buffalo, State University of New York	CAS/MA	Full
North Carolina		
Appalachian State University	SSP, MA	Full
East Carolina University	CAS, MA	Full
University of North Carolina–Chapel Hill	MA/MEd	Full
Western Carolina University	MA	Full
North Dakota		
Minot State University	EdS	Full

(cont.)

TABLE 4.1. *(cont.)*

University	Master's/ Specialist degree	NASP/ NCATE
Ohio		
Bowling Green State University	EdS, MA	Full
Cleveland State University	PsyS	Full
John Carroll University	CAGS, MEd	Full
Kent State University	EdS	Full
Miami University	EdS, MS	Full
Ohio State University	MA	Full
University of Cincinnati	EdS	Full
University of Dayton	EdS, MS	Full
University of Toledo	EdS, MA	Full
Oklahoma		
East Central University	MS	
Oklahoma State University	EdS	Full
University of Central Oklahoma	MA	Full
Oregon		
George Fox University	MS	
Lewis and Clark College	MA	Conditional
University of Oregon	MS	
Pennsylvania		
Bryn Mawr College	Certificate	
Bucknell University	MA	
California University of Pennsylvania	EdS, MS	Full
Duquesne University	CAGS, MSEd	Full
Eastern University	MS	
Edinboro University of Pennsylvania	CAGS, MEd	Full
Immaculata University	MA	
Indiana University of Pennsylvania	MEd, EdS	Full
Lehigh University	EdS	Full
Marywood University	EdS	
Millersville University of Pennsylvania	MA	Full
Philadelphia College of Osteopathic Medicine	Eds, MS	Full
Temple University	MEd + 45	Full
Rhode Island		
Rhode Island College	CAGS, MA	Full
University of Rhode Island	MS	Full
South Carolina		
Francis Marion University	MS	Conditional
The Citadel	EdS, MA	Full
Winthrop University	SSP, MS	Full
South Dakota		
University of South Dakota	EdS	Full
Tennessee		
Middle Tennessee State University	EdS	Full
Tennessee State University	EdS, MS	
Tennessee Tech University	EdS, MA	
University of Memphis	EdS, MA	Full
University of Tennessee–Chattanooga	EdS	Full
University of Tennessee–Knoxville	EdS	

(cont.)

TABLE 4.1. *(cont.)*

University	Master's/Specialist degree	NASP/NCATE
Texas		
Abilene Christian University	MS	Full
Baylor University	EdS	Full
Our Lady of the Lake University	MS	
Sam Houston State University	MA	Conditional
Stephen F. Austin University	MA	Full
Tarleton State University	MS	
Tarleton State University–San Marcos	MS	
Texas A&M University–Commerce	MS	Full
Texas State University–San Marcos	MA	Full
Texas Women's University	SSP	Full
Trinity University	MA	Conditional
University of Houston–Clear Lake	MA	Full
University of Houston–Victoria	MA	
University of Texas–Pan American	MA	
University of Texas–Tyler	MS	
West Texas A&M University	MA	
Utah		
Brigham Young University	EdS	Full
University of Utah	MS	
Utah State University	EdS	Full
Virginia		
College of William and Mary	EdS, MEd	Conditional
George Mason University	MA, CAGS	Full
James Madison University	EdS, MA	Full
Radford University	EdS	Full
Washington		
Central Washington University	MEd	Full
Eastern Washington University	MS	Full
Seattle University	EdS	Full
University of Washington	MEd	Full
West Virginia		
Marshall University	EdS	Conditional
Wisconsin		
University of Wisconsin–Eau Claire	EdS, MSE	Full
University of Wisconsin–La Crosse	EdS, MSE	Full
University of Wisconsin–Milwaukee	EdS	Conditional
University of Wisconsin–River Falls	EdS, MSE	Full
University of Wisconsin–Stout	EdS, MSEd	Full
University of Wisconsin–Whitewater	EdS, MSE	Full
Canada		
McGill University	MA	
Mount St. Vincent University	MA	
University of British Columbia	MA/MEd	
University of Calgary	MEd/ MS	
University of Saskatchewan	MEd	
University of Toronto	MA	

TABLE 4.2. Listing of Doctoral-Level School Psychology Training Programs in the United States and Canada

University	Doctoral degree	APA accreditation	NASP/ NCATE
Alabama			
Auburn University	PhD		
University of Alabama	PhD		Full
Arizona			
Argosy University/Phoenix	PsyD		
Arizona State University	PhD	Full	Full
Northern Arizona University	PhD		Conditional
University of Arizona	PhD	Full	Full
Arkansas			
University of Central Arkansas	PhD	Full	
California			
La Sierra University	EdD		
University of California–Berkeley	PhD	Full	
University of California–Riverside	PhD	Full	Full
University of California–Santa Barbara	PhD[a]	Full	Full
University of the Pacific	PhD		
Colorado			
University of Denver	PhD		
University of Northern Colorado	PhD	On probation	Full
Connecticut			
University of Connecticut	PhD	Full	
Delaware			
University of Delaware	PhD		Full
District of Columbia			
Howard University	PhD		Full
Florida			
Florida State University	PhD[a]	Full	
University of Florida	PhD	Full	Full
University of South Florida	PhD	Full	Full
Georgia			
Georgia State University	PhD	Full	Full
University of Georgia	PhD	Full	Full
Hawaii			
Argosy University–Hawaii	PsyD		
Illinois			
Illinois State University	PhD	Full	Full
Loyola University of Chicago	PhD		Full
National-Louis University	PhD		
Northern Illinois University	PhD	Full	

(cont.)

TABLE 4.2. *(cont.)*

University	Doctoral degree	APA accreditation	NASP/ NCATE
Indiana			
Ball State University	PhD	Full	Full
Indiana State University	PhD	Full	Full
Indiana University–Bloomington	PhD	Full	Full
Iowa			
University of Iowa	PhD	Full	Conditional
Kansas			
University of Kansas	PhD	Full	Full
Kentucky			
University of Kentucky	PhD	Full	Full
Louisiana			
Louisiana State University–Baton Rouge	PhD	Full	Full
Tulane University	PhD	Full	
Maine			
University of Southern Maine	PsyD		
Maryland			
University of Maryland–College Park	PhD	Full	Full
Massachusetts			
Northeastern University	PhD[a]	Full, inactive	
University of Massachusetts–Amherst	PhD	Full	Full
Michigan			
Andrews University	PhD/EdD		
Central Michigan University	PhD	Full	Full
Michigan State University	PhD	Full	Full
Wayne State University	PhD		
Minnesota			
Minnesota State University–Mankato	PsyD		
University of Minnesota	PhD	Full	Full
Walden University	PhD		
Mississippi			
Mississippi State University	PhD	Full	Full
University of Southern Mississippi	PhD	Full	Full
Missouri			
University of Missouri–Columbia	PhD	On probation	
Montana			
University of Montana	PhD		
Nebraska			
University of Nebraska–Lincoln	PhD	Full	Full
Nevada			
University of Nevada–Las Vegas	PhD		
University of Nevada–Reno	PhD/EdD		

(cont.)

TABLE 4.2. *(cont.)*

University	Doctoral degree	APA accreditation	NASP/ NCATE
New Jersey			
Fairleigh Dickinson University	PsyD		
Rutgers, The State University of New Jersey	PsyD	Full	Full
New York			
Alfred University	PsyD	Full	
City University of New York, Graduate Center	PhD	Full	
Columbia University, Teachers College	PhD/EdD	Full	Full
Fordham University–Lincoln Center	PhD	Full	Full
Hofstra University	PsyD	Full	Full
New York University	PhD/PsyD	Full, inactive	Full
Pace University	PsyD [a]	Full	Full
St. John's University	PsyD	Full	Full
Syracuse University	PhD	Full	
University at Albany, State University of New York	PsyD	Full	
University at Buffalo, State University of New York	PhD[a]	Full	
Yeshiva University	PsyD[a]	Full	Full
North Carolina			
North Carolina State University	PhD	Full	Full
University of North Carolina–Chapel Hill	PhD	Full	Full
Ohio			
Kent State University	PhD	Full	Full
Ohio State University	PhD		Conditional
University of Cincinnati	PhD		Full
Oklahoma			
Oklahoma State University	PhD	Full	Full
Oregon			
University of Oregon	PhD	Full	Full
Pennsylvania			
Bryn Mawr College	PhD		
Duquesne University	PhD	Full	Full
Indiana University of Pennsylvania	EdD		Full
Lehigh University	PhD	Full	Full
Pennsylvania State University	PhD	Full	Full
Philadelphia College of Osteopathic Medicine	PsyD		Full
Temple University	PhD	Full	Full
Widener University	PsyD		
Rhode Island			
University of Rhode Island	PhD	Full	Conditional
South Carolina			
University of South Carolina	PhD	Full	Full
South Dakota			
University of South Dakota	PhD		Full

(cont.)

TABLE 4.2. *(cont.)*

University	Doctoral degree	APA accreditation	NASP/ NCATE
Tennessee			
Tennessee State University	PhD		
University of Memphis	PhD		
The University of Tennessee–Knoxville	PhD	Full	Full
Texas			
Texas A&M University–College Station	PhD	Full	Full
Texas Women's University	PhD		Full
University of Houston	PhD	Full	Full
University of Texas–Austin	PhD	Full	Full
Utah			
University of Utah	PhD	Full	Full
Utah State University	PhD[a]	Full	
Virginia			
James Madison University	PsyD[a]	Full	
University of Virginia	EdD/PhD		Conditional (PhD only)
Washington			
University of Washington	PhD	Full	Full
Wisconsin			
University of Wisconsin–Madison	PhD	Full	Full
University of Wisconsin–Milwaukee	PhD	Full	Full
Canada			
McGill University	PhD	Full	
University of Alberta	PhD		
University of British Columbia	PhD		
University of Calgary	PhD		
University of Toronto	PhD		

[a]School psychology training provided within a combined program in professional-scientific psychology that also includes a clinical and/or counseling psychology focus.

Models of Training

Although there are many commonalities among the various school psychology training programs, each program has unique characteristics and a unique identity and tradition. Even two training programs that claim to use the same broad training model and have similar training philosophies may differ substantially. As prospective students research various training programs and make decisions regarding where to apply, the array of choices can be overwhelming, particularly if one is not exclusively focused on a specific location or region. One of the ways to distinguish training programs is to identify the model of training they utilize as well as the specific focus or philosophy to which they adhere. In this regard, there are existing models of training that provide a framework for looking at the similarities and differences among programs.

The APA has supported numerous efforts since the 1940s to articulate and define models of training for doctoral programs in professional areas of psychology. The best known of these is the *scientist-practitioner* training model which is presumed to describe programs that provide students a solid foundation in research and scientific aspects of psychology, enabling them to apply these foundations to the professional practice or application of the discipline. This model was initially articulated in a 1949 clinical psychology training conference held in Boulder, Colorado (Frank, 1984). Hence, the scientist-practitioner model of training is sometimes referred to as the "Boulder model."

In addition to the well-known scientist-practitioner model, other models of training emerged beginning in the 1970s. The *professional* or *practitioner* model of professional psychology emerged from the Vail conference on graduate training in psychology in 1973, partially as a result of dissatisfaction with the scientist-practitioner model, which some trainers and practitioners contended did not provide sufficient attention to the preparation of practitioners in psychology and did little to alleviate personnel shortages during that era. The practitioner model of training places the primary focus of graduate education on professional or clinical practice and may not emphasize conducting independent research (e.g., an original dissertation or thesis) as an integral aspect of preparing psychologists. In this respect, the professional/practitioner model is more similar to the training that physicians receive during medical school, which is typically built on a foundation of basic science and clinical practice but does not require the completion of a research dissertation or extensive research methodology courses for receipt of the MD degree.

In addition to these two best known training models, newer models have emerged within American psychology since the 1980s. The *clinical science* model of training focuses on training scientists who have interests in clinical problems, such as childhood psychopathology or prevention science. The more recent *practitioner-scholar* model seeks to bridge the difference between the scientist-practitioner and practitioner models of training. Within this model, the primary focus is on training graduate students to become practitioners, with more emphasis placed on the production of scholarly work than would be expected in a practitioner model program.

These four training models just described are not specific to school psychology. Rather, they have evolved from the broad area of professional psychology doctoral training, which includes many more training programs in clinical psychology and counseling psychology than in school psychology. Within school psychology doctoral programs, there is probably a smaller variety of training models currently in use. We are not aware of any PhD programs in school psychology that claim to follow the clinical science model, and the practitioner-scholar model, although promising, has not yet been formally adopted by many programs (although we suspect that many doctoral programs that list "scientist-practitioner" as their model are actually more closely aligned to the practitioner-scholar model). Most doctoral programs in our field tend to list either the scientist-practitioner or practitioner model as the training model they follow.

Because a majority of school psychology programs are at the specialist rather than doctoral level of training, it is doubtful that the four training models that have emerged in American psychology apply as much to them as they do to doctoral programs. Within a specialist-level program (which typically consists of at least 60 semester or 90 quarter hours of coursework), it is simply not as feasible to be as highly specialized as within a doctoral program (which typically consists of about 100 or more semester hours or 150 or more quarter hours). We doubt that the clinical science model of training fits outside of doctoral-level training. Rather, the specialist-level programs in school psychology tend to fit within the practitioner, practitioner-scholar, and, in some cases, scientist-practitioner models. Fagan and Wise (2000, 2007) have presented a fifth model of training, the *pragmatic* model, which is considered to be a relevant option for nondoctoral programs. The pragmatic model reflects an orientation toward meeting accreditation requirements and standards (of NASP and state departments of education) and is highly prescriptive in terms of specific courses and competencies that must be covered for someone to become a practicing school psychologist. This "can result in a high degree of similarity among programs" (Fagan & Wise, 2007, p. 201), which is considered to be an unavoidable trade-off with the specificity inherent in accreditation standards. Certainly, there is something to be said for this pragmatic model of training, although we believe that it is still quite possible for specialist-level programs to focus on one of the general training models, particularly the practitioner-scholar and practitioner models. The five training models are summarized in Table 4.3.

Curricula

Although individual training programs may establish whatever curricula and course-work requirements they deem to be appropriate, there is a great deal of similarity among programs in this regard because of the need to adhere to prescribed standards from national accrediting bodies and from state departments of education (which often use national accrediting standards as a basis for their internal requirements for school psychology licensure or certification). As a result, training programs may vary substantially in terms of their models of training and the philosophical underpinnings of the program faculty, but there tends not to be much difference in terms of credit hour requirements, general curriculum domains, and, in many cases, even the content and title of specific courses.

The specialist-level training standard advocated by NASP (and adopted with few changes by numerous state departments of education for program approval) requires a minimum of 60 semester credits or 90 quarter credits and includes a full-time internship (1,200 clock hours). The complete criteria for this standard are found in NASP's *Standards for Graduate Preparation of School Psychologists* (NASP, 2010c). Students in specialist-level programs typically are required to complete 2 years of full-time study on campus, in which they complete 12 to 16 credit hours of coursework each semester or term and also engage in practicum or field training requirements. In terms of specific coursework

TABLE 4.3. Overview of Five General Training Models in School Psychology

Training model	Brief description
Scientist-practitioner	Emphasizes research and scientific aspects of psychology and application of these foundations to the professional practice or application of the discipline
Practitioner (professional practice)	Emphasizes professional or clinical practice of discipline; does not include substantial requirements for research
Practitioner-scholar	Primary emphasis on professional or clinical practice of discipline, but also has extensive expectations for production of scholarly work, such as dissertation research
Clinical scientist	Emphasizes scientific research in areas of psychology that have direct application to clinical practice, such as developmental science, prevention science, and child psychopathology
Pragmatic	Main emphasis is on alignment with state department of education and/or NASP training standards to ensure that program meets all relevant criteria and receives program approval

required, NASP has adopted a general approach wherein several content domains are specified and programs are required to demonstrate that their curricula sufficiently cover these domains. In some instances, state departments of education are more prescriptive of specific coursework requirements and may require the completion of specific courses rather than general domains. The following 10 domains of training practice are included in the NASP (2010c) standards:

- Data-based decision making and accountability
- Consultation and collaboration
- Interventions and Instructional support to develop academic skills
- Interventions and Mental Health Services to develop social and life skills
- Schoolwide practices to promote learning
- Preventive and responsive services
- Family–school collaboration services
- Diversity in development and learning
- Research and program evaluation
- Legal, ethical, and professional practice

At the conclusion of the 2 years of coursework and practicum training, students in specialist-level programs complete a full-time internship for 1 academic year (1,200 clock hours minimum) under the supervision of a licensed or certified school psychologist. NASP training standards also allow students to complete the internship on a part-time basis over a 2-year period and provide some flexibility in the settings in which the internship may be completed. At least 600 of the 1,200 clock hours must be completed in a school setting, a requirement that allows students to complete their remaining hours in a non-school setting (such as a clinic or research center) under the supervision of an appropriately credentialed professional. While not all training programs are NASP approved, few training programs purposefully adopt curriculum requirements below the NASP standard, because doing so would preclude them from pursuing NASP program approval and because graduates of programs with lower standards may have difficulty obtaining jobs outside of the state in which the training program is located.

Separate standards for doctoral-level training in school psychology have been developed by both NASP and APA. The doctoral standards advocated by NASP include the basic standards for all training programs and coverage of the 10 domains listed above but also specify that doctoral programs provide "greater depth in one or more school psychology competencies identified by the program in its philosophy/mission of doctoral-level preparation and reflected in program goals, objectives, and sequential program of study and supervised practice" (NASP, 2010c, p. 4). In addition, the NASP standards stipulate that doctoral programs must include a minimum of 4 years of full-time training at the graduate level, consisting of a minimum of 90 semester credits (or the equivalent) and a minimum of 1,500 clock hours for the internship. For doctoral students, programs can allow up to half of these 1,500 hours to be from "prior, appropriately supervised specialist-level internship or equivalent experiences in school psychology" (NASP, 2010c, p. 8). Students must have previously completed a specialist-level internship in school psychology in accordance with NASP standards in order to do this. In this case, the student may complete the doctoral internship in a non-school setting, such as a clinic, residential treatment facility, or child guidance center. Otherwise, the same rule for a minimum of 600 clock hours in a school setting during the internship holds true for doctoral internships.

The doctoral program training standards espoused by APA and required for accreditation from this organization differ from NASP's in terms of specificity and design but are otherwise similar in terms of general expectations and credit hour requirements. APA does not have separate accreditation requirements for doctoral programs in clinical, counseling, school, and combined professional-scientific psychology. Rather, the accreditation standards, which are detailed in *Guidelines and Principles for Accreditation of Programs in Professional Psychology* (APA, 2007b), are generic, but they specify that programs have the right to be evaluated in terms of their unique education and training philosophy, models, goals, objectives, and methods, so far as they are consistent with those generally accepted as professionally appropriate.

It is assumed that doctoral programs in school psychology that seek APA accreditation will adhere to the general psychology training guidelines and will also be consistent with what is generally deemed to be appropriate specialty training in school psychology. Like NASP's doctoral training standards, the APA guidelines specify that doctoral programs must include at least 3 years of full-time academic study beyond the bachelor's degree plus an additional year of full-time internship training. The APA domains that are expected to be covered through coursework and other training experiences include the following areas (APA, 2007b):

- Biological aspects of behavior.
- Cognitive and affective aspects of behavior.
- Social aspects of behavior.
- History and systems of psychology.
- Psychological measurement.
- Research methodology.
- Techniques of data analysis.
- Individual differences in behavior.
- Human development.
- Dysfunctional behavior or psychopathology.
- Professional standards and ethics.
- Theories and methods of assessment and diagnosis.
- Effective intervention.
- Consultation and supervision.
- Efficacy of interventions.
- Issues of cultural and individual diversity relevant to all of the areas just listed.

In comparing the NASP and APA standards and domains for doctoral training programs, there are certainly some identifiable differences but also many similarities. Regardless of whether doctoral programs in school psychology are accredited by APA, approved by NASP, or have joint program approval, students who enter these programs can expect that their training will take at least 4 years beyond the bachelor's degree (5 years, including the internship year, is more typical, and 6 years is not uncommon); that their coursework will include broad coverage of scientific, theoretical, and professional practice issues; that they will engage in extensive practicum or fieldwork experiences during the years in which they complete their coursework; and that their experience will culminate in a full-time internship for 1 year in a school setting or a related youth-serving setting. Doctoral students can also typically expect to complete a dissertation research project toward the end of their program. Some programs (particularly PsyD, EdD degree programs and programs that adhere to a professional training model) may require a comprehensive or terminal project in lieu of the doctoral research dissertation, but the dissertation requirement seems to be much more typical than the alternatives.

Specialist or Doctoral Training? Where?

As well-qualified prospective school psychology students consider applying to graduate programs, they face a bewildering array of choices concerning which programs to target. One of the first decisions that must be considered is whether to pursue training at the doctoral level or at the specialist level. There is no question that the specialist level of training will continue to serve as the entry level into the field in most, but not all, respects. The large majority of practitioner positions within public school systems do not require more training than the master's/specialist degree, and in many systems there is no financial incentive for investing the additional time and money required to obtain a doctoral degree. However, there are some very good reasons to consider doctoral-level training. One cannot become a core faculty member in a school psychology training program without a doctoral degree, and this level of training is also usually required for school psychologists who desire to work in clinic or medical practice settings. Although some states allow school psychologists with specialist degrees and appropriate credentials to engage in independent or private practice, most do not have such a provision and require the doctoral degree and a state-issued psychology license (through a board of psychological examiners or similar entity) for this role. In addition, some supervisory positions in larger school systems, such as school psychology coordinator, director of pupil personnel services, or director of student services, may require a doctoral degree.

Aside from these practical considerations, there are other reasons for prospective students to consider doctoral-level training. Although the 2 years of university-based training and the additional year of internship training required for the specialist degree may provide an excellent foundation for a career as a school psychologist, the additional 2 to 3 years of training that are typically required for doctoral degree programs may greatly enhance one's background and competence in research methods, specialized assessment and intervention techniques, and clinical expertise with specialized populations. These benefits may be important to consider in selecting the level of training to which one aspires. In addition, we have observed that many of our students in master's- or specialist-level programs have the desire to obtain a doctoral degree but decide that it would be best first to work for 3 to 5 years or so and then return to graduate school. Although having such professional experience can be a great asset to students in a doctoral program, the reality is that there are many potential barriers that can obstruct one's return to graduate school once full-time employment is attained. Not the least of these barriers to returning to the role of a full-time student (with its accompanying lifestyle changes) are the practical issues of, for example, becoming accustomed to a full-time professional income, starting a family, taking on greater financial obligations, and so forth. For these reasons, graduate students interested in pursuing doctoral-level training may want to think twice before deciding to work for a few years after the specialist degree and then returning to school. Although some doctoral programs in school psychology are tailored to the needs of working professionals who decide to pursue the doctoral program while maintaining their employment, such programs are still the exception and are not available in most regions of the United States, particularly outside of large urban areas.

The other choice that prospective students must make is which specific institutions or programs to consider. Certainly, there are practical issues to consider in this regard, such as relocation to a distant state or region, the cost of tuition, availability of financial assistance, and so forth. There are also important professional and conceptual issues to consider in the selection of a program. Although a great deal of similarity exists among various training programs in terms of training and curricula offered, there are also many important differences. Typically, each program has its own unique philosophical orientation and training model. Thus, programs may vary greatly in their approach to teaching assessment and intervention techniques, in their view of the role of school psychologists, in the types of training settings available, and so forth. Prospective students would be wise to carefully research potential graduate programs and apply to programs that have the type of training model, course offerings, and practice or research specialties they are seeking. Another important element in program selection is to learn about the faculty who staff particular programs. What are their research, teaching, and clinical interests? How many are there, and what is the faculty-to-student ratio? What is the availability of faculty for advising students? For students who enter doctoral programs and are considering the possibility of becoming a school psychology faculty member, the selection of a program with faculty who can provide them with the appropriate mentoring and experiences in research and publication may be especially critical. Finally, there is an important climate or environmental element to consider when selecting admission offers to training programs. Given that one is investing 3 to 6 years of his or her life in the program, it is wise to consider such issues as level of collegiality among faculty and students, how satisfied and positive current students seem to be, and what it would be like to live in the community where the program is located. These are important issues, and we consider them so essential that we advise potential graduate students to do whatever they can to visit the program and community in person if possible before making a decision.

Characteristics of Faculty and Students

For the same reasons that it is difficult to obtain a highly accurate picture of school psychology training programs, it is quite complicated to accurately portray the characteristics of graduate students in school psychology training programs as well as the faculty (or "trainers" as they are commonly called) who staff these programs. In many respects it is even more difficult to gather highly accurate data on students and faculty, because the numbers are so much greater than the numbers of programs and because there is not a common metric or reporting system for programs to provide this information. Given these caveats, accurate representation of the graduate students and faculty in school psychology training programs is of great worth to the field, because the faculty serve as the gatekeepers and socializing agents into the profession, and the current student population represents an important part of the future of the profession.

Students

The most recent data available from NASP that supplied specific categorical breakdowns of its members by work category during the time this volume was being prepared (from a 2000 membership survey and a 2004 listing of NASP membership) indicates that there were just over 5,000 members of NASP in the "student" and "student in transition" categories. The most recent complete membership data available from APA's Division 16 (the 2004 membership list) indicate more than 600 student affiliates of the division. Although there is some overlap between the student membership of the two organizations, we can assume that these data underestimate the total number of students preparing to enter the field of school psychology because not all students become student members or affiliates of the professional organizations. A very conservative estimate, then, would be approximately 6,000 students currently in graduate training programs in school psychology in the United States and Canada. If we look at this estimate as a percentage of our estimate of 39,000–43,000 school psychologists in the United States and Canada that we presented in Chapter 1, the implications are revealing: if these figures are reasonably close, then about 15% of the individuals who are currently aligned with the profession of school psychology are students who are at some stage of preparation. A small percentage of these students are undoubtedly going back to school for doctoral degrees after having previously worked full time as school psychologists, but even taking this possibility into account, the percentage of students affiliated with the field is both sizable and healthy. These data give us reason to believe that there is a continual infusion of new talent into the field, with new generations of school psychologists continually emerging.

Previous efforts to analyze the demographic characteristics of graduate students in school psychology (such as Thomas's 1998 training directory) have indicated that a large majority of school psychology students at all levels—80% or more—are female. As has been discussed in earlier chapters, a strong shift in gender balance in the field has been noticeable since about the 1970s, and the percentage of female school psychologists surpassed the percentage of male school psychologists in about 1980 (Curtis, 2002). Since then, the percentage of female students and practitioners in the field has been rising and may continue to do so slightly. The other two fields of professional psychology—clinical psychology and counseling psychology—have also experienced a similar gender shift among graduate students in recent decades. When considering only doctoral training programs, some interesting comparative data are available. A National Science Foundation (2010) report on doctoral recipients from U.S. universities indicates that in 2009 (the most recent reporting year when the report was issued) 71% of all doctoral degree recipients in psychology were women, and women made up 75% of counseling psychology doctoral recipients, 76% of clinical psychology doctoral recipients, and 76% of school psychology doctoral recipients, respectively. Over time, as graduate students enter the field and older members retire, the gender composition of the field will look increasingly more like the current composition of graduate students.

In terms of race or ethnicity, the field of school psychology is also quite dissimilar to the population of children served by professionals within the field and to American society in general. Although members of racial or ethnic minority groups currently make up 35% or more of the general population within the United States (U.S. Bureau of the Census, 2001), they made up only about 20% of 2009 doctoral graduates from school psychology programs and about 24% of doctoral graduates from psychology programs (National Science Foundation, 2010). A recent report from the APA Center for Workforce Studies (APA, 2010a) on ethnicity of psychology graduate students (not broken down by specialty area) indicated that for the most current reporting year (2008–2009) ethnic minority group members constituted 24% of all students in doctoral programs at public universities, 33% of all students in master's programs at public universities, and 22% of all students in master's programs at private universities. We note that, while we were in the process of preparing this edition of the volume, the 2010 decennial U.S. Census was underway, and it is generally expected that when the results are available, they will show that the proportion of Americans who are members of ethnic minority groups will have grown since the 2000 census.

NASP, APA, various state-level organizations, and many university training programs have enacted initiatives during the past two decades to increase the racial/ethnic diversity of school psychologists, and it is important to recognize that the current student data represent an increased percentage of members of ethnic minority groups from early periods of time in the field and that the racial/ethnic proportionality of the current graduate student population is substantially more diverse than that of the field in general, in which only about 7% are from a racial or ethnic minority group (Curtis, Lopez, et al., 2008). However, even though the percentage of school psychologists who are members of racial or ethnic minority groups may continue to increase as the more diverse graduate student population enters the field, the diversity of the field is not growing nearly as fast as the diversity of the U.S. population in general. These demographics illustrate a significant challenge for the field: Even with the increasing diversity of individuals entering the field, the profession of school psychology is not currently on track to achieve anything like ethnic or racial similarity to the larger population in the foreseeable future.

What characteristics make for a successful graduate student and ultimately a successful school psychologist? Although a few attempts have been made over the past decades to describe the desirable personal attributes of school psychology students and practitioners, no consensus, overarching survey, or scientific findings exist. However, based on some of the common elements of lists compiled by previous authors (e.g., Bardon, 1986; Bardon & Bennett, 1974; Fagan & Wise, 1994; Fireoved & Cancelleri, 1985), as well as our own take on what is required for a successful educational and professional experience in school psychology, we view the following characteristics as being highly desirable (and essential in many respects) for school psychology graduate students and practitioners to possess:

- Strong academic aptitude.
- Intellectual curiosity and the ability and desire to apply scientific methods in conceptualizing and solving problems.
- Excellent interpersonal and social skills.
- The ability to communicate clearly and effectively, both verbally and in writing.
- A sense of personal, social, and ethical responsibility.
- Intrapersonal strength, including insight into one's own behavior and motivations, emotional stability, and the ability to persist and persevere when circumstances are difficult.
- A strong desire to assist and support children, their families, and other professionals through educational and psychological processes.
- Understanding of and respect for persons from diverse backgrounds and with varying experiences and worldviews.
- The ability to provide leadership and facilitate effective problem solving within small groups.
- The ability to adapt successfully to changing conditions and expectations and to be resilient in stressful situations.
- The ability to be well organized and to complete a high volume of tasks in a timely manner.

To some extent, these skills and personal characteristics may be taught, learned, or refined within a graduate training program in school psychology. There is also the reality that many of these attributes are developed and refined over one's lifetime and that it may be difficult to simply "teach" the characteristics during the graduate training years; over time, these characteristics tend to become more like a trait than a state of behavior. For example, if a new graduate student begins his or her training with noticeable deficits in social and interpersonal skills, there may be limits to how much these characteristics can be improved during a 3- to 5-year period of graduate education. Thus, school psychology training program faculty are likely to carefully consider an applicant's possession of these desired personal attributes during the admission process for graduate school.

Faculty

Each school psychology training program must have faculty to teach courses, admit and advise students, administer the program, supervise student research and field training, and assist students in their transition from internship to regular employment, including endorsing them for licensure or certification after they have completed all program requirements. This list is only partial. School psychology trainers do not operate independently or within a vacuum (although they may sometimes feel that this is the case!). Rather, they are typically part of a broader faculty within a college of education or department of psychology and as such have faculty responsibilities within the larger context outside of the program. School psychology faculty may teach undergraduate courses or other graduate courses outside of the school psychology program. They may have departmental, college, or university committee responsibilities, such as serving on the faculty senate or being on a personnel, curriculum, or facilities committee. They may have administrative responsibilities outside of the program, such as budget planning, program development, and review of personnel decisions, such as tenure and promotion or hiring. In addition, school psychology faculty members are typically expected to contribute to their field outside of the college or university context. They may provide leadership or other service in state or national school psychology organizations and collaborate with state departments of education in developing the standards for the profession within that state. School psychology faculty may be asked to serve as editorial board members or editors of professional journals or newsletters within the field. Faculty who work at institutions in which research and the production of scholarly work are considered primary activities are expected to conduct research, publish articles in peer-reviewed journals, and present their research at professional meetings. They may also be expected to write books, develop products (e.g., assessment tools and intervention programs) for use in the field, and secure funding for their research or training efforts through submitting grant proposals to government agencies or private foundations. In some cases, school psychology faculty may provide professional services in schools or clinics on a part-time basis or work as consultants to school districts or other organizations. Indeed, the roles and expectations of school psychology faculty are many and varied, and this role requires creativity and the ability to juggle multiple responsibilities.

Faculty in school psychology programs typically work full time for the institutions in which the programs are housed, although many programs hire part-time or "adjunct" faculty to teach courses and assist in supervising the training of students in other ways. In many cases, these adjunct faculty members are full-time practitioners or administrators in school districts and clinics. Given that there are more than 200 institutions of higher education in the United States and Canada that support school psychology training programs, a very conservative estimate is that at least 600 full-time school psychology faculty and many adjunct faculty are employed at these institutions. We reach this conclusion by examining the training and accrediting standards of the national organizations and through our own experience examining what is typical practice in training programs. According to NASP's *Standards for Graduate Preparation of School Psychologists*

(NASP, 2010c), each approved program must have "faculty who are designated specifically as school psychology program faculty members and total at least three full-time equivalents" (p. 3). APA's *Guidelines and Principles for Accreditation of Programs in Professional Psychology* (APA, 2007b) do not have a specific requirement in terms of number of faculty in accredited programs, but instead state that programs must have "an identifiable core faculty responsible for its leadership who ... are sufficient in number for their academic and professional responsibilities" (p. 10). In practice, programs differ in the number of faculty they have, a figure that is usually correlated with the number of students in a program. Usually, the more students a program admits, the more faculty members the program has. Data from a 2003 policy clarification document from APA indicated that at that time APA-accredited PhD programs in school psychology had an average of 4.5 core faculty per program and a mean ratio of 8.8 students for each faculty member in the program (APA, 2003). We are not aware of any more recent analyses in this area, and assume that those figures are close to what is currently reflected in school psychology programs.

As training standards and professional expectations have evolved over the years, the doctoral degree has become the entry-level educational attainment to work as a school psychology faculty member, at least on a full-time basis (some programs may employ specialist-level adjunct faculty to assist in supervising students or teaching courses). The few surveys of characteristics of school psychology trainers that have been published in the past two decades (e.g., Reschly & Wilson, 1995; Thomas, 1998) indicate that the demographic characteristics of school psychology faculty differ to some extent from those of graduate students and the field in general. For example, although women make up over 70% of school psychologists, they account for only 60% of school psychology trainers (Curtis, Lopez, et al., 2008). For whatever reason, the percentage of women in school psychology faculty positions has lagged behind that of the field in general. However, the percentage of women who enter faculty positions has appeared to increase substantially from the 18% reported in 1969–1970 (Curtis, 2002), and we believe that this trend will continue to the point at which the percentage of female trainers will be considerably larger than the percentage of male trainers within the next decade or two as the number of new graduates continues to be approximately 75–80% female. However, it has also been our observation that the gender representation of trainers is related to more than just the demographics of doctoral graduates entering the field. In our collective experience as trainers, we have observed that a smaller percentage of female than male doctoral graduates aspire to obtain full-time faculty appointments or even view this role as desirable. This trend mirrors the percentage of female faculty members in psychology fields in general: The percentage of female students does not match the percentage of female faculty members. Perhaps this trend will change in future years as more women enter faculty positions and become role models and mentors for graduate students.

In terms of ethnicity, no recent estimates of the percentage of ethnic minority faculty members could be located. Thomas (1998) reported about 15% of program faculty are members of racial or ethnic minority groups, a figure somewhat lower than the percentage of minority graduate students in school psychology training programs but more than the percentage of minority school psychologists in general and considerably lower than the 35% for racial or ethnic minority group members in U.S. society in general. It is our observation that diversity of school psychology faculty helps greatly to enhance diversity within student recruitment and retention. Programs that specifically emphasize multicultural diversity within their curricula and mission statements and that have faculty members of color are often more successful in recruiting minority students to their training programs. In terms of other demographic characteristics of school psychology faculty, such as age and prior experience as school psychology practitioners, no national or comparative data exist of which we are aware.

There appear to be a substantial number of school psychology program faculty approaching retirement age within the next several years, which in some respects portends for a very strong employment market for well-qualified doctoral graduates who desire to become trainers. That said, there is plenty of evidence that the market for hiring school psychology faculty has shrunk—we believe temporarily—as a result of the global economic recession that began in 2007. Prior to the 2008–2009 academic year, we observed that there were as many as 80 to 100 faculty positions being posted per year. The financial crisis that become evident in October 2008 led to a rapid succession of freezes and cuts in higher education budgets, stimulated by losses in university endowments and reductions in state revenues to public institutions. As a result of all of these economic factors, many institutions of higher education that anticipated hires in the area of school psychology have either put a freeze on those positions or temporarily filled them by increasing the number of part-time adjunct faculty. We have also noted that some veteran school psychology trainers who are approaching retirement age have put their plans for retirement on hold because of losses in their equities-based retirement savings. Despite the current conditions as we are preparing this edition, we anticipate that the long-term prospects for doctoral graduates who desire careers in higher education are still solid, and that there will be an eventual increase in hiring in this area, which may move slowly but is almost certain to respond to the combination of continued need for school psychologists and the pending retirements of veteran trainers.

It was common for faculty who joined training programs two decades ago or more to have had several years' experience as school psychologists in practice settings before becoming trainers. Certainly, there is much to be said for the mentoring and role modeling qualities of school psychology trainers who have extensive experience as practicing school psychologists. It is our observation that it is becoming increasingly typical for new program faculty to enter their first academic jobs directly out of graduate programs, with only practicum and internship experiences as practitioners, and less common for new faculty members to have had several years' prior experience as practitioners. Perhaps the increased demands on academicians in recent years to establish prominent research and publication records, regardless of the type of institution at which they work, has been responsible in part for this perceived trend. The "publish or perish" nature of faculty positions at many research-oriented institutions certainly may drive this phenomenon.

What are the personal characteristics or attributes necessary to help one become a successful faculty member in a school psychology training program? To start with, the characteristics we have previously noted as desirable for graduate students and practicing school psychologists would be of great value in making an excellent trainer. To these qualities we add a few more that we believe are especially relevant to the unique demands and expectations of being a faculty member:

- A desire to mentor graduate students into the profession and to serve as a professional guide and role model for them.
- The ability to juggle multiple, and often conflicting, role demands and expectations (e.g., staying current in practice within the field while also establishing a strong program of scholarly work).
- The ability to think creatively and establish innovative programs of teaching, scholarly work, and clinical training.
- The ability and desire to stay current on trends and findings within the field of

school psychology and to continually incorporate new ideas into teaching and scholarly work.

- The ability to work effectively and positively within systems that often have what we call a "lean schedule of reinforcement," understanding that some important efforts and roles required to be a good trainer and faculty member will not necessarily be rewarded or highly valued by the institution.
- For faculty who work at research universities or other institutions at which research and scholarly work is an essential expectation, it is absolutely necessary for one to have the desire to engage in these activities on a continual basis and to produce the expected results (publications, products) at regular intervals and sometimes in large volume.
- Increasingly, the desire and ability to garner resources through state and federal funding mechanisms for research and training purposes (e.g., student and program support) are highly desired and necessary for school psychology faculty, particularly in the current era of fiscal retrenchment in public higher education.

After reading this list of desired characteristics (and some of the implications), graduate students may wonder why one would want to become a faculty member in the first place! Although there are certainly some aggravations and frustrations built into the role of a trainer, just as there are the role of a practitioner, we in no way want to discourage graduate students from considering careers as faculty members. On the contrary, we view this role as exciting, tremendously rewarding, and usually quite enjoyable. Having the opportunity to shape the future of the field and to mentor graduate students into the profession is a great privilege, and we believe that being a school psychology trainer is a great career path for those graduate students who are so inclined and have the necessary characteristics.

Practicum and Internship Training

In the applied or professional areas of psychology and education, students develop expertise in the practice of their particular field through supervised field experience. The field of school psychology has particularly strong traditions and practices in this area. Both NASP and APA have been active in shaping experience standards for the field and have addressed expectations for practicum and internship training at length in their respective guidelines for training and credentialing (APA, 2007b; NASP, 2010c). Although there are some differences in the standards of the two organizations with respect to field training (especially with regard to differences between specialist- and doctoral-level training standards), there is also a great deal of similarity.

Practicum Training in School Psychology

Practicum training generally begins early during the graduate training experience. It is not unusual for school psychology training programs to have students begin a limited practicum placement during their first year in the program. Practicum training provides an opportunity for students to receive an orientation to the culture and expectations of schools and related systems, to become familiar with professional practice in the field through observing and shadowing a practicing school psychologist, and to take on gradually increasing responsibilities for providing professional services. Professional services provided during the practicum experience may include assessment, consultation, and direct interventions conducted under the supervision of an experienced credentialed professional.

Training programs vary in terms of their specific expectations and opportunities for practicum training. Some programs maintain university-based clinics or service centers in which students practice their clinical skills by providing direct services to the public under the supervision of program faculty. Other programs do not maintain such clinics but place their students in practicum settings in the community. These settings are primarily in public schools, but they are not limited to such settings, particularly in doctoral programs. For example, training programs that are located in universities with medical centers may also provide practicum opportunities for their students in specialty medical clinics under the supervision of licensed psychologists. In addition, training programs that have relationships with child guidance, mental health, or residential treatment facilities may create practicum opportunities for their students in these agencies.

By definition, practicum training occurs on a time-limited basis while students also complete academic coursework, research, and other program requirements. A practicum experience may be tied to a specific academic course (such as a consultation or assessment course), or it may be broader in scope. In a typical arrangement, practicum placements require anywhere from 6 to 10 hours per week, and they might be done in one or more time blocks per week. Practicum experiences typically include time for on-site supervision with the field supervisor, but by definition they are conducted under the direction of the training program and may include weekly supervision and training seminars with program faculty. The best available survey on the practicum requirements of school psychology training programs is found in Thomas's (1998) NASP-published directory of training programs. Although this survey is now somewhat dated, we are not aware of any more recent efforts in this area. This resource indicates a median of 225 clock hours of practicum training for master's-level training programs, 360 clock hours for specialist-level programs, and 600 clock hours for doctoral-level programs, with a wide variation in clock-hour requirements within each level. Our observation is that current practicum requirements in training programs are still generally similar on average to what Thomas identified from the previous survey.

Internship Training in School Psychology

Internship training differs from practicum training in four major ways. First, rather than being integrated within the academic coursework, internships are conducted at the end of a student's program of study, after all coursework, practica, and other program requirements have been completed. Second, rather than being a part-time experience with limited involvement, internships require a full-time commitment over the course of an academic or calendar year (although both NASP and APA allow for internships to be conducted on a half-time basis over 2 years). Third, whereas supervision of practicum experiences is usually the direct responsibility of faculty within the training program (with assistance from field supervisors on site), internship training is conducted under the direct supervision of a field supervisor, with the training program playing a more limited role, such as progress monitoring, communicating with the student and supervisor, and student evaluation. Fourth, although practicum training experiences may focus on limited types of professional skills, interns are expected to provide a comprehensive range of professional services, using and integrating a broad range of skills. In essence, the internship is a capstone experience of student's graduate training in school psychology, one of the final steps toward independence as a professional. Definitions of what constitutes a full-time internship in school psychology vary somewhat based on training programs, organizational training standards, and level of training. As long as they meet the training standards of relevant professional associations, and assuming they satisfy the credentialing requirements of the states or provinces in which they are located, training programs may establish their own unique guidelines for internship training in order to make this experience appropriate to the specific objectives of the program. Some of the primary general principles and guidelines for internship training in school psychology are as follows:

- For specialist-level internships, NASP requires that the internship must be at least 1,200 clock hours, which is equivalent to full-time work for an academic year or half-time work over a 2-year period.
- For doctoral-level internships, both APA and NASP require a minimum of 1,500 clock hours. Some predoctoral internships (particularly those in non-school settings or consortiums) may require as many as 2,000 clock hours.
- NASP training standards stipulate that approximately half of the internship time (600 hours minimum) must be conducted in school settings. APA has no such setting-specific requirement, a difference that has been a point of contention between the two organizations with respect to doctoral training programs.
- Internships must be conducted under the supervision of an appropriately credentialed school psychologist or, in the case of non-school settings, a board-licensed psychologist. Supervision duties may be split among two supervisors if needed. Supervisors of specialist-level interns are expected to hold at least a specialist degree, whereas supervisors of predoctoral interns are expected to hold a doctoral degree.
- A minimum of 2 hours per week of individual, face-to-face supervision between interns and their supervisors is the general expectation.
- The internship experience is considered to be a training experience, not just full-time employment. Thus, the internship should be based on a written internship plan and include a broad range of activities, including activities such as group supervision seminars, professional development workshops, opportunities for observation of supervisors, and so forth.
- The training program monitors the student's internship experience to ensure that the objectives of the program are realized. The internship supervisors and training program faculty communicate as needed for problem solving and evaluation of the student's progress.

The process of securing an internship placement is as variable as the training and internship programs. NASP has yet to adopt any accreditation or approval program for specialist-level internships, so there is no central clearinghouse for posting internship positions. School psychology training programs typically develop their own network of internship settings on an informal basis, and it is not unusual for students from particular training programs to intern at these sites. Information on internship opportunities is often sent to training program directors and then posted for potential interns to consider. Attending state school psychology association conferences and networking with psychologists and administrators from potential internship sites is a time-honored way to get one's foot in the door for an internship. If a student is willing to look nationally rather than regionally for internship opportunities, attendance at a national convention

(NASP or APA) often provides similar networking opportunities on a broader scale, and such national opportunities are sometimes advertised in professional newsletters such as the NASP *Communiqué* or APA *Monitor on Psychology*. In addition, students who desire to stay or to relocate in a particular geographical area are often successful in securing internships by contacting school psychologists and administrators early in the year prior to their internships, letting them know of their interest and availability and initiating a dialogue.

Potential interns in doctoral programs in school psychology often secure their internships through the same methods as were discussed for specialist-level internships. However, for many doctoral-level internships, an established network is available for accreditation and posting of internships. APA accredits predoctoral internships and posts a listing of accredited sites on its website (*www.apa.org*) and in each December issue of the *American Psychologist*. APA-accredited internships operate their posting, applications, and notification process through the Association of Psychological Postdoctoral and Internship Centers (APPIC; *www.appic.org*). APPIC listings include APA-accredited internships as well as many other doctoral-level internships that are not APA accredited but that agree to operate under the conditions established by APPIC, which are similar to those of APA. Although many of the internship opportunities in this network are not appropriate or relevant for school psychology students (i.e., those that focus exclusively on adult populations), this system includes a considerable number of other internship opportunities that are appropriate for school psychology students. These opportunities include a limited number of school districts, consortiums between school districts and community agencies, child guidance centers, residential treatment centers for youth, children's medical centers, and some community mental health agencies that work extensively with schools and children. The advantage for students to securing internships through this established network is that all sites have agreed to provide training opportunities and appropriate supervision, areas that are sometimes problematic when a student develops his or her own internship.

In recent years the APPIC system has consistently had more applicants for its internships than could be placed. In other words, a supply-and-demand issue has emerged for doctoral-level internships in professional psychology. A brief article on this problem that appeared in the April, 2010 *Monitor on Psychology* by Munsey noted that for the February 2010 APPIC selection process approximately 23% of doctoral students seeking internships did not match with an internship. This figure is similar to the 2009 selection data, when a record 24% of doctoral students seeking internships did not match through APPIC. Our observation of this phenomenon is that it is related more to a continual increase in the number of doctoral students and doctoral training programs in professional psychology rather than any actual reductions in available internships, which seem to be staying stable or even increasing slightly. In other words, the supply of internships seems to have stayed stable or increased slightly, but the demand for them has continually increased. Match rates vary greatly by program, and prospective students should be encouraged to look at match rates (which APPIC publishes and which APA-accredited programs are required to post on their websites) when making decisions regarding graduate school. For doctoral students in school psychology programs, there may be a "silver lining" in this regrettable supply–demand problem. Unlike doctoral students in counseling and clinical psychology, school psychology students are less dependent on or locked into the APPIC system, despite its many advantages when one is successful in obtaining an internship through it. Doctoral students in school psychology, even if they are not successful in finding an internship match through APPIC, still have many other avenues available for finding appropriate internships in school settings. That being said, there are certain career paths that school psychologists might take that would make an APA-accredited internship more important. Doctoral students should explore their career options early and know the associated requirements so that they are in the best position to be competitive for the internships and jobs they will be seeking in the future.

Finding a good internship placement is a critically important element of becoming a successful school psychologist. A carefully planned and supervised internship experience will help a student move into the field appropriately prepared and well positioned for future success. Internships that do not meet one's expectations for training and supervision may prove to be disappointing and may even discourage a student from working in the field. As school psychology trainers, we have seen both results and much prefer the former outcome to the latter. With careful planning and a willingness to go where the best training opportunity is available, a positive outcome is more likely. Selection of the best internship site is dependent to some extent on whether a student is geographically mobile and able to go to where the better opportunities are. For students who are bound to location, opportunities must be secured within a limited locale, and in some cases the fewer choices involved in such situations means that extra planning and effort are required for a good internship experience. Almost all full-time internships in school psychology are paid experiences. Although accepting unpaid internships is sometimes a reality for students who are not willing or able to relocate to sites that offer paid opportunities, we do not encourage unpaid full-time internship situations and believe that some of these situations border on exploitation. The rate of pay varies greatly by state and region. It has been our experience that the lower paying internships typically pay a student about half of what a fully credentialed beginning school psychologist would earn in that setting, although it is more typical for interns to earn maybe five eighths to three fourths of the salary of a beginning credentialed professional in that setting. Some interns may even be able to negotiate for full salary, especially in districts in which interns are hired to fill vacant school psychologist positions rather than to fill position specifically allotted to interns. In addition to salary, it is important for interns to consider whether the district provides benefits, such as health care insurance. Particularly for interns with families, it may make monetary sense to take a lower paying internship that comes with benefits rather than a higher paying internship with no attached benefits. One's personal circumstances and needs will be important in determining how much the financial remuneration aspect of the internship will influence the selection of a training site.

Credentialing in School Psychology: Certification and Licensure

Completing the internship and receiving the graduate degree or completion certificate in a school psychology program is a necessary but insufficient step toward working as a school psychologist. To work as a practitioner in a public school or independent-practice setting, one not only must have the necessary academic preparation but must also possess an appropriate credential. In some cases, getting the necessary license or certificate credential following completion of the program and endorsement by the training program faculty is mostly a formality: The training institution certifies that the individual who is applying for the credential has completed all essential program requirements, the applicant completes the paperwork process (including providing information for a criminal background check to be performed) and pays a fee, and the credential soon appears in the mail. However, in many cases, the process is more complex and in some instances downright intimidating. A more lengthy application process, a rigorous transcript evaluation, a challenging written exam, and in some cases an oral exam with licensing board members may all be required. This section provides a brief overview of the three most common credentialing processes that school psychologists are likely to encounter: state department of education certification/licensure, the NCSP credential from NASP, and licensing for independent practice as a psychologist from state psychology licensing boards.

State Department of Education Certification/Licensure

Each of the 50 U.S. states has particular processes for credentialing professional educators and related service professionals (e.g., school administrators, speech–language pathologists, school counselors, school psychologists) to work in the public school systems of that state. Prior to about the 1980s, this process was almost always referred to as *certification*, and it culminated in the receipt of a certificate allowing one to work in public school settings. After some of the educational reform activities that were typical in U.S. states in the 1980s and 1990s, some states changed the title of the credential they awarded from certificate to *license*, but the intent and meaning were the same: to allow the holder of that credential to work within his or her specialty area within the public schools. The Canadian provinces have similar procedures for credentialing individuals to work as education professionals within public school systems. The purpose of state or provincial credentialing is quality control. The state legislature sets minimum preparation standards that must be attained for one to work as a teacher, counselor, school psychologist, and so forth and then verifies that these standards have been met prior to issuing the practice credential.

The typical route to receiving a credential within the state in which one's training program is located is to obtain an endorsement from the training program, which is then accepted by the state or provincial department of education as evidence that the training criteria have been met. States may have additional requirements, such as evidence of satisfactory scores on general skills and communication tests (such as the National Teacher Exam Core Battery or the California Basic Skills Test) and specialty knowledge tests specific to school psychology (such as the Praxis II Educational Specialty Area Test for School Psychologists). Although some states have entered into reciprocal certification compacts with other states, for applicants who are applying for a state department of education credential following completing of a training program in another state or upon demonstrating that they are similarly credentialed in another state, the process may be more complicated. Because out-of-state institutions are not approved by that particular state department of education, a detailed transcript evaluation process may be required to ensure that the standards of the state have been met. In addition, the state credentialing body may require the applicant to demonstrate evidence of completion of their out-of-state training program through an additional endorsement process. As school psychology trainers, we have all had the experience of receiving such requests from graduates of our training programs, some of whom completed the program years before we were employed there. Because there is variability in the training and credentialing standards adopted by individual states and provinces, an individual may complete a training program in one state, obtain experience working as a school psychologist in that state, and still not meet the credentialing requirements of another state in which he or she is attempting to gain employment. In such instances, additional specific coursework is sometimes necessary, although states may issue a temporary credential and allow the applicant a period of 1 or 2 years to show evidence of completing the additional requirements. Because credentialing requirements may vary considerably across states and provinces, we advise that individuals who are considering practicing in a state other than the one in which they were trained research carefully the specific requirements of that state and ensure that they complete the necessary expectations prior to completion of their training program, if possible. In general, graduates of NASP-approved training programs are likely to meet credentialing requirements across different states. However, there may be situations in which this is not the case.

Nationally Certified School Psychologist Credential

In 1988, NASP established the National School Psychology Certification Board (NSPCB), which administers the process of awarding the Nationally Certified School Psychologist (NCSP) credential. The board and the NCSP credential were established to provide a national standard that can be used as a measure of professionalism by interested agencies and individuals and to recognize school psychologists who meet this national standard. Additional purposes for establishing the NCSP program include the promotion of continuing professional development among school psychologists and a desire to foster cooperation and commonality among groups that recognize school psychologists. Among the circumstances surrounding the creation of the NCSP was the fact that so much variation exists across states with regard to the criteria for being considered for school psychology certification or licensure (Batsche & Curtis, 2003). Although NASP has made it clear that it is not the intent of the NSPCB to certify school psychologists for employment nor to impose personnel requirements on agencies and organizations (NASP, 2004), an implicit goal in the development of the NCSP is to promote the NASP standard of the 60-semester-hour specialist-level graduate training program, including a 1,200 hour internship, as the entry level for practice as a school psychologist.

Awarding of the NCSP requires the following:

- Completion of a minimum 60-semester-hour graduate-level training program in school psychology with training across the 10 NASP domains of professional service.
- Completion of an internship of at least 1,200 clock hours as part of the training program under the supervision of an appropriately credentialed school psychologist and including a minimum of 600 clock hours in a school setting.
- Receipt of a passing score (currently 165) on the Praxis National School Psychology Examination administered by Educational Testing Service.

Graduates of NASP-approved training programs automatically qualify to apply for the NCSP credential and to take the exam without a transcript review following completion of their graduate programs. However, the NCSP is not limited to graduates of NASP-approved programs. Individuals who graduate from any recognized school psychology graduate training program may be approved to take the national exam and ultimately receive the NCSP credential if they can demonstrate that their program included the appropriate amount and types of coursework, practicum, and internship experiences. Coursework requirements are explicit in the NCSP criteria, based on NASP professional service domains noted earlier in this chapter. The process for making a determination of eligibility in such cases is the responsibility of the NSPCB.

According to Hunley (2004), the NCSP enjoyed an initial burst of popularity following its establishment in 1988, but interest appears to have leveled off, with only about half of NASP members currently possessing the credential; these members are disproportionately older than the NASP membership in general. Apparently, a majority of school psychologists who are relatively new to the field do not view the credential as something that is essential for them to pursue. We believe that the possible leveling off of interest described by Hunley masks what appears to be steady interest in the NCSP as well as its increasing influence and viability. Despite the less than universal interest in the NCSP, there are some practical reasons that recent graduates may wish to pursue the NCSP credential. It may be viewed favorably as an indication of one's commitment to professionalism when seeking employment or advancement in the field. Perhaps more important, the NCSP has slowly emerged as a standard for many state departments of education to accept when applicants from other states apply for a license or certificate to practice in that state. According to Hunley's 2004 analysis, 21 state departments of education accepted at that time the NCSP credential as evidence of meeting or exceeding their requirements for school psychology credentialing. As of 2010, NASP's website listing for NCSP reciprocity (see *www.nasponline.org/certification/statencsp.aspx*) indicates that 31 states now accept the credential as the basis for granting their own license or credential, and that more than 11,000 professionals now hold this credential. Although the total number of school psychologists with the NCSP is a relatively small percentage overall, we see this 48% growth in NCSP reciprocity in only 6 years as solid evidence of the influence of the NCSP credential and that it will will likely become the *de facto* standard across most states within another decade.

State Board of Examiners in Psychology License

Obtaining licensure for the independent practice of psychology and for use of the title *psychologist* (not *school psychologist*) requires that one have a doctoral degree in psychology and meet the specific application and approval requirements of a state board of examiners in psychology. Independent practice as a psychologist is sometimes confused with the term *private practice*. Although it is true that psychologists in private practice settings are independently practicing as psychologists, independent practice is not limited to these situations. Psychologists who work in public and private hospitals, clinics, health maintenance organizations, community mental health centers, college and university counseling centers, and various other settings are also engaging in the independent practice of psychology. That is, they are using the term *psychologist,* offering psychological services to the public, and are not required to work under the supervision of another licensed mental health professional in order to engage in these activities. By contrast, the term *school psychologist* is recognized in the psychology licensing laws of most states as applying to those who have a state department of education credential in school psychology and whose practice is limited to school settings. As described in Chapter 2, these licensing and terminology differences have long been a point of contention between NASP (which advocates for specialist-level school psychologists being able to engage in independent practice) and APA (which advocates that independent practice be limited to those holding a doctoral degree).

It is important to understand that neither NASP nor APA "owns" or regulates the terms *school psychologist* or *psychologist,* nor are there any federal laws dictating how these terms are to be used. Rather, legal regulation is the domain of states and provinces. Aside from contacting specific licensing boards, the best source for general information on state licensure for independent practice is the Association of State and Provincial Psychology Boards (ASPPB; P.O. Box 2125, Montgomery, AL 36124-1245; phone: 334-832-4580; *www.asppb.net*), an organization that coordinates and supports board licensing efforts among the states and provinces and that maintains an extensive website. Although there is some variation in the licensure requirements established by specific state boards, there are also many similarities. In most cases, being recognized as a licensed psychologist for independent practice requires:

- A doctoral degree in psychology.
- Completion of at least 2 years of supervised (by a licensed psychologist) psychology practice experience; in most cases at least 1 of the years must be at the postdoctoral level. However, an increasing number of states are not requiring supervised post-doctoral hours as long as the applicant has sufficient supervised experience at the predoctoral level.
- A passing score on the Examination for Professional Practice in Psychology (there is no universal standard for passing scores; each state or province establishes its own criteria for passing).
- A passing score on a state or provincial jurisprudence (law and ethics) exam administered by the board and, in some cases, an oral exam or case presentation to the board.

Despite the commonalities in requirements among state and provincial licensing boards, it is not a given that psychologists who are licensed in one state will automatically qualify for licensure elsewhere, and the process of obtaining licensure in a new area is sometimes complex and time consuming. However, a recent effort of ASPPB has been to establish a procedure for making license reciprocity among states and mobility for psychologists easier than it has been in the past. This procedure involves registering one's credentials with ASPPB and obtaining their Certificate of Qualification in Professional Psychology (CPQ), which is currently accepted for licensure in 39 states or Canadian provinces, accepted to a more limited extent by nine states or provinces, and under consideration by seven other states or provinces. An early-career licensed psychologist who anticipates the possibility of needing to have geographic mobility for several years may find the CPQ to be a useful credential.

Given the apparent complexity of obtaining licensure for independent practice as a psychologist, why would a doctoral-level school psychologist who already has a state department of education credential in school psychology want to go through this process? The major benefit is that an independent practice license allows school psychologists to practice in nontraditional or non-school settings (e.g., clinics, hospitals, community health centers, private practice groups) where their training in school psychology may allow them to provide unique services. Other benefits include the role expansion that such opportunities provide to school psychologists and the impact that school psychologists may be able to make in settings in which they may be the only professionals trained in their specialty.

Specialty Credentialing

In addition to the basic licensure and certification types just described, various additional opportunities exist for school psychologists to receive recognition of their particular areas of competence, especially at the doctoral level of training. For example, the

American Board of Professional Psychology (see *www.abpp.org* for more information) has established processes for board certification in 13 different specialty areas of doctoral-level training, including school psychology. Some school psychologists with particular skills and interests in applied behavior analysis have obtained certification from the Behavior Analyst Certification Board (see *www.bacb.com* for more information), a credential that is available to master's- and specialist-level practitioners as well as doctoral-level practitioners (and that includes fields other than psychology) and that requires specific coursework and supervised experience in behavior analysis. Some school psychologists who have gone through training programs with a strong emphasis on counseling skills have earned the National Board Certified Counselor credential (see *www.nbcc.org* for more information) in recognition of having developed specific expertise in the area of counseling. Other specialty credentials and recognition programs are also available. Specialty credentials are usually not required for specific employment, but they can serve as evidence to potential employers and the public that one has acquired specialized expertise.

Continuing Professional Development

Given the great effort required to get admitted to a graduate program in school psychology, to successfully complete the program, to complete a 1-year supervised internship, and to receive a certificate, license, or other credentials for the practice of school psychology and specialty areas, it is often surprising to new school psychologists that they are not really "done" with their educational training and professional development. On the contrary, continuing professional development is an important part of being a school psychologist. It is not only considered to be an important value within the profession but, in many cases, is required for maintaining practice credentials. In thinking about the importance and necessity of continuing professional development, consider that new knowledge and techniques are constantly emerging in the field of school psychology and that what may have been best practice 10 or 20 years ago may currently be considered obsolete.

State boards of education vary in their specific requirements for renewal of school psychology certificates or licenses. These credentials are typically issued for a specified number of years—for example, 3 to 5—with the stipulation that the recipient must show evidence of meeting specified professional development requirements before the credential is renewed for another period of time. Some states require a minimum number of years of professional employment during the credential period for it to be renewed. Some states require completion of a specified minimum number of clock hours of approved continuing professional development activities (such as workshop or conference attendance). Some states have both experience and training requirements for credential renewal. NASP's NSPCB requires renewal of the NCSP certificate every 3 years, a process that requires documentation of 75 clock hours of continuing professional development activities during the 3-year time period. State and provincial psychology licensing boards vary somewhat in terms of their requirements for license renewal, but a typical approach is to require documentation of a minimum of 40 clock hours of approved professional training activities (e.g., graduate coursework or approved professional training workshops) for every 2-year renewal cycle. In each of these instances, credential renewal requires not only documentation of the required activities but also completion of an application form and payment of a renewal fee.

Continuing professional development activities can take a variety of forms, and each credentialing body has its own specific rules governing what activities are acceptable. The most common activities include attending professional workshops or taking graduate-level continuing education courses from school psychology programs or related professional training programs. The annual NASP and APA conventions provide a wealth of opportunities for professional training and development, as do most state affiliates of NASP and APA at their own annual or semiannual conferences. Many areas, particularly large metropolitan areas, have numerous opportunities available for attending privately sponsored professional training workshops in the education and mental health fields. In addition, independent study programs are available for continuing professional development from some national and state professional associations and from some of the same private organizations that sponsor professional training workshops.

DISCUSSION QUESTIONS AND ACTIVITIES

1. If you are currently a graduate student in a school psychology training program and are using this text as part of an introductory school psychology course, discuss your own process of learning about the field and making the decision to apply to graduate training programs in the field. Why did you select school psychology over other areas of professional psychology (clinical or counseling) or over other professions within the field of education? Why did you choose to enter the particular graduate training program where you currently study?

2. Using the Internet, locate the standards for training programs in school psychology in the documents from APA and NASP that are referenced in this chapter. Review and evaluate the requirements for specific areas of coursework and field experience for accredited programs. Do you consider these requirements to be sufficient? Do you think that the requirements should be more specific or more general than they are currently?

3. Although the debate regarding the appropriate entry level of training required to become a school psychologist (specialist level or doctoral level) has raged for years, there has not been a substantial increase in the percentage of doctoral-level school psychologists, who currently make up only about 25% of the professionals in the field. What are the issues and practical considerations that have resulted in little change in the entry-level debate or status of the field over the years?

4. Go to the APPIC website (*www.appic.org*) or to recent issues of the NASP *Communiqué* or other professional newsletters and study the internship opportunities available to specialist-level and doctoral-level students in school psychology. What are the elements of postings that make them attractive or unattractive to potential applicants?

5. Increasingly, school psychologists are required to engage in specified continuing professional development activities to keep their practice credentials current. What are the advantages and disadvantages of typical methods of professional development training (e.g., attending workshops and conferences)? Are there possible alternative methods of continuing professional development for school psychologists that should be considered as evidence of meeting recredentialing requirements?

CHAPTER 5

Working as a School Psychologist
Employment Trends, Opportunities, and Challenges

In the previous chapters, we outlined general issues regarding what school psychologists do, the history of the field of school psychology, and the broader field of education, and provided information on training to become a school psychologist. In this chapter, we focus more specifically on the job of a school psychologist and address the following questions: How does one obtain a job as a school psychologist? In what settings are school psychologists employed? What functions or roles do school psychologists serve? Who are school psychologists? What is the job outlook in the field of school psychology? As when we wrote the previous edition of this book, there are some encouraging as well as discouraging trends in the field of school psychology. On the encouraging side, the job market in school psychology remains quite favorable for those seeking employment in the field. Particularly in certain areas of the country the shortage of school psychologists that became evident in the 1990s shows few signs of remitting. However, the economic climate in the United States has certainly impacted education in a less than desirable manner, with many states forced to make cuts (or not add money even with a growing student body population) to their education budgets. Another encouraging trend is the expansion of the function of school psychologists. In line with the problem-solving model discussed in Chapter 7, more and more school psychologists are actively involved in implementation of problem solving/RTI models in their schools, and by all appearances this is a role that is continuing to expand. The traditional "gatekeeper"/test-and-place role, although still present, appears to be on the decline as education and psychology in general both move more toward an evidence-based practice (EBP) model, using data to guide decisions. Given these changes, we believe it is an exciting time to be a school psychologist.

Obtaining a Job as a School Psychologist

Upon completion of graduate school, individuals with specialist-level degrees (including those with EdS degrees as well as those with MA/MS/MEd degrees who have completed a program that consists of 60 credit hours as required in most states) and doctoral degrees in school psychology are prepared to enter the workforce. Those with specialist-level degrees are most commonly employed in public school districts as school psychologists. Prior to obtaining a job as a school psychologist, an individual must obtain certification or educator licensure through the state's office of education (see Chapter 4 for more details on this process). The search for a job typically begins toward the end of a student's internship year. Many students may desire to continue to work in the districts in which they completed their internships. For such students, it should be easy to identify who to contact within the school district to inquire about job opportunities. For students wishing to find employment in a different district or to relocate to another state, the process of locating districts with open jobs and contact individuals within those districts can be somewhat daunting.

Unfortunately, there is no national posting of all jobs available in the field of school psychology. However, there are some resources students can use to attempt to locate districts with open positions. The NASP *Communiqué* (the official NASP newsletter), which is published eight times per year, publishes job announcements, and some school districts will advertise open positions in this publication. However, the number of open jobs listed in the *Communiqué* is very small, so students should not rely solely on this method to help them locate possible positions. Increasingly jobs are be advertised online (often in lieu of in print), and NASP also maintains a career center as part of its website (*jobs. naspcareercenter.org*) on which employers can post jobs and job seekers can search the listed postings. However, as with the *Communiqué*, only a small number of jobs are actually posted on this website. In fact, in several recent searches of this site, we found only 13 to 17 open positions listed (several of which were not even for school psychology jobs), a figure that certainly represents only a very small fraction of the total number of jobs available. Although there are a variety of other online sites where one can search for school psychology jobs, these also return few truly school psychology positions. For those seeking employment who know the state in which they would like to work, the websites of the state school psychology association or individual school districts may be some of the best places to locate open jobs. A quick perusal of several of these sites revealed that all had sections in which jobs were posted and all had multiple job postings. In addition, school psychology program training directors are often sent job announcements to share with their students, and many of these announcements are also sent to college or university career planning centers. However, even taking into account all these different methods, many jobs are secured through more informal avenues. Thus, it is crucial that students be proactive in their job searches.

Students often locate open professional positions by contacting individuals in school districts in which they are interested in working and inquiring as to whether there are open positions within the district or whether it is *anticipated* that there may be open positions for the following school year. However, determining who one should contact can be confusing, and this contact person often varies by school district. In many school districts, it is the special education director or coordinator who will be able to provide this information. In other school districts, it may be someone in the human resources or personnel office. In still other districts, especially those that are quite small, it may be the superintendent or someone in the superintendent's office. If a prospective job applicant is unsure who the best person is to contact initially, a good course of action is to make contact with one of the district's school psychologists. This person can then, it is hoped, direct the student to the appropriate person who will know about job openings.

Contacting current school psychologists also can be beneficial to applicants who are interested in obtaining more information regarding the practice of school psychology in a particular district. For example, applicants might ask about expected school loads, adoption of the RTI model, typical number of assessments completed, ability to engage in intervention and consultative services, and general work atmosphere of the district. Generally, students can contact a district's school psychologists by calling the school district office or searching the district's website. Some school psychologists may be housed in a central district office location. Others may have offices in their schools. Even for those with school-based offices, district office personnel should be able to provide information on how to best reach a school psychologist.

After finding the appropriate contact person in a school district, the applicant will likely be able to ask about the procedures involved in applying for a job in that district. Typically, an application form must be completed. Along with this form, the applicant should provide a curriculum vita or resume as well as names of references. School districts will often, although not always, want formal letters of recommendation from individuals with whom the applicant has worked. In addition, some school districts have their own recommendation forms, which must be completed by the applicant's references. These recommendations should be completed by professional contacts who can attest to the applicant's skills and potential for excellence in school psychology. For individuals just out of graduate school, we recommend that the applicant seek one reference letter from his or her internship supervisor. Other recommendations will likely be obtained from graduate school instructors. If a recent graduate has formed a good working relationship with a school administrator at his or her internship site, such as a building principal, it may be useful to seek a letter of reference from that person as well.

In addition to the paper application and recommendations, school districts typically conduct interviews with job applicants. Applicants must treat these interviews seriously, arrive well prepared, and present themselves in a professional manner. In a pool of applicants in which many may be equal on paper, the interview can be the deciding factor in terms of who is offered the job. Interviews vary widely in terms of formality and questions asked. However, all applicants should be prepared to answer basic questions regarding their background in school psychology, perceived strengths and weaknesses, and their view of school psychology. Interviewers may ask applicants to respond to case scenarios. These can be intimidating for applicants, and, unfortunately, there is no specific way to prepare for such questions. By being familiar with best practices, applicants should be able to successfully answer questions of this nature.

In addition to the difficulty of knowing who to contact regarding job openings in a given school district, knowing when to look for jobs can also be a bit confusing. We recommend that individuals begin contacting school districts in mid-winter to early spring. However, many school districts will be unsure of their funding situations and vacancy status at that time. Thus, they will not be in a position to make job offers until later in the year. Many school districts will not even begin interviewing until later in the year; some may not begin the interview process until as late as May, when the school year is ending. Some districts may interview earlier in the year but then not make job offers for several months. Because this process is so variable by district, we recommend contacting districts earlier rather than later so as to not miss out on applying for a job simply because application materials were not submitted early enough. That being said, applicants should not worry if they are told that a district is unsure of its ability to hire and will not know if there are open positions until later in the spring or even early summer. Although this type of response can be anxiety provoking for students who want to know if they are going to be gainfully employed the following year, such a response is typical in many districts. As discussed later in this chapter, there has been an ongoing nationwide shortage of school psychologists. The shortage has perhaps slowed somewhat with the recent economic downturns and associated cuts to education spending in many states. However, the shortage still appears to exist and also appears likely to continue. Given that shortage, it is highly likely that applicants who are not completely place-bound (i.e., in need of a job in one specific district or geographical region) will be able to locate a job. In fact, our experience is that well-qualified, geographically mobile applicants often receive several job offers.

Obtaining a Job in a Non-School Setting

Individuals with doctoral degrees have more options than those with specialist-level degrees in terms of where they can find employment. Obviously, the K–12 schools are one common source of jobs for doctoral-level school psychologists as well as specialist-level school psychologists. For doctoral-level school psychologists wishing to work in the schools, the process of locating a job is identical to that previously described. In most school districts, there is no differentiation in the hiring process between those with PhDs and those with specialist-level degrees.

Doctoral-level psychologists may also find employment in university training programs and clinical settings, including medical centers, hospitals, and community mental health agencies. In addition, these individuals may elect to pursue practice independently as a psychologist. Because most graduates of school psychology programs seek employment in public school settings, finding employment in each of these other areas is only briefly addressed.

University Training Programs

A few of the best places to look for postings of open faculty positions are APA's *Monitor on Psychology* and its online career center (PsycCareers: *jobs.psyccareers.com/jobs*) as well as NASP's *Communiqué* and online career center (*jobs.naspcareercenter.org*). Other web-based searchable job sites geared toward academic positions, such as *higheredjobs.com*, may also be good places for job seekers to search. In addition, prospective trainers would do well to stay in touch with their university training directors, who often receive postings for academic positions from other programs and job announcements, which are increasingly being sent via e-mail lists (e.g., the Trainers of School Psychologists mailing list). However, the majority of faculty positions in the United States and Canada, particularly those at research universities, have traditionally been advertised in the APA *Monitor on Psychology* and on APA's website; thus, this is one of the best sources of information for such positions. Individuals interested in jobs in nonresearch universities may also find it helpful to look in the *Chronicle of Higher Education*. Unlike school-based positions, which often do not open up until later in the school year, university faculty positions are advertised early (generally in the fall and early winter of the year before the position is to begin). So, for an individual seeking a faculty position directly out of his or her doctoral program, the job search process begins almost immediately after beginning the internship year. Within each ad or announcement for a faculty position is a list of materials applicants must submit in order to apply for the position. A letter of application and a curriculum vita are standard materials that are requested. Universities may also want transcripts, copies of published articles, teaching evaluations, or other materials that demonstrate the potential for excellence as a faculty member. Most universities now utilize online application programs. Applicants should be sure to submit the materials requested in the format requested when applying for jobs. Letters of recommendation are typically required and may need to be uploaded to a job site by the recommender or sent directly to the search committee chair. However, some universities may simply want names of references, who the search committee members will then contact via phone.

University positions typically involve a combination of research and teaching and service activities, but different universities place different weight on these domains. Typically, specialist-level programs place less emphasis on research than do doctoral-level programs. Because of the decreased emphasis on research, teaching loads in specialist-level programs may be higher than teaching loads in doctoral programs. In addition, service expectations may vary greatly depending on the university and individual departments. Although all universities have some service expectations (e.g., sitting on university and departmental committees, providing service to the local community), the extent of service expected varies greatly from department to department. Applicants should consider these differences and apply for positions that they believe are most suited to their interests and strengths.

Applicants for faculty positions should also keep in mind that "fit" (in terms of program philosophy and program needs) is an important quality in applying for academic jobs. It is important that applicants state clearly in their letters of application how they fit with the training program to which they are applying for a faculty position. Individuals should not apply for positions for which they perceive they are a poor fit. For example, if a job announcement indicates that the university is looking for a faculty member whose research involves behaviorally based interventions in the schools, it is unlikely that an individual whose research involves neuropsychological assessments for children with traumatic brain injury would be a good fit for the program. It is important that applicants consider fit not just in terms of whether they would be competitive for the job but also in terms of whether they would enjoy the job. Teaching outside of one's area or working within a department in which the program philosophy differs substantially from one's own philosophy can make for a difficult job experience.

When evaluating academic positions, applicants should also seek to understand the supports available to them in the programs to which they are considering applying. As mentioned in Chapter 4, the demands on a university trainer can be many and are often not overtly rewarded. It is imperative that new faculty have good sources of support. This support may be partially provided by individuals outside of the university (e.g., a former graduate school advisor), but applicants for faculty positions should also assess support from within the program they are considering joining. For example, are colleagues friendly and easily accessible? Are administrative personnel (e.g., department head, dean) supportive of the program and its mission? Are new faculty assigned an experienced faculty mentor to help them navigate the complexities of academic life? Although these questions can be difficult to answer, taking time to investigate these supports can be invaluable to an applicant in choosing the position that is right for him or her.

Clinical Settings

For individuals who desire to work in a clinical setting, such as a community mental health center, children's hospital, or specialty clinic, it may be important to first complete a postdoctoral fellowship. To practice independently in such settings, a license as a psychologist is necessary. In most states this requires the completion of supervised postdoctoral hours, although increasingly states are allowing all supervised hours to be completed at the predoctoral level (including Utah, Washington, Ohio, North Dakota, Arizona, and Alabama). Thus, individuals who have just graduated from a PhD program may not yet be eligible for licensure. For current information on licensing requirements in all U.S. states and Canadian provinces, see the licensure requirement handbook on the website of the ASPPB (*www.asppb.net*). Some clinical settings may hire a person and provide the supervision necessary to complete postdoctoral hours if needed, but other settings will want applicants to have already achieved licensure. A postdoctoral fellowship is one way to obtain these hours and be eligible for licensure prior to applying for a full-time clinical position. Not only do postdoctoral positions allow individuals to accrue supervised hours toward licensure, but such positions also allow individuals to obtain specialty training in certain areas (e.g., child neuropsychology, pediatric obesity). Although postdoctoral positions are by no means a required part of training, they do seem to be becoming more common in the applied fields of psychology, including school psychology.

Jobs in clinical settings, as well as postdoctoral positions, may be advertised in the APA *Monitor on Psychology* and APA's website or the NASP *Communiqué*. In addition, APA has begun accrediting postdoctoral programs (as they accredit doctoral training programs and predoctoral internships). A listing of postdoctoral programs accredited by APA can be found on APA's website (see *www.apa.org/ed/accreditation/programs/accred-postdoc.aspx*). Because APA's accrediting of postdoctoral programs is relatively new, there are a limited number of programs accredited currently but we expect this to continue to grow. The Association of Psychology Postdoctoral and Internship Centers (APPIC) also maintains a searchable list of postdoctoral programs approved by APPIC (see *www.appic.org*). Although listings of postdoctoral programs are growing, informal networking (via faculty and internship mentors as well as their contacts) may be needed to locate positions. Because clinical positions tend to be year-round jobs, there are no specific times of the year when most jobs are advertised, although for postdoctoral positions posted on the APPIC website, most application deadlines are in January or February (to start in the summer of fall of that year). We recommend that individuals who desire a clinical position begin searching for these positions in the late winter or early spring of their internship years.

Although there are no specific qualifications (other than licensure) to work in most clinical settings, as with university positions, applicants should consider their "fit" with positions and how their prior training and interests match with the described job. For example, if applicants have no prior training working with children with autism, it is highly unlikely that they would be hired to fill a position in which this population was a large focus of the clinical work. Individuals should take care to the tailor their practicum, internship, and postdoctoral experiences (if any) so that they receive both the breadth and depth of experience that will prepare them for clinical jobs in their areas of interest following graduation.

The Work Setting

Although school psychologists, particularly those trained at the doctoral level, have the credentials to work in a number of different settings, the majority of school psychology graduates work in the public schools. According to data obtained from the 2004–2005 NASP membership survey (Curtis, Lopez, et al., 2008), the vast majority (83.1%) of school psychologists report working in public school settings. School psychologists not in the public schools report working in a variety of other settings, including colleges or universities (6.5%), private practice (4.1%), private (5.2%) or faith-based (2.1%) schools, hospital or medical settings (1.3%), and state departments of education (0.8%). A small number of individuals (2.8%) reported being employed in a setting other than one of these listed.

As would be expected given the employment settings of most school psychologists, the majority of these individuals report working as school psychologists. According to the NASP membership data (Curtis, Lopez, et al., 2008), of those school psychologists who reported their function, 80.4% reported working as school psychologists. The next most common function reported was that of a university faculty member (6.0%) followed by administrator (5.4%), and state education personnel (0.6%); 7.6% reported another primary position other than those listed.

It should be acknowledged that these numbers likely underestimate the percentage of school psychologists working outside of school settings and those working in roles other than that of school psychologists, given that these numbers are based on responses to an NASP membership survey. It seems likely that individuals trained as school psychologists but no longer functioning in a school psychology-related role would be less likely to maintain their membership in NASP. In addition, although this survey was completed by 1,748 NASP members, this is still a small percentage of total NASP members. However, it is clear from this list of employment settings and roles that school psychologists are working in a number of areas in addition to the traditional school setting.

Even within the school setting, a great deal of variability exists in the work settings (as well as the roles and functions, discussed later) of school psychologists. For example, most school psychologists serve multiple schools. These school psychologists are frequently based out of a central district office (where they typically have their own office space) rather than having school-based offices. However, some school psychologists are school based and serve just one school, allowing them to become a part of that school's daily workings and culture.

School psychologist-to-student ratios also vary considerably and will affect the services that a school psychologist is able to provide. Currently, NASP recommends a school psychologist-to-student ratio of 1:1,000. However, as reported from the NASP membership survey (Curtis, Lopez, et al., 2008), the mean ratio was 1:1,482, with 40% of respondents indicating a ratio of 1:1,000 or less. Based on 2004 estimates by Charvat (Charvat, 2005), most states saw a decrease in their ratios from 1999 to 2004, although some states saw notable increases (e.g., Mississippi's ratio increased from 1:3,505 in 1999 to 1:7,946 in 2004; New Mexico's jumped from 1:951 to 1:1,922).

School Psychologists in Nontraditional Settings

As noted earlier, a small portion of individuals trained as school psychologists do not work in school settings or are not employed as school psychologists. However, it is almost impossible to obtain data specifically on what these individuals are doing given most surveys of school psychologists are geared toward those working in more traditional settings and that most survey samples are drawn from NASP's membership list. As discussed in previous chapters and later in this chapter, increasing emphasis has been given to the expansion of the role of the school psychologist. With this role expansion, and as school psychologists become increasingly recognized as providers of comprehensive educational and mental health services rather than simply being psychometricians, it is likely that the number of school psychologists working in "nontraditional" (i.e., non-school) settings will expand. Obviously, this role expansion will also allow school psychologists to provide more comprehensive services within school settings. An example of this role expansion is the emergence of pediatric school psychology as a relatively new subspecialty within the field of school psychology. Pediatric school psychologists specialize in meeting the needs of children with medical conditions, including collaborating with medical providers about optimal treatments, working with educators to meet the needs of individual children with health problems, and developing primary and secondary prevention programs to promote healthy behaviors (Power, DuPaul, Shapiro, & Parrish, 1995).

The likelihood of doctoral-level school psychologists working in non-school settings is probably, in part, related to the settings in which the individuals completed their predoctoral internships. It seems likely that school psychology students who complete their predoctoral internships in non-school settings will be more likely to choose such settings for their permanent employment. Such individuals may also be more competitive for non-school positions than those who completed school-based internships, so students should be thinking ahead as they apply for internships in terms of the type of career they would eventually like to have. However, it can be more difficult for school psychology students (compared with clinical or counseling psychology students) to obtain internships in non-school settings, because many non-school-based internship sites do not consider applicants from school psychology programs. According to a searchable internship directory available on the website of the APPIC (*www.appic.org*), 457 APA-accredited predoctoral internship sites (and 210 non-APA-accredited sites) consider applicants from clinical psychology programs, 424 accredited (and 195 nonaccredited) sites consider applicants from counseling psychology programs, and only 137 accredited (and 84 nonaccredited) sites consider applicants from school psychology programs. Of course, it should be acknowledged that these figures are for all internship sites (including those that focus on adults as well as children) and school psychologists will most likely apply to those that focus on services to children. Narrowing the search of internships to those that have a major rotation with children, 171 sites (114 APA accredited) accept applications from individuals in school psychology programs, 280 (179 APA accredited) accept applications from counseling psychology program students, and 315 (204 accredited) accept applications from clinical psychology program students. Although completing a school-based internship is in no way a negative and we want to encourage school psychologists to seek internship and employment opportunities in the schools, the relative lack of alternative internship sites is concerning. It is likely that this furthers the perception that school psychologists predominately engage in assessment activities and are not prepared to undertake other types of activities more often associated with clinical and counseling psychologists.

One study provides support for the notion that school psychology students may have more difficulties locating non-school-based internships than students from clinical or counseling programs. Gayer, Brown, Gridley, and Treloar (2003) conducted an analogue study in which they sent internship training directors simulated internship application materials. The materials were identical, with the exception that one-third of the "applicants" were identified as being from clinical psychology programs, one-third from counseling psychology programs, and one-third from school psychology programs. The internship training directors were asked to indicate whether they would accept, reject, or hold the student. Clinical psychology students were most likely to be accepted, whereas school psychology students were most likely to be rejected. The acceptance rates were 66% for clinical, 48% for counseling, and 31% for school psychology students. The rejection rates were, respectively, 2%, 7%, and 40%. Findings such as these support the notion that the opportunities for school psychologists outside of the school setting may be more limited than for clinical and counseling psychologists. It is imperative that those within the field of school psychology increasingly advocate for themselves and their profession. We believe that schools and education should be the prominent focus within school psychology training programs, but at the same time we advocate for school psychologists being able to work in a variety of other settings and decry stereotypes and biases against school psychology that limit such opportunities.

A potential reason for the lower acceptance rates may be the perceptions of strengths and weaknesses of school psychology students by internship directors. In a survey of internship training directors of sites that stated they accepted applications from individuals from school psychology training programs (Brown, Kissell, & Bolen, 2003), 31% of directors perceived individual and group counseling as a weakness for school psychology students even though this was the activity in which interns spent the most time. Educational assessment was perceived as strength of school psychology interns by 56% of directors. Given this, it may be important for school psychology students who desire to complete an internship and/or work in a "nontraditional" setting to ensure they obtain sufficient intervention experience while in graduate school.

Salaries and Time Spent Working

It is well known that school psychology is not the field to enter if one's sole desire is to become wealthy. That being said, salaries for school psychologists are not abysmal, and they compare favorably with those of other service-oriented professions, especially when one considers that most school psychologists work on 9- or 10-month contracts. The most recent comprehensive analysis of salary data is from the United States for the 2004–2005 school year (Curtis, Lopez, Batsche, & Smith, 2006; Curtis, Lopez, Batsche, Minch, & Abshier, 2007). Data from this survey are presented on the NASP website (*www.nasponline.org/about_sp/salaryinfo.aspx*). As reported here, the mean annual salary for school psychologists was $60,581. University faculty averaged slightly more ($65,398) than school psychology practitioners ($62,513 for 200-day contracts; $56,262 for 180-day contracts). Regional differences existed in salaries (as well as average contracted days). The average annual salary for a 200-day contract by region ranged from a low of $50,400 in the West South Central region (consisting of Arkansas, Louisiana, Oklahoma, and Texas) to a high of $70,600 in the mid-Atlantic region (consisting of New Jersey, New York, and Pennsylvania). Overall, school psychologists with their PhD had a slightly higher daily salary ($350.03) than those with their specialist-level degree ($287.03). The average number of days in a school psychologist's contract range from a low of 186 (in the Northeast region) to a high of 208 (in the South Atlantic region). Overall, 50.4% of the NASP members who responded to the survey reported having contracts of 180 to 190 days and 33.6% reported having contracts of 200 days or more.

The Role and Function of School Psychologists

In addition to variations in the work setting and environment, there are also likely to be differences in the role and function of the school psychologist from state to state and even from district to district within the same state. As discussed in Chapter 1, the definition of school psychology, as well as the role of the school psychologist, has changed over time. However, changes in practice may occur at varying paces and often lag behind philosophical changes regarding the practice of school psychology. The purpose of this section is to provide an overview of some of the stated roles and functions of school psychologists as well as to provide some data on what school psychologists are actually doing.

School psychologists engage in a wide variety of activities; however, three activities are consistently identified as the main activities school psychologists perform. These include (1) assessment, (2) consultation, and (3) intervention. School psychologists can also engage in a variety of other activities or activities that may be considered subcategories of these. In the NASP brochure titled *What Is a School Psychologist?* (available online at *www.nasponline.org/about_sp/whatis.aspx*), some of the numerous activities school psychologists may engage in with students, families, teachers, administrators, and community providers are outlined. These services include helping students with learning and behavior problems via direct interventions as well as working with parents and teachers to implement interventions. Preventive activities such as promoting wellness and resiliency, creating positive classroom environments, and implementing schoolwide prevention programs are also mentioned.

Assessment has long been identified as a primary function of school psychologists. As discussed in the historical context in Chapter 2, the role of assessment increased substantially for many school psychologists following the passage of Public Law 94-142 in 1975. With the advent of this law, guidelines were put into place that required certain assessment procedures to be followed prior to placing children in special education programs. School psychologists provided these assessments, and quickly this function took over all other functions for many school psychologists. Because federal and state laws required assessments to be completed, when resources were scarce in districts school psychologists were often required to first complete these required activities before engaging in other activities. Unfortunately, school psychologists quickly began to be seen simply as psychometricians. Although school psychologists did engage other professional activities, the vast majority of most school psychologists' time was spent in assessment activities.

More recently, especially with the changes in special education law with the Individuals with Disabilities Education Improvement Act (IDEIA) passed in 2004 regarding the identification of learning disabilities (discussed in more detail in Chapter 6), school psychologists have seen some changes in their roles that we regard as positive. For many years, some school psychologists as well as a number of school psychology trainers advocated for school psychologists to function as comprehensive educational and mental health service providers (e.g., NASP, 2008). However, in reality many school psychologists continued to engage predominately in standardized assessment activities for the purpose of classification for special education services. With the passage of IDEIA-2004 and the possibility that an RTI model could be used to identify students with a learning disability (LD), the field has increasingly moved toward the RTI model. Although many trainers and some practitioners had been advocating for this model for some time (e.g., Deno, 1986; Fuchs, 2003; Good & Kaminski, 1996; Tilly, 2008), it really was not until this term appeared in law that this process became more widely utilized in schools throughout the country (Spectrum K12 School Solutions, 2010). Although certainly not all schools have adopted an RTI model, there has been a dramatic increase in the use of this model since we wrote the first edition of this book.

Data presented by the Spectrum K12 group (2010) indicates that as of 2010 more than 60% of school district administrators who responded to a web-based survey reported that their districts were either fully implementing RTI or were in the process of a districtwide implementation. This figure is up from numbers in previous years (54% in 2009, 32% in 2008, 24% in 2007). Reading was the area in which RTI was implemented with the greatest frequency; 90% of elementary schools implemented RTI procedures for reading, 59% for math, and 48% for behavior (numbers were considerably lower for middle schools and high schools). However, because this model is still relatively new in terms of wide practice in the field, it is difficult to know at this time just how much the role of the "average" school psychologist has changed. In the Spectrum K12 survey, special education directors were reported most frequently as the person who initiated RTI implementation (36%), but school psychologists' involvement in the RTI process was not addressed in this survey. In a survey of practicing school psychologists regarding their districts' experiences with RTI and LD classifications (Cangelosi, 2010), only 22% of participants indicated that their assessment and diagnostic practices had *not* changed at all following their state's adoption of the IDEIA-2004 regulations. More than 40% indicated that RTI information was taken into account "always" or "almost always" when evaluating a child for an LD (with 10% indicating it was "never" taken into account). Interestingly, 83% indicated that results of cognitive assessment measures were "always" or "almost always" considered in making LD determinations and almost 70% indicated that a severe discrepancy between IQ and academic achievement was considered "always" or "almost always."

It is important to point out that, although we see the move toward the RTI model as a positive one, this does not mean that we see assessment as unimportant. Indeed, assessment is very important within the RTI and problem-solving models we espouse in this book. However, the type of assessment is different than the standardized intellectual ability and achievement testing that have historically been associated with school psychology. Ideally, assessment should be conceptualized not as one specific activity but as a problem-solving *process*, as discussed in Chapter 7. School psychologists receive referrals regarding children who are struggling academically, emotionally, or behaviorally. Prior to implementing an intervention, the school psychologist must conduct an assessment to determine what the problem is and what methods might be effective in remediating the problem. In some cases, the assessment may be utilized to help determine whether a student is eligible for special education services. In all cases, the assessment should help identify the specific difficulties that are present and that preclude the child from learning or behaving as expected.

Assessment is an extremely valuable task that school psychologists perform. Without an appropriate assessment, it is difficult to know what intervention to use and whether the implemented intervention is having the desired effect. However, assessment has received a bad rap because historically many people (including many school psychologists) have seen assessment as simply the administration of a standardized measure or two and have failed to see it as part of the broader problem-solving context. We believe it is imperative that school psychologists develop a broader view of assessment, and with the recent emphasis on the RTI model we believe that this is starting to happen. As discussed in much more detail in Chapter 7, school psychologists who engage in the problem-solving model of practice are continually using assessment in order to obtain the needed data to guide decision making at each stage of the problem-solving process. This type of assessment bears little resemblance to the standardized testing traditionally associated with school psychology. Assessment as part of the problem-solving process is key in guiding effective practice, and we are encouraged to see more and more school psychologists engaged in this type of assessment activity.

Consultation has also historically been a key part of school psychologists' roles, although to a lesser extent than assessment. Consultation is an intervention method that is usually conceptualized as a triadic relationship. The professional (in this case, the school psychologist) works with a third party in the interest of changing the behaviors of the targeted client (i.e., the child referred). Within the school setting, the third party is typically a teacher or parent. School psychologists engage in teacher consultation more frequently than in parent consultation, likely due in part to the fact that teachers are there at the schools and are easier to access than parents. Consultative activities with teachers include assisting in the development of a classroom behavior management plan or helping develop an academic intervention for a student who is struggling in reading. Parent consultation may involve working with parents on issues related to effective parenting and assisting parents in setting up programs at home to reinforce homework completion.

Some school psychologists also conduct systems-level consultation. In this form of consultation, the school psychologist does not work with one individual to promote changes in one child but instead works to bring about broader change. For example, the school psychologist may assist the school district in developing a new prereferral intervention process. This type of consultation (discussed further in Chapter 11) has great potential to bring about changes that affect more than just one individual child. In addition, systems-level work is essential in developing prevention efforts that address the needs of all students at a universal level. Unfortunately, school psychologists have traditionally spent most of their time consulting with parents and teachers regarding the individual needs of students who are already experiencing difficulties. Although this level of consultation should not be ignored, we are encouraged to see that school psychologists are beginning to expand their roles to consult at classwide, small-group, and schoolwide levels to address primary and secondary prevention needs in addition to tertiary prevention and intervention efforts (e.g., Barnett, Ihlo, Nichols, & Wolsing, 2006; Reinke, Lewis-Palmer, & Merrell, 2008).

Within the intervention domain, school psychologists may engage in indirect interventions or direct interventions, and these interventions may be conducted in group or individual settings. Indirect intervention is conducted via collaboration with important "others" in the child's life (e.g., parents, teachers), as we described previously. For example, a school psychologist may run parenting groups concerning effective management of child behavior problems. School psychologists also may provide services directly to students. For example, a school psychologist may work one on one with a student to alleviate symptoms of depression that student is exhibiting. Another intervention activity may involve running a social skills group to increase appropriate social behaviors in a group of elementary school children. As part of their intervention efforts, school psychologists may also engage in prevention activities. Obviously, it is better to prevent problems from occurring than to treat problems once they have occurred. Prevention efforts may include running groups for children identified as being at risk for emotional and behavioral problems, developing schoolwide programs to decrease problems such as bullying, and implementing early literacy programs. Although prevention activities are often conceptualized as occurring before any problems are noticed, prevention activities are probably most frequently put into place after problems are first identified but before they have reached a clinically significant level.

Ideal and Actual Roles

Although school psychologists are trained to practice assessment, consultation, and intervention, as well as other activities such as research and program evaluation, historically there has been a disparity between the amount of time school psychologists report engaging in these activities and the amount of time they would like to spend engaged in these activities. Although school psychologists' roles do seem to be changing, it is difficult to know at this point how much they will change and how closely they will align with school psychologists' ideal role, which may also change as RTI becomes more common place in K–12 schools.

Surveys of school psychologists' activities prior to the passage of IDEIA-2004 all document that school psychologists spent more time in assessment-related activities than in any other activities. For example, in a survey of approximately 400 school psychologists conducted in 1999, school psychologists reported spending on average 46% of their time in assessment-related activities. Consultation was reported to take 16% of their time and intervention (including interventions, counseling, and parent training) 22% of their time (Bramlett, Murphy, Johnson, Wallingsford, & Hall, 2002). The other 16% of their time was divided between conferencing (7%), supervision (3%), inservice activities (2%), research (1%), and other, unreported activities (3%). These findings are consistent with an earlier study completed in the 1991–1992 school year (Reschly & Wilson, 1995) in which school psychologists reported that they spent most of their time in assessment-related activities. In this study, school psychologists reported spending an average of 22 hours a week (55% of their time) in assessment activities, 8.3 hours (21%) in direct interventions, 8.8 hours (22%) in consultative activities, and 0.8 hours (2%) in research and program evaluation activities. However, in this same study, school psychologists reported that their preferred role would involve less assessment and more intervention work. The practitioners in this study indicated their preferred role breakdown would be to spend 12.9 hours a week (32%) in assessment activities, 11.3 hours (28%) in direct intervention activities, 13.1 hours (33%) in consultative activities, and 2.7 hours (7%) in research and program evaluation activities. Although practitioners in this study were not engaged in intervention and consultative activities to the extent they wished to be, they still reported a relatively high level of job satisfaction. However, it should be noted that respondents were most satisfied with their colleagues and slightly less satisfied with other aspects of their jobs.

In a similar study, Hosp and Reschly (2002) examined actual and preferred roles of school psychologists across the United States in spring 1997. The findings from this study are consistent with those from Reschly and Wilson (1995). Overall, school psychologists reported spending 22.2 hours per week (55% of their time) in assessment activities but indicated that they would prefer to spend only 12.8 hours per week (32%) in such activities. They indicated that they spent 7.6 hours a week (19%) in intervention activities but would prefer to spend 11.4 hours (29%) involved in intervention work. In terms of consultation, school psychologists reported spending 9.2 hours a week (23%) but would prefer to spend 13.3 hours (33%) in these activities. Overall, the school psychologists in this sample reported that they spent about 60% in eligibility-related services (e.g., conducting evaluations, attending individualized education program team meetings).

In addition to looking at nationwide responses, Hosp and Reschly (2002) examined their data for differences based on geographic region. Although there was some variability in terms of actual and preferred role by geographic location, on average respondents from all areas of the United States indicated they would prefer to engage in less assessment and more intervention and consultation. School psychologists in the Northeast (Connecticut, Massachusetts, Maine, New Hampshire, Rhode Island, Vermont), mid-Atlantic (New Jersey, New York, Pennsylvania), West South Central (Arkansas, Louisiana, Oklahoma, Texas), and Mountain West states (Arizona, Colorado, Idaho, Montana, New Mexico, Nevada, Utah, Wyoming) reported engaging in assessment activities 20 hours per week or less, whereas those in other regions reported engaging in assessment activities more than 20 hours per week, with those in the East South Central (Alabama, Kentucky, Mississippi, Tennessee) area reporting that they spent an average of 26.5 hours a week in assessment activities. School psychologists in all areas of the United States reported that at least half of their time was spent in eligibility-related activities.

With regard to job satisfaction, Hosp and Reschly (2002) obtained findings similar to those of Reschly and Wilson (1995). The school psychologists in Hosp and Reschly's study reported being at least moderately satisfied with their jobs, even given the disparity between their actual and preferred roles. On a scale of 1 to 5, with 5 indicating greater satisfaction, the respondents rated their satisfaction with colleagues as 4.0 and their satisfaction with work duties as 3.6. There were no differences in job satisfaction based on geographic region.

In a more recent study looking at job satisfaction over time but still prior to the implementation of IDEIA-2004, Worrell, Skaggs, and Brown (2006) noted that there had been a slight increase in job satisfaction over time. In 2004 83.7% of school psychologists reported being satisfied with their jobs (compared with 80.7% in both 1982 and 1992) and 6.9% reported being very satisfied (compared with 5.0% in 1982 and 5.3% in 1992).

In the most recent survey of school psychologists regarding their professional practices, Curtis, Lopez, et al. (2008) provide data on practices of school psychologists from the 2004–2005 year. Although these are the most recent data we could locate, it should be noted that, for the purposes of this discussion and given what seems to be a relatively rapid change over the past 5 to 6 years, these data likely do not adequately capture the school psychologist's role today.

School psychologists who responded to Curtis, Lopez, et al.'s (2008) survey reported that they spend approximately 80% of their time in special education-related activities and completed an average of 34.7 initial special education evaluations in a year (and 34.3 reevaluations). Curtis, Lopez, et al. did note a downward trend in the number of initial evaluations completed from a similar survey conducted in the 1999–2000 school year. During that earlier time, 33.4% of school psychologists reported completing between 1 and 25 evaluations per year compared with 42.7% who reported completing between 1 and 25 evaluations in the 2004–2005 year. In a survey conducted in the 1994–1995 year, only 29.8% reported completing 25 or fewer initial evaluations. As RTI procedures become more widely implemented and more children's difficulties are remediated through Tier 1 and Tier 2 interventions, we expect that there will continue to be a downward trend in the number of evaluations that are completed by school psychologists. For example, Torgesen (2009) noted significant decreases in the percentage of children identified as having learning disabilities in grades K–3 following the implementation of a reading RTI program. (Torgesen also noted that, although end-of-year reading improved, these improvements do not fully account for the decrease in LD identification.)

The majority of school psychologists (96.4%) surveyed by Curtis, Lopez, et al. (2008) reported being involved in consultative activities. Most school psychologists (71.4%) also reported being involved in individual counseling with students and 39.9% reported conducting group interventions with students. Interestingly, these numbers do not appear to have changed much since 1994–1995, when 97.4% of school psychologists reported engaging in consultative activities and 82.2% reported being involved in individual counseling (and 53.5% involved in group counseling). The rate of consultation in 1994-95 also appears to be similar to the more recent reports: in 1994–1995, 45.9% reported serving 1 to 25 students in consultative activities and 25.6% reported serving 50 or more. In 2004–2005, 47.9% reported 1 to 25 children served via consultative and 28.5% reported serving more than 50.

Overall, the results from the Curtis, Lopez, et al. (2008) survey indicate that, although time in assessment activities seems to be decreasing, school psychologists are still spending the majority of their time in special education-related activities. It will be interesting to see whether this percentage declines as more school psychologists (it is hoped) begin to engage more with RTI procedures in the regular education environment. Our hypothesis is that as RTI procedures become more widely adopted, the school psychologist's role will continue to evolve. A 2008 doctoral dissertation by Larson found some support for this notion. In this study, 122 school psychologists were asked about the percentage of time they spent in varying professional activities pre- and post-IDEIA-2004. Although assessment remained the top role, the time these school psychologists estimated they spent in assessment activities decreased from 55% pre-IDEIA 2004 to 47% post IDEIA-2004. Time spent in intervention, preventive services, consultation, and team collaboration increased but only slightly (1–2%).

In another doctoral dissertation, the notion that school psychologists are increasingly being trained for roles that involve more consultation and assessment was supported (Daly, 2007). Current graduate students in school psychology programs ($n = 144$) and recent graduates ($n = 67$ [within the past 3 years]) estimated the percentage of time they spent in field placements in different domains while in training. Recent graduates estimated they spent 56.8% of their time in assessment activities compared with current students' estimate of 43.1%. Current students reported more time in intervention (23.7% vs. 19.1%), consultation (18.3% vs. 14.1%), systems/organizational work (6.7% vs. 2.8%), and research/evaluation (5.4% vs. 3.6%) compared with recent graduates.

Since the passage of IDEIA-2004, there have been increased discussions in forums such as the NASP *Communiqué* on the role of the school psychologist in the RTI process (e.g., Canter, 2006; Ern, Head, & Anderson, 2009). In addition, a rapidly increasing number of scholarly articles on the implementation of RTI (as well as perceived problems with RTI) have appeared in the professional journals in school psychology. Based on the limited data currently available, it does appear that there have been some changes in school psychologists' roles. However, it remains to be seen how much change there is and how sustained these changes are over time.

Demographic Characteristics of School Psychologists

Now that we have considered what school psychologists do, we turn to the topic of who school psychologists are. The information presented here expands on sections of Chapter 4, in which the demographic characteristics of school psychology trainers and students were briefly discussed. Although the children and families served by school psychologists are an increasingly diverse group, school psychologists as a group are not very diverse. In general, school psychologists are predominately female and European American and hold specialist-level degrees. School psychologists are also increasingly an aging population (on average), leading, in part, to shortages of school psychologists as a result of retirements.

Gender

According to data from the 2004–2005 NASP membership survey, 74% of school psychologists who are NASP members are female. However, the gender ratio has not always been so lopsided. Reschly (2000) reported that the number of women in school psychology has gradually increased since the early 1970s, when the gender ratio was tipped toward men (about 60:40). By the mid-1970s the gender ratios were equal, and since the mid-1980s the field has become increasingly dominated by women. This trend is not unique to the field of school psychology but, rather, seems to be reflective of an increased feminization of the field of psychology in general. As reported from the 2009 Survey of Earned Doctorates (National Science Foundation, 2010), 71% of psychology doctoral graduates were female compared with 47% of all doctoral recipients. Women are even more predominant in school psychology; of the 121 school psychologists who earned their doctoral degrees in 2009, 92 (76%) of these were women.

Interestingly, the gender ratios have been significantly different for university trainers of school psychologists compared with the general population of school psychologists. Although women are increasingly represented in faculty positions, women do not outnumber men in these positions at the same rate as they do in practitioner positions. In the early 1970s fewer than 20% of school psychology faculty positions were filled by women (Reschly, 2000). That percentage has changed over time so that currently trainers are more likely to be female – although still not at the percentages of women in practitioner positions. Curtis, Lopez, et al. (2008) report that based on 2004–2005 data, 60% of trainers are female (up from 51% in 1999–2000). Although it is not clear why the gender ratios have been so different for trainers versus students and practitioners, Reschly indicates that historically fewer women have applied for academic positions than have men, with only about 40% of the applicants for faculty positions being female. However, this appears to be changing. In Demaray, Carlson, and Hodgson's (2003) survey of programs with assistant professor openings and faculty members who filled these positions, of the 39 new hires who responded to the survey, 28 (72%) were female. As with the general trend for women in psychology, we expect that trainer positions will be increasingly filled with women.

Age

The median age of school psychologists has been steadily increasing over the past two decades. The median age of practitioners increased from the mid- to late 30s in the late 1980s to the mid- to late 40s in the late 1990s (Reschly, 2000). The mean age of all school psychologists who responded to the 2004–2005 NASP membership survey (Curtis, Lopez, et al., 2008) was 46.2, with practitioners being slightly younger (mean = 45.2). The percentage of school psychologists 50 and older has also been increasing over time (from 1989–1990 to 1999–2000 to 2004–2005; Curtis, Lopez, et al., 2008; Curtis, Hunley, & Grier, 2004), with more than 40% of all school psychologists 50 years or older. Curtis, Hunley, and Grier (2004) presented additional data demonstrating that the average number of years of experience of school psychologists has also increased from 1989–1990 to 1999–2000. In 1989–1990, only 23% of school psychologists had been practicing for more than 15 years. However, in 1999–2000, that percentage increased to 40%. The mean number of years of experience reported by those who responded to the most recent NASP membership survey (Curtis, Lopez, et al., 2008) was 14.8. As Curtis, Hunley, and Grier (2004) noted, and as discussed later in this chapter, this increase in median age has resulted in a shortage of school psychologists as older school psychologists retire and an insufficient number of younger school psychologists are available to step in and take their place.

Ethnicity

Practitioners in school psychology tend to be overwhelmingly European American. According to the 2004–2005 NASP membership data (Curtis, Lopez, et al., 2008), approximately 92.6% of school psychologists are European American. This figure is consistent with findings from surveys of school psychologists indicating that, although the number of Latino/a school psychologists is increasing slightly (from 1.5 to 3.1% in a decade; Curtis, Hunley, & Grier, 2004), individuals from ethnic minority backgrounds are still substantially underrepresented in the field of school psychology.

Educational Level

Despite predictions that the field of school psychology would become increasingly populated with individuals with doctoral degrees, the specialist-level degree (EdS or a 60-credit master's degree or the equivalent) is still by far the most common highest degree that school psychologists report obtaining. According to the 2004–2005 NASP membership survey, 32.4% of school psychologists have doctoral degrees. As Reschly (2000) points out, this percentage is unlikely to change significantly any time soon given that the majority of school psychology training programs do not grant doctoral degrees. Of graduate training programs in school psychology, only about 40% have programs at the doctoral level (Miller, 2008). Miller (2008) also reports that about 30% of school psychology graduate students in 2006 were enrolled in doctoral programs. However, the graduation data for the 2005–2006 school year indicate that only about 18% of all school psychology graduates received doctoral degrees. Thus, it seems likely that those prepared at the specialist level will continue to dominate the field of school psychology.

Job Supply and Demand

As mentioned earlier, a shortage of school psychologists—of both practitioners and university faculty—has existed for a number of years. Such a shortage also existed in the late 1980s; it seemed to briefly remit but began increasing again in the mid-1990s. It showed no signs of remission through the late 1990s and early 2000s (Curtis, Grier, & Hunley, 2003; Curtis, Hunley, & Grier, 2004). Curtis and colleagues (2003; Curtis, Hunley, & Grier, 2004) evaluated a variety of data and estimated, based on these data, that the shortage of school psychologists would peak in about 2010. They also indicated that the shortage would be particularly acute for doctoral-level school psychologists and predicted a large number of unfilled positions in university training programs.

Although the negative economic climate since the global recession that started in 2007 has certainly had an impact on positions in K–12 schools as well as university settings, the job outlook for school psychologists still appears to be quite positive. Concrete data are hard to obtain given the recent economic difficulties; however, *U.S. News & World Report* listed school psychology as one of the best careers for 2011 (*money.usnews. com/money/careers/articles/2010/12/06/best-careers-2011-school-psychologist.html*). This article notes that the number of jobs held by school, clinical, and counseling psychologists is likely to increase over time and that "growth is expected to be particularly strong in schools ... thanks to increased efforts to provide mental health services to students."

In the discussion of job prospects for psychologists in general, the U.S. Department of Labor notes in its 2010–2011 *Occupational Outlook Handbook* that "employment of psychologists is expected to grow as fast as average. Job prospects should be best for people who have a doctoral degree from a leading university in an applied specialty, such as counseling or health, and those with a specialist or doctoral degree in school psychology." The report goes on to note that employment for all psychologists is expected to grow 12% from 2008 to 2018. Estimates specific to school psychologists were not reported; however, it was noted that "increased demand for psychological services in schools" was one reason for this expected growth, and for clinical, counseling, and school psychologists in the "educational services" industry jobs were projected to increase by 10.4% from 2008 to 2018.

Not only is there a good outlook for practitioner jobs, but the outlook remains very positive for those school psychologists seeking jobs in academic settings as school psychology trainers. In the late 1990s to early 2000s, jobs in university programs were frequently going unfilled, with surveys indicating that one-quarter or more of school psychology training programs nationwide had openings for faculty members (Demaray et al., 2003; Little & Akin-Little, 2004). Of course, some of these openings are created by individuals switching jobs but staying within the academic sector. As Little and Akin-Little (2004) point out, just because there are a large number of job openings does not necessarily mean there is a shortage of trainers. However, both anecdotal and formal survey data make it clear that not all of the advertised open positions were filled. Of the training directors who responded to Demaray et al.'s (2003) survey regarding assistant professor positions in 1998, 45 of the 60 job openings (75%) were reported to have been filled. In a survey of program directors (Clopton & Haselhuhn, 2009) looking at faculty openings in school psychology over 3 academic years (2004–2005, 2005–2006, and 2006–2007), 79% of program directors reported at least one opening in their program during those years. The mean number of openings across the 3 years was 1.84. The majority of these positions (88%) were reported to be filled, but the number of unfilled positions increased each year from eight in 2004–2005 to 11 in 2005–2006 to at least 13 in 2006–2007. Of course, the responses to these surveys do not represent all programs (91 program directors responded to the job opening portion of Clopton & Haselhuhn's survey; 126 responded to Demaray et al.'s survey). However, based on the consistency of these findings as well as discussions among school psychology program directors, it seems safe to conclude that there are still many faculty positions in school psychology that are going unfilled.

The reasons for the shortage of trainers seem to involve several factors. Because of the rapid growth of the field in the 1970s and early 1980s, many of the faculty who have been with their programs since their inception are of retirement age. Thus, a number of individuals are leaving the field. However, this is only part of the problem. In both Demaray et al.'s (2003) survey and Clopton and Haselhuhn's survey (2009), about one-third of the open positions were reportedly new positions. These positions may have been created as part of the increasing efforts of training programs to obtain NASP approval and/or APA accreditation (Little & Akin-Little, 2004). Another difficulty is that not all doctoral-level training programs focus on preparing students for possible academic careers. Of the 99 doctoral training programs identified by Little and Akin-Little (2004), 82 had at least one graduate in an academic position. However, since 1990 only 19 programs had more than one graduate in an academic position. Clearly, programs must do a better job of preparing and encouraging students to enter the academic world if the shortage of trainers is to remit. One difficulty that Little and Akin-Little (2004) hypothesize may influence the lack of interest in faculty positions is the perception that an academic job is much more difficult and demanding than a school-based job. Particularly when pay levels may not be all that different (and may, in fact, be higher for school-based professionals who have earned doctoral degrees), graduates of doctoral programs simply may not be interested in entering the academic world. Little and Akin-Little (2004) suggest that both adequate financial support in graduate school and increased mentoring may help create a more favorable outlook on academic jobs for potential future trainers.

The shortage of practitioners is likely tied, in part, to the shortage of university trainers. Without fully staffed programs, it becomes difficult for programs to maintain their student numbers, and increasing their numbers becomes even more difficult. Given the many impending retirements among practitioners, programs need to increase their numbers of graduates if there is to be any hope of filling the vacant positions created by these retirements. Curtis et al. (2003) estimated that more than half of the individuals employed as school psychologists were expected to retire within the next 12 years and that those with doctoral degrees were expected to retire at a rate disproportionate to those with specialist-level degrees. In fact, they estimated that by 2020 75% of doctoral-level school psychologists employed in 1999–2000 will be retired compared with 52% of those with specialist degrees and 67% with master's degrees. Curtis et al. (2003) reported that, largely as a result of these retirements, there would likely to be a shortage of close to 9,000 school psychologists from 2000 to 2010. This projection then drops off to approximately 3,000 for the next decade. Although this shortage is likely to be a nationwide phenomenon, data suggest that different regions of the country will not be equally affected by the shortage. Historically, the mid-Atlantic and New England regions have had more consistency in the supply and demand for school psychologists, whereas the West South Central region (Arkansas, Louisiana, Oklahoma, and Texas) has reported more shortages (Lund, Reschly, & Martin, 1998).

The shortage of school psychologists has not gone unnoticed by NASP or by Division 16 of APA. NASP has collected some anecdotal data on the shortage and has also begun efforts to address it. Examples of activities in which NASP has begun to attempt to increase the pool of school psychologists include coordinating with trainers and universities to expand school psychology programs, strengthening the NCSP credential, communicating with Division 16 of APA to develop ideas to protect school psychology, and working for loan forgiveness programs through the federal government (Charvat, 2003). In addition, Division 16 of APA and NASP (as well as other school psychology organizations) held a Future of School Psychology Conference in November 2002. One of the key areas of discussion at the conference was the shortage of school psychologists and how this shortage will affect service delivery to children, their families, and schools.

Two options for addressing the shortage of school psychologists are to retrain psychologists who were not initially trained as school psychologists and to allow licensed clinical and counseling psychologists to practice in the schools without obtaining their school credentials. These options are increasingly being seen as viable ones because of the continuing shortage of school psychologists as well as what seems to be an oversupply of clinical psychologists. However, there is significant debate regarding how these options could be carried out. One possibility would be to require clinical or counseling psychologists who wish to work in the schools to return to school for specific training in school-based issues. This retraining would include coursework related to the climate of the school and education-specific issues (e.g., special education law, curriculum). The second possibility would be to allow licensed clinical or counseling psychologists to practice in the schools without becoming certified as school psychologists. They would be able to provide mental health services to children under their state psychologist licensure. At one time, Division 16 of APA and NASP were working to develop a joint position statement regarding some of these issues (Tharinger & Palomares, 2004). However, to the best of our knowledge, nothing has moved forward with this. It remains to be seen what will happen with the school psychology shortage. It is likely that additional options for hiring school psychologists, as well as perhaps a change in the duties of school psychologists, will need to occur to deal with this ongoing problem. However, in the meantime, this shortage may be good news for students wondering about job possibilities. Given that shortages are expected to hit almost every region in the United States, students will likely be able to find jobs without significant difficulty and may be able to be selective, choosing a job in which the role of the school psychologist matches their desired role.

DISCUSSION QUESTIONS AND ACTIVITIES

1. Search for school psychology jobs using the NASP Career Center (*jobs.naspcareercenter. org*) and state school psychology association websites. Locate jobs in your current state as well as in states where you may wish to work in the future. How many jobs are listed? What are the differences in jobs in terms of salaries, requirements, stated duties, and so forth?

2. Talk with school psychologists who have been working in the field for some time. Have their roles changed over time? What percentage of their time is spent in traditional, standardized assessment activities?

3. School psychology as a profession is dominated by European American individuals. How might this affect the provision of services to children in our public schools?

4. There has been a shortage of school psychologists for some time now. What is the job market like for school psychologists in your area? If possible, talk with school district personnel to find out whether local districts have experienced budget cuts and how this has impacted school psychologists in districts in your area.

CHAPTER 6

Legal and Ethical Issues in School Psychology

Numerous legal and ethical statutes guide the practice of school psychology. Within the legal realm of the United States, for example, federal legislation affects the provision of school psychology services at a national level. In addition, state legislation and case law based on rulings from civil lawsuits (which may eventually be codified into state law) can affect the provision of services at the state level. Even services mandated by federal legislation can be delivered somewhat differently in different states because states have some flexibility in how they implement federally mandated services. For example, states can require that reevaluations for students in special education be conducted every 2 years, even though the federal guidelines indicate that they can be done every 3 years. However, states cannot be less restrictive than the federal law (so states could not require reevaluations to be completed every 4 years). Because of this flexibility, as well as the numerous laws that are made at the state level regarding the provision of educational and psychological services, there will always be some practice differences among states. Therefore, it is imperative that school psychologists become familiar with laws in the state (or province) in which they are employed. In particular, they should become familiar with their state's interpretation of federal special education legislation as well as their state's statutes on the practice of psychology. At a federal level, school psychologists should be familiar with the laws that govern the provision of special education and other services within the schools as well as those that cover general educational issues.

In addition to legal mandates, school psychologists must be familiar with ethical codes that apply to the practice of school psychology and of psychology in general. Ethical codes outline expected conduct in professional activities. Although ethical codes are not enforceable by law, ethical violations may result in dismissal from professional organizations or revocation of professional licensure and may be the basis for civil malpractice lawsuits.

This chapter provides an overview of the federal U.S. legislation as well as the ethical codes with which school psychologists practicing within the United States should be familiar. We have chosen to focus on U.S. legislation to illustrate how school psychology practice is influenced by ethical codes and legislation. Although it is beyond the scope of this book to cover laws and their structures in other countries, we encourage international readers to consider how legislation influences the practice of school psychology within their home country and/or province and also how governing laws might be similar or different from the U.S. laws described in this chapter. School psychologists practicing outside of the United States should take care to review the laws applicable in their countries. All school psychologists should recognize that laws frequently change and ethical codes are updated. Because of this, it is important that school psychologists engage in continuing education activities to ensure that they are familiar with the most recent laws and ethical guidelines and that they are practicing in a legal, ethically responsible manner.

Individuals with Disabilities Education Improvement Act–2004

The Individuals with Disabilities Education Improvement Act (IDEIA)–2004 is the federal special education legislation that mandates the provision of free and appropriate public education services to students with disabilities. This law was originally passed as Public Law 94-142 in 1975 and titled the Education for All Handicapped Children Act. Since that time the law has gone through several major reauthorizations, including one in 1990 in which the name of the law was changed to the Individuals with Disabilities Education Act. In the following section, we provide background information on the development of IDEIA and its current provisions. Table 6.1 provides a summary of the federal legislation discussed here. For those looking for a more comprehensive overview of some of these issues, Jacob and Hartshorne's (2007) *Ethics and Law for School Psychologists* is an excellent source.

Background on Special Education Law

Under the U.S. Constitution, education is not a fundamental right of the citizens of the United States. However, the 10th Amendment to the Constitution provides that "powers not delegated to the United States by the Constitution, nor prohibited by it to the States, are reserved to the States." Thus, the duty of education has been left to individual states, which provide education as an entitlement: All children have a right to an education provided by the state within which they reside. States must provide this education in a manner that is consistent with the principles outlined in the U.S. Constitution. In particular, the 14th Amendment to the U.S. Constitution provides for both *equal protection* (states cannot deny a person equal protection under state law) and *due process* (states cannot "deprive a person of life, liberty, or property, without due process of law") to all citizens. States may not enact laws that infringe on the rights of citizens, including their right to an education, which is considered a property right. Furthermore, if a state does intend to take away any rights, there must be a procedure in place to guarantee that the rights of the person are not being violated (due process). However, historically (prior to the passage of Public Law 94-142), many students with disabilities were excluded from public schools without any consideration of their rights. Children who were considered to be unable to benefit from a public education (including those with significant disabilities) were prevented from enrolling in school. Many of these children remained at home with their parents, others were institutionalized, and a small portion received education in a private school setting (Jacob & Hartshorne, 2007).

TABLE 6.1. Timeline of Major Special Education and Related Legislation

1965   Public Law 89-10   Elementary and Secondary Education Act (ESEA)

Under Title I of this Act, school districts were provided with federal financial assistance primarily intended to assist in the education of children who were economically disadvantaged. Four other Titles provided funding for other aspects of education, but children with handicaps were not specifically mentioned.

1965   Public Law 89-313   Elementary and Secondary Education Act Amendments of 1965

Established grant programs for state-run schools and institutions for children with disabilities.

1966   Public Law 89-750   Elementary and Secondary Education Act Amendments of 1966

Amended Public Law 89-10 to include a Title VI to assist states in developing programs for students with disabilities.

1970   Public Law 91-230   Education of the Handicapped Act (EHA)

Replaced Title VI of ESEA. Provided grant programs for states to provide services to children with disabilities.

1973   Public Law 93-112   Rehabilitation Act of 1973

Included Section 504, which prevents discrimination by public agencies based on a disability. Mandates that schools provide free, appropriate education to students with disabilities. No funding attached to this mandate.

1974   Public Law 93-380   The Education Amendments of 1974

Reauthorized ESEA and EHA. Increased financial assistance to states to provide services to children with disabilities. Federal aid for programs for students with disabilities was dependent on states enacting plans to educate students with disabilities.

1974   Public Law 93-380   Federal Educational Rights and Privacy Act (FERPA)

Protects the privacy of children's educational records. (Part of Education Amendments of 1974.)

1975   Public Law 94-142   The Education for All Handicapped Children Act

The landmark federal legislation that guaranteed children with disabilities the right to a free, appropriate public education.

1986   Public Law 99-457   The Education of the Handicapped Act Amendments of 1986

Mandated special education services for children ages 3–5 with disabilities and provided financial incentives for states to provide services to children with disabilities ages birth–3.

1990   Public Law 101-476   Individuals with Disabilities Education Act (IDEA)

Amendment and reauthorization of EHA. Name changed to IDEA. Mandated transition services. Added autism and traumatic brain injury as disability conditions.

1990   Public Law 101-336   Americans with Disabilities Act (ADA)

Prohibited discrimination against individuals with disabilities by public and private organizations.

1997   Public Law 105-17   Individuals with Disabilities Education Act

Amendment and reauthorization of Public Law 101-476 (IDEA). Strengthened rights of parents.

2001   Public Law 107-110   No Child Left Behind Act

Reauthorization of ESEA. Increased school accountability.

2004   Public Law 108-446   Individuals with Disabilities Education Improvement Act

Amendment and reauthorization of IDEA.

2010   S. 2781   Rosa's Law

Amended a variety of educational laws (including IDEIA) to strike "mental retardation" and replace with "intellectual disabilities."

In 1954 the U.S. Supreme Court ruled in the landmark case of *Brown v. Board of Education* that separate educational facilities for racial minority children were "inherently unequal." The court ruled that state laws that required or permitted segregation of students in schools based on race were unconstitutional because they violated the equal protection clause of the 14th Amendment. Based on this ruling, states were required not to limit access to particular schools based on race. Although this case did not mention students with disabilities, following the *Brown* ruling, parents of children with disabilities filed lawsuits using the same argument: that the denial of a public education to children with disabilities was a violation of their constitutional rights based on the equal protection clause of the 14th Amendment.

Two important court cases—*Pennsylvania Association for Retarded Children (PARC) v. Commonwealth of Pennsylvania* (1971, 1972) and *Mills v. Board of Education of the District of Columbia* (1972)—were key in the eventual granting of educational rights to all students regardless of their disability status. We briefly review these cases here.

In the *PARC* case, attorneys for the parents of 13 children with intellectual disabilities (termed "mental retardation" at the time) who had been excluded from the public schools argued that the exclusion of these children violated their constitutional rights under the 14th Amendment. In a consent decree (i.e., the involved parties consented to a court-approved agreement), the Commonwealth of Pennsylvania agreed to provide "access to a free public program of education and training appropriate to his learning capacities" to every child between the ages of 6 and 21 with intellectual disabilities. The state also agreed that school districts would provide services to children younger than age 6 if the district already provided preschool services to children without intellectual disabilities. The consent decree also stated that a placement in the regular public classroom for children with intellectual disabilities was preferable to a placement in any other setting (including a special classroom setting within the school). This decree further mandated that educational placements of and programs for children with intellectual disabilities be reevaluated every 2 years.

The *Mills* case was filed by attorneys on behalf of seven students with varying disabilities (including intellectual disabilities, behavior problems, and brain injuries). In the consent decree for this case, the court once again agreed that not providing these children with an appropriate education violated their constitutional rights. However, the District of Columbia failed to comply with the directives set forth in the consent decree, in part because it argued that the financial costs were prohibitive, and the case ended up back in court. In the *Mills* ruling, the District of Columbia was ordered to provide "each child of school age a free and suitable publicly supported education regardless of the degree of the child's mental, physical, or emotional disability or impairment. Furthermore, defendants shall not exclude any child resident in the District of Columbia from such publicly supported education on the basis of a claim of insufficient resources." The right of school districts to expel or suspend students with disabilities was also limited by the *Mills* case.

Following these rulings, as well a number of other, similar rulings, the momentum for a national special education law increased. Even prior to the *PARC* and *Mills* cases, there had been some federal legislation that assisted states in providing services to children with disabilities. In 1965, the Elementary and Secondary Education Act (ESEA; Public Law 89-10) was signed into law. Title I of this legislation was intended to provide school districts with federal financial assistance to help meet the needs of students who were disadvantaged primarily as a result of economic circumstances. Four other titles provided funding for other aspects of education, but children with disabilities were not specifically mentioned. Later in 1965, this law was amended to include money for grant programs for state-run schools and institutions for children with disabilities. This law was amended again in 1966 and included a Title VI, which authorized funds to assist states in developing programs for students with disabilities. In 1970 a new law (Public Law 91-230; the Education of the Handicapped Act [EHA]) replaced Title VI of the ESEA and provided grant programs for states to provide services to children with disabilities. In 1974 amendments to ESEA and EHA were passed (Public Law 93-380) that increased financial assistance to states to provide services to children with disabilities. This law also included language that informed school districts that federal aid for programs for students with disabilities would be dependent on states developing plans for adequate services for children with disabilities. Finally, in 1975, the landmark Education of All Handicapped Children Act (EHA; Public Law 94-142) was passed. This law required that all students have access to a free and appropriate public education (FAPE) that is provided in the least restrictive environment (LRE).

Under Public Law 94-142, schools were required to provide services only for children of school age. In 1986, Public Law 99-457 (the EHA amendments) was passed. This law mandated special education services for children ages 3 to 5 and provided financial incentives to states to provide services for children from birth to age 3. In 1990, EHA was amended and its name changed to the Individuals with Disabilities Education Act (IDEA; Public Law 101-476). In 1997 IDEA was amended and reauthorized (Public Law 105-17). This version of the special education law is often referred to as IDEA-97. The most recent reauthorization of the law occurred in 2004 with the passage of the IDEIA (Public Law 108-446). The final rules and regulations for Part B of this law (which applies to students ages 3–21) were issued by the U.S. Department of Education in August 2006. However, as of fall 2010, the final rules of regulations for Part C (the portion of the law covering services to infants and toddlers from birth to age 3) had still not been issued. We next present a brief discussion of IDEIA-2004. Readers are also encouraged to look at the federal rules and regulations as well as their state regulations.

IDEIA-2004: Part B

There are four parts to IDEIA-2004: Part A, General Provisions; Part B, Assistance for Education of All Children with Disabilities; Part C, Infants and Toddlers with Disabilities; and Part D, National Activities to Improve Education of Children with Disabilities. Parts B and C are key in terms of service provision to children with disabilities. Part B is discussed in more detail in this section, and Part C services are discussed in a later section.

IDEIA requires that each state have a policy to ensure that all children with disabilities between the ages of 3 and 21 have a right to a FAPE. The law specifies that services provided to children with disabilities must meet all of their special education needs as well as related service needs, and that the services provided must be based on the unique needs of each child (34 C.F.R. § 300.1). Students with disabilities who have been suspended or expelled from school also have a right to a FAPE. Although all children have a right to a FAPE, students who are placed by thei parents in private schools do not have "an individual right" to receive special education services (34 C.F.R. § 300.137). In these instances, the local educational agency (LEA), in collaboration with the private school, decides who is provided with what services. Children placed in a private school by their LEA (as opposed to parental placement) retain all of their rights under IDEA (34 C.F.R. § 300.146).

According to IDEA, a child with a disability is one who has been evaluated and determined to have one of 13 specific handicapping conditions, listed in Table 6.2 along with brief definitions of each. In addition to these specific disabilities, children between the ages of 3 and 9 can also be identified as having a developmental delay. To be so classified, a child must exhibit delays in one or more of the following areas: physical development, cognitive development, communication development, social or emotional development, and adaptive development (34 C.F.R. § 300.8).

One of the changes from IDEA-97 to IDEIA-2004 that has received significant attention and has had a direct impact on the practice of school psychology is the language regarding evaluation of LDs. According to IDEIA-2004, states "must not require the use of a severe discrepancy for determining whether a child has a specific learning disability" and "must permit the use of a process based on the child's response to scientific, research-based intervention" (34 C.F.R. § 300.309). This language is a significant change from previous versions of special education law, which specified that a severe discrepancy between a child's intellectual abilities and academic achievement had to be present to give an LD classification.

Not only are states required to provide services to all children with disabilities, but they must also proactively seek to find children who could benefit from special education services. The Child Find provision of IDEIA (34 C.F.R. § 300.111) requires that states have a plan to ensure that all students with disabilities are "identified, located, and evaluated" to determine whether they are in need of special education services. When children who may benefit from special education services are identified, states are required to complete a "full and individual evaluation," the purpose of which is to determine whether the child qualifies for services and, if so, what educational needs the student has (34 C.F.R. § 300.301). Students must be reevaluated at least every 3 years unless the parents and the school agree that a reevaluation is not necessary (although this reevaluation does not necessarily need to involve complete retesting of the child; 34 C.F.R. § 300.303, 300.305). Evaluation procedures must be technically sound and nondiscriminatory and must be provided in the child's native language (or other mode of communication). The evaluation should be thorough enough to identify all of the student's special education and related needs (34 C.F.R. § 300.304).

The results of the evaluation are used to develop a written individualized education program (IEP) for each child with a disability. The IEP must be reviewed at least once a year by an IEP team that includes: the child's parents; at least one regular education teacher of the child; at least one special education teacher of the child; a representative of the public agency (e.g., school principal); an individual who can interpret the instructional implications of the evaluation results; other individuals deemed appropriate by the parents or school personnel; and the child, if appropriate (34 C.F.R. § 300.321). Parent participation in the IEP process is emphasized (34 C.F.R. § 300.322). Parents must be notified of an IEP meeting sufficiently ahead of time so that they are able to attend, and the meeting must be scheduled at a time that is convenient for them. Schools may conduct IEP meetings without parents only if they have made multiple, documented attempts to try to secure the attendance of the parents. IDEIA-2004 did make some minor modifications regarding IEP meetings and IEP reviews. Some members of the IEP team can now be excused from attending meetings if no modifications are being made to their area or if they provided input prior to the meeting. However, parents must agree to this (34 C.F.R. § 300.321). In addition, changes to the IEP (after the annual IEP) can be made without holding a meeting if the school and the parents agree (34 C.F.R. § 300.324).

TABLE 6.2. Definitions of Disabilities from IDEIA-2004 (34 C.F.R. § 300.8)

Autism

A developmental disability significantly affecting verbal and nonverbal communication and social interaction, generally evident before age 3, that adversely affects a child's educational performance. Other characteristics often associated with autism are engagement in repetitive activities and stereotyped movements, resistance to environmental change or change in daily routines, and unusual responses to sensory experiences.

Deaf-blindness

Concomitant hearing and visual impairments, the combination of which causes such severe communication and other developmental and educational needs that they cannot be accommodated in special education programs solely for children with deafness or children with blindness.

Deafness

A hearing impairment that is so severe that the child is impaired in processing linguistic information through hearing, with or without amplification, that adversely affects a child's educational performance.

Emotional disturbance

(i) A condition exhibiting one or more of the following characteristics over a long period of time and to a marked degree that adversely affects a child's educational performance:

(A) An inability to learn that cannot be explained by intellectual, sensory, or health factors.

(B) An inability to build or maintain satisfactory interpersonal relationships with peers and teachers.

(C) Inappropriate types of behavior or feelings under normal circumstances.

(D) A general pervasive mood of unhappiness or depression.

(E) A tendency to develop physical symptoms or fears associated with personal or school problems.

(ii) The term includes schizophrenia. The term does not apply to children who are socially maladjusted, unless it is determined that they have an emotional disturbance.

Hearing impairment

An impairment in hearing, whether permanent or fluctuating, that adversely affects a child's educational performance.

Intellectual disability (previously Mental retardation)

Significantly subaverage general intellectual functioning, existing concurrently with deficits in adaptive behavior and manifested during the developmental period, that adversely affects a child's educational performance.

Multiple disabilities

Concomitant impairments (such as intellectual disability-blindness, intellectual disability-orthopedic impairment), the combination of which causes such severe educational needs that they cannot be accommodated in special education programs solely for one of the impairments.

Orthopedic impairment

A severe orthopedic impairment that adversely affects a child's educational performance. The term includes impairments caused by congenital anomaly, impairments caused by disease (e.g., poliomyelitis, bone tuberculosis, etc.), and impairments from other causes (e.g., cerebral palsy, amputations, and fractures or burns that cause contractures).

(cont.)

TABLE 6.2. *(cont.)*

Other health impairment

Limited strength, vitality, or alertness, including a heightened alertness to environmental stimuli, that results in limited alertness with respect to the educational environment, that—

(i) Is due to chronic or acute health problems such as asthma, attention deficit disorder or attention deficit hyperactivity disorder, diabetes, epilepsy, a heart condition, hemophilia, lead poisoning, leukemia, nephritis, rheumatic fever, and sickle cell anemia and Tourette syndrome; and

(ii) Adversely affects a child's educational performance.

Specific learning disability

(i) **General**. The term means a disorder in one or more of the basic psychological processes involved in understanding or in using language, spoken or written, that may manifest itself in an imperfect ability to listen, think, speak, read, write, spell, or do mathematical calculations, including conditions such as perceptual disabilities, brain injury, minimal brain dysfunction, dyslexia, and developmental aphasia.

(ii) **Disorders not included**. The term does not include learning problems that are primarily the result of visual, hearing, or motor disabilities, of intellectual disability, of emotional disturbance, or of environmental, cultural, or economic disadvantage.

Speech or language impairment

A communication disorder, such as stuttering, impaired articulation, a language impairment, or a voice impairment, that adversely affects a child's educational performance.

Traumatic brain injury

An acquired injury to the brain caused by an external physical force, resulting in total or partial functional disability or psychosocial impairment, or both, that adversely affects a child's educational performance. Traumatic brain injury applies to open or closed head injuries resulting in impairments in one or more areas, such as cognition; language; memory; attention; reasoning; abstract thinking; judgment; problem solving; sensory, perceptual, and motor abilities; psychosocial behavior; physical functions; information processing; and speech. Traumatic brain injury does not apply to brain injuries that are congenital or degenerative, or to brain injuries induced by birth trauma.

Visual impairment including blindness

An impairment in vision that, even with correction, adversely affects a child's educational performance. The term includes both partial sight and blindness.

The IEP must include the following information (34 C.F.R. § 300.320):

- A statement of the child's current educational and functional performance and how the disability affects the child's involvement in the general education curriculum.
- A statement of measurable annual goals.
- Information on how a child's progress toward these goals will be measured.
- A statement of special education and related services and supplementary aids to be provided to the child as well as a statement of program modifications or supports for school personnel to be provided to the child. These services and supports should allow the child to advance toward annual goals, be involved and progress in the general curriculum as appropriate, and be educated with other children with and without disabilities.
- A explanation of the extent to which the child with a disability will *not* participate in educational activities with children without disabilities.

- A statement of any modifications in state or districtwide testing that are needed for the child to participate in these assessments and, if the IEP team determines that the child will not participate in an assessment, an explanation of why the assessment is not appropriate and how the child will be assessed.
- Dates services are to be provided as well as their frequency, location, and duration.
- When the child reaches age 16, a statement of postsecondary goals and transition services needed to meet these goals.

As indicated, the IEP must include information regarding involvement with children without disabilities. A key part of IDEIA, dating back to the original legislation, is the provision of services within the LRE. As stated in IDEIA, "To the maximum extent appropriate, children with disabilities, including children in public or private institutions or other care facilities, are educated with children who are nondisabled" (34 C.F.R. § 300.114). The law goes on to state that children can be removed from the regular education environment "only if the nature or severity of the disability is such that education in regular classes with the use of supplementary aids and services cannot be achieved satisfactorily" (34 C.F.R. § 300.114). Schools must provide a continuum of placements for students with disabilities so that the individual needs of each student can be met. This continuum includes regular classes at one end of the spectrum and special schools, institutions, or home instruction at the other end (34 C.F.R. § 300.115). The placements of children with disabilities should be as close as possible to their homes, and children should not be "removed from their age-appropriate classrooms solely because of needed modifications in the general education curriculum" (34 C.F.R. § 300.116).

IDEIA-2004 does place greater emphasis on pre-referral interventions than did previous versions of special education law by allowing local education agencies to spend up to 15% of their IDEIA funds to assist students who are not yet identified with disabilities but who need additional academic and behavioral supports to be successful in the general education setting. Although these services can be provided to children in all grades, the focus is intended to be on children in grades K–3.

To ensure that each child is receiving a FAPE and that the rights of the child, as well as his or her family, are not violated, IDEIA also outlines *procedural safeguards*. These safeguards highlight the importance of involving parents in the special education process. Parents have a right to be present at all meetings in which educational placement decisions regarding their child are made and to review their child's educational records (34 C.F.R. § 300.501). Parents also have a right to seek an independent evaluation of their child if they desire. If a parent requests such an evaluation, the school district may choose to hold a hearing to show that its evaluation was appropriate, or the district can simply agree to pay for the requested independent evaluation. If a hearing is held and the evaluation completed by the school district is determined to be appropriate, the parents can still seek an independent evaluation but at their own expense (34 C.F.R. § 300.502). Before school district personnel can conduct an assessment, parents must provide consent for the evaluation to occur (34 C.F.R. § 300.503), and the parents must be given a copy of the procedural safeguards, which explains their rights in understandable language (34 C.F.R. § 300.504). In addition to requiring parental consent for testing, IDEIA also requires consent for placement in special education programs (34 C.F.R. § 300.503). If a child's parents and the school district disagree on testing and/or placement issues, mediation can help resolve those differences. School districts must have a mediation process in place (34 C.F.R. § 300.506). However, if mediation does not resolve the differences, a due process hearing may occur. A due process hearing is conducted by an impartial hearing officer. If one party is dissatisfied with the outcome of the due process hearing, the next course of action is to file a civil lawsuit. If parents prevail in a lawsuit, they can be awarded attorney's fees (34 C.F.R. § 300.507–300.517).

Discipline procedures (34 C.F.R. § 300.530–300.537) are also an important topic addressed under procedural safeguards. School districts are allowed to suspend children with disabilities, as they would children without disabilities, for no more than 10 consecutive school days. A school district may also place a child in an interim alternative education setting for up to 45 school days if the child carries a weapon to school; possesses, uses, or sells illegal drugs while at school or at a school function; or has caused "serious bodily injury" to another person at school or a school function. If a child is removed for more than 10 consecutive school days, the removal is considered to be a change in placement. A child who has been removed for a total of more than 10 school days across the academic year would also be considered to have had change in placement (34 C.F.R. § 300.536). When a change in placement occurs, an IEP meeting must be convened and the IEP reviewed. If no functional behavioral assessment had been completed prior to this time, and if there is no written behavioral intervention plan for the student, these must be completed. In addition, if the disciplinary action being considered is a result of a weapons or school code violation resulting in a recommended suspension of more than 10 school days, then a manifest determination review must be held. The child's behavior is considered to be a manifestation of the child's disability if the behavior is determined to be caused by or had a direct and substantial relationship to the child's disability or if the behavior was the result of a failure to implement the IEP. If the review finds that the behavior was *not* a manifestation of the student's disability, then the student can be subjected to the same disciplinary procedures as students without disabilities. However, the student must still be provided with a FAPE. In such case, a student could be suspended but would still need to be provided with educational services to allow the child to progress toward achieving his or her educational goals. If the behavior is determined to be a manifestation of the child's disability, the IEP team must conduct a functional assessment and implement a behavioral intervention plan (if it has not already done so) or review an existing plan and modify it to address the behavior of concern. In addition, the child should be returned to his or her educational placement unless the parents and LEA decide on a change of placement or unless the violation involves weapons, drugs, or serious bodily injury (34 C.F.R. § 300.530).

Since the passage of the initial federal special education law in 1975, numerous court cases have dealt with its implementation. We review some of the key cases in the following sections; however, these cases are too numerous to review in this chapter. Jacob and Hartshorne (2007) as well as Rothstein (2010) and Yell (2005) provide a more comprehensive overview of case law and IDEIA.

LRE and Court Cases

The idea of educating all children in the least restrictive environment (LRE) has been the subject of several court cases. In *Daniel R. R. v. State Board of Education* (1989), the parents of Daniel, a young child with Down syndrome, wanted him to be placed in a regular PreK class. However, after a short time in such a class, the teacher reported concerns regarding Daniel's placement and believed that he was not able to benefit from being in the regular classroom. Daniel's placement was changed; however, his parents believed that his right to an education in the LRE had been violated. The hearing officer, as well as a district court, agreed that the school district had appropriately placed Daniel. In upholding the district court's ruling, the court of appeals proposed two criteria to evaluate the appropriateness of a child's educational placement: (1) whether education in the regular classroom, with the use of supplementary aids and services, can be achieved satisfactorily and (2) if placement outside of a regular classroom is needed, whether the school has mainstreamed the child to the maximum extent possible.

A similar but expanded test of whether a placement is appropriate was created in a series of later cases. In the *Board of Education, Sacramento City Unified School District v. Holland* (1992), the parents of Rachel, a 9-year-old girl with moderate intellectual disabilities, requested her full-time placement in a regular education classroom, whereas the school district believed that half time in a regular classroom and half time in a special education classroom was the best placement. A hearing officer agreed with the parents, but the school district appealed this decision to the district court. The school district lost the case in district court but appealed. In the appeal decision, *Sacramento City School District v. Rachel H.* (1994), the court upheld the district court's decision and outlined a four-part test for whether the district had proposed an appropriate placement for Rachel:

1. The educational benefits to Rachel in a regular classroom, supplemented with appropriate aids and services, compared with the educational benefits of a special education classroom.
2. The nonacademic benefits of interaction with children who did not have disabilities.
3. The effect of Rachel's presence on the teacher and other children in the classroom.
4. The cost of mainstreaming Rachel in a regular classroom.

Similarly, in *Oberti v. Board of Education of the Borough of Clementon School District* (1993), the court proposed that when deciding whether a child with disabilities can be educated in the regular classroom, the following should be considered:

1. Whether the school district has made reasonable efforts to accommodate the child in the regular classroom.
2. The educational benefits available to the child in a regular class, with appropriate supplementary aids and services, compared with the benefits provided in a special education class.
3. The possible negative effects of the inclusion of the child on the education of other students in the class.

In this case, the court ruled that the school district failed to comply with IDEA when they placed Rafael Oberti, a young child with Down syndrome, in a segregated special education classroom.

Several court cases have upheld school districts decisions to place children in more restrictive settings (e.g., *DeVries v. Fairfax County School Board*, 1989; *Hartman v. Loudoun County Board of Education*, 1997), citing the fact that special education law encouraged mainstreaming "but only to the extent that it does not prevent a child from receiving educational benefit." Thus, if a school district can document that the less restrictive setting does not allow the child to benefit from his or her education (with supplementary aids and services) the child can be placed in a more restrictive setting.

Based on these court cases, schools can place children in more restrictive settings. However, they must ensure that they have considered the appropriateness, including the benefits and possible negative outcomes, of both more restrictive and less restrictive settings prior to placing a child in the more restrictive setting.

Appropriate Education and Court Cases

Although IDEIA and its predecessors mandated that all children are entitled to a free and appropriate public education, the meaning of "appropriate" is not clearly defined. A number of court cases have attempted to provide clarity on this matter. The *Board of Education of the Hendrick Hudson Central School District v. Rowley* (1982) was the first case in which the U.S. Supreme Court addressed the issue of what constitutes an appropriate education. In this case, Amy Rowley, a Deaf student with excellent lip-reading skills and some residual hearing, was placed in a regular kindergarten class and provided with an FM hearing aid system. At the IEP meeting before her first-grade year, it was decided that Amy would remain in a regular class and continue to use the FM system. In addition, Amy was to receive instruction from a tutor for the Deaf 1 hour a day and services from the speech–language pathologist for 3 hours per week. Amy's parents argued that she also needed an interpreter full time in the classroom. An interpreter had been provided on a trial basis for 2 weeks in her kindergarten class, but the interpreter reported that Amy did not need those services. In a hearing initiated by Amy's parents, the district's decision was upheld. Amy's parents then brought suit in a district-level court. The court ruled that Amy was not being provided with an appropriate education, and this ruling was upheld by a court of appeals. However, the U.S. Supreme Court ruled in favor of the school district and reversed the earlier rulings. In making their decision, the Supreme Court reviewed Public Law 94-142 and held that the IEP should be "reasonably calculated" to allow a child to progress; however, it does not require the state to "maximize the potential" of each student with a disability. Therefore, if the state has complied with special education law procedures and developed an IEP that is "reasonably calculated to enable the child to receive educational benefits," then the school district has met the requirements of the law.

Since the *Rowley* case, there have been a number of other court cases in which parents have argued that their children were not receiving an appropriate public education. Specific outcomes have varied, but in general the courts have ruled that schools must provide services that are likely to result in meaningful educational benefits to the child (e.g., *Polk v. Central Susquehanna Intermediate Unit 16*, 1988). In a recent case (*J.L. and M.L. and their minor daughter K.L. v. Mercer Island School District*, 2006) the Western U.S. District Court found that the Rowley standard "set the bar too low" for children with disabilities. The court argued that the school district had not adequately focused on "progressing K.L. toward self-sufficiency (i.e., independent living) and her desired goal of post-secondary education" and that this was "a failure to confer the benefit contemplated by the IDEA." The court further argued that with IDEA-1997, legislation had moved from granting "access" to educational to being an "outcome-oriented process." However, the Ninth Circuit Court of Appeals reversed the District Court's decision (*J. L., M. L., K. L., their minor daughter, v. Mercer Island School District*, 2009), indicating that the Rowley standards of whether a FAPE was provided continued to apply and that the District Court had "misinterpreted Congress' intent," stating that if the Congress had meant to change the FAPE meaning in IDEA-1997 related to the educational benefit standard, "it would have expressed a clear intent to do so."

Several FAPE cases have dealt with the issue of related services. For example, in *Irving Independent School District v. Tatro* (1984), the U.S. Supreme Court ruled that clean intermittent catheterization was a needed related service for an 8-year-old with spina bifida. The Court ruled that this service was needed to allow the child to stay in school during the day to benefit from her education. In a similar case, a school district was required to provide nursing care as a related service for a student who was wheelchair bound and ventilator dependent so that he could benefit from the educational environment (*Cedar Rapids Community School District v. Garrett F.*, 1999).

As a whole, these cases suggest that school districts should ensure that the services they provide allow children to benefit from their educational services. Services do not have to be the best available, but they do need to be adequate to allow children to access and benefit from their public educational experiences.

In the context of providing a FAPE, increasingly parents of students with disabilities have been seeking reimbursement for services provided in private school settings. In *Florence County School District Four v. Carter* (1993), the U.S. Supreme Court held that parents who had withdrawn their child from public school and placed him in a private school were entitled to compensation for the costs of the private school because the district did not provide a FAPE. In a case focusing on services to a young child with autism (*L. B., and J. B., on behalf of K. B. v. Nebo School District*, 2004), the Court of Appeals concluded that K. B. had not been provided an education in the LRE (and, therefore, also not provided a FAPE) and allowed that parents could be reimbursed for the 40 hours/week of applied behavior analysis services they had elected to provide to K. B.

In a more recent case (*Forest Grove School District v. T.A.*, 2009), the U.S. Supreme Court granted parents' request for private school tuition after they had unilaterally placed their son in a private school and requested an administrative hearing on his eligibility only after the private school placement was made. The district found him ineligible for services but the parents sued saying he had been denied a FAPE. Although the district court initially sided with the school, indicating that parents could not be reimbursed when the child had not previously received special education services, this decision was overturned on appeal and affirmed by the U.S. Supreme Court.

IDEIA-2004: Part C

Part C of IDEIA-2004 contains the regulations applicable to early intervention programs for infants and toddlers from birth through age 3. Unlike Part B of IDEIA, which requires a FAPE for all students, Part C provides grants to states to assist them in developing early intervention services for children up to age 3. However, states are not required to apply for funds to implement these programs (although all states are currently providing Part C services), and states can charge parents for a portion of the services provided under Part C. The final regulations of Part C were released by the U.S. Department of Education in September 2011 (as 34 C.F.R. § 303). Part C services require that states identify a lead agency responsible for the provision of early intervention services (34 C.F.R. § 303.120). This lead agency then submits an application that outlines how early intervention services will be provided. In many states the lead agency is not the state's department of education but another state agency, such as the state's department of health. In addition to an identified lead agency, Part C regulations require that an interagency coordinating council be developed to assist the lead agency in the coordination and provision of services to children and their families (34 C.F.R. § 303.600).

Under Part C, children up to age 3 may be eligible for early intervention services if they have delays in one or more of the following areas: cognitive development, physical development (including vision and hearing), communication development, social and emotional development, and adaptive development. Children who have diagnosed physical or mental conditions that have a high probability of resulting in delays are also eligible for services. In addition, states can choose to provide services to children who are determined to be at risk for delays (34 C.F.R. § 303.21).

Children who receive Part C services are provided with a service coordinator. The coordinator's role is to help parents access and coordinate services for their children (34 C.F.R. § 303.34). Early intervention services are required to be provided in the "natural environments" to the maximum extent that is appropriate (34 C.F.R. § 303.126). A child receiving early intervention services is required to have an individualized family service plan (IFSP). This plan is essentially a downward extension of the IEP but should include more family-focused goals and objectives. IFSP meetings, as with IEP meetings, must include the parents of the child. The IFSP must be reviewed every 6 months (at a minimum), and annual meetings must occur to evaluate the IFSP (34 C.F.R. § 303.340–303.344).

In addition to having a Child Find program (as with Part B of IDEIA), Part C requires that states have a public awareness program that focuses on the purpose of the early intervention program and how referrals can be made to it (34 C.F.R. § 303.300–303.301). After a child has been referred and the parents have consented to an evaluation, the state has 45 days to complete the evaluation and develop an IFSP for the child (34 C.F.R. § 303.310). In the assessment and evaluation process, the inclusion of the family is emphasized. This process includes supports and services necessary to help the family meet the needs of the child (34 C.F.R. § 303.321). Under Part C, states may elect to impose a sliding-scale fee, requiring parents to pay a portion of the costs of the early intervention services (34 C.F.R. § 303.500 and 303.521). Procedural safeguards specified in Part C are much the same as those specified in Part B of IDEIA (see 34 C.F.R. § 303.400–303.449).

One of the new aspects of IDEIA Part C is that states can elect to continue to provide early intervention services to children over the age of 3 (up until the child enters kindergarten). If states elect this option, parents would be provided with notice regarding their options for services once the children turn 3 (34 C.F.R. § 303.211).

Section 504 of the Rehabilitation Act of 1973 and the Americans with Disabilities Act

In addition to IDEIA, the Rehabilitation Act of 1973 promoted the development of services for children with disabilities. The Rehabilitation Act prevents discrimination on the basis of disability in programs that receive federal support. Section 504 of this act specifically states that "no otherwise qualified individual with a disability ... shall, solely by reason of her or his disability, be excluded from the participation in, be denied the benefits of, or be subject to discrimination under any program or activity receiving Federal financial assistance" (29 U.S.C. § 794). Subpart D of Section 504 refers specifically to preschool, elementary, and secondary education. This subpart specifies that all children have a right to a FAPE. Although many students with disabilities will be covered under IDEIA, some students with disabilities may not be eligible for IDEIA services but are still eligible for accommodations under Section 504. Section 504 is broader and less specific than IDEIA. The definition of a "handicapped" person (and, therefore, one qualifying for services under Section 504) is "any person who (1) has a physical or mental impairment which substantially limits one or more major life activities; (2) has a record of such impairment; (3) is regarded as having such impairment." Physical or mental impairment is broadly defined, with no specific definitions of disability conditions as is found in IDEIA. Children with medical conditions such as diabetes, as well as those with mental illnesses, are covered under Section 504.

Unfortunately, when the Rehabilitation Act was passed, it included no provisions for how the law should be implemented or enforced or how remedies should be decided on in cases in which the law was violated. A 1976 lawsuit (*Cherry v. Mathews*) resulted in a court order that the government create guidelines for the implementation of Section 504. In 1977, the first guidelines regarding Section 504 were issued (Jaeger & Bowman, 2002). However, even following the issuance of Section 504 guidelines, schools were somewhat slow to respond to the mandates of this law. There were several reasons for this time lag, including confusion about who qualified for Section 504 services versus special education services. In addition, Section 504 has no funding attached to it as does IDEIA. Although Section 504 lacks funding, school districts are required to comply with this law, and the Office of Civil Rights (OCR) is charged with investigating violations of Section 504 policy. If OCR finds that a school district is not compliant with Section 504, certain federal funds may be removed from the school district. In 1991 a memorandum from the U.S. Department of Education clarified school districts' responsibilities under Section 504 to children diagnosed with attention-deficit/hyperactivity disorder (ADHD) who did not qualify for special education services. (This memo also clarified how students with ADHD could be served under IDEA.) It was after this that schools began to attend more closely to the appropriate development of Section 504 plans (Jacob & Hartshorne, 2007). Interestingly, Jacob and Hartshorne (2007) predicted that with some of the recent changes in special education law the need for Section 504 services may decline. They cited several changes that they believe will allow more children to be served through other avenues, including (1) the specific mention of ADHD in the Other Health Impaired category beginning with IDEA-1997; (2) the allowance in IDEIA-2004 that districts can use up to 15% of their IDEIA money to develop early intervening services; and (3) the removal of the requirement in IDEIA-2004 that children must have a severe discrepancy between their achievement and intellectual abilities to receive services within the LD category. In addition, they cited growing concerns that students may be overidentified as having disabilities under Section 504 and that an increasing awareness of this may contribute to a decline in such services.

Under Section 504, schools must provide reasonable accommodations to students with disabilities. However, schools do not have to provide the best possible education, only one that is reasonably designed to meet the needs of the individual student. In order to comply with Section 504, school districts must appoint a 504 coordinator, who ensures that students with disabilities (as defined under Section 504) are appropriately evaluated and that appropriate accommodations are made for students who have a need. Students receiving services under Section 504 should have written plans (similar to an IEP) that address their individual needs (Jaeger & Bowman, 2002).

The Americans with Disabilities Act (ADA) of 1990 is similar in many ways to Section 504. However, whereas Section 504 applies only to organizations receiving federal assistance, ADA applies to employment and schooling organizations regardless of whether they receive federal financial assistance. The definition of a person with a disability remains the same as the definition cited previously from Section 504. Because elementary and secondary public schools, as entities that receive federal assistance, were already required to comply with Section 504, ADA had minimal impact on services provided in preschool, elementary, and secondary schools (Jaeger & Bowman, 2002).

Other Important Federal Legislation

In addition to federal legislation (and related case law) dealing specifically with disability issues, there are pieces of legislation that deal with school-related issues in general. These acts are important to understand for everyone involved in education, but because they are less relevant to the day-to-day practice of school psychologists, we review them only briefly.

Family Educational Rights and Privacy Act

The Family Educational Rights and Privacy Act of 1974 protects the privacy of students' educational records. Parents have a right to review the school records of their children and request corrections if they believe there are errors in the records. This law also requires that parents provide consent in order for a school district to release a child's educational records to a third party. There are certain exceptions to this last provision. Schools may disclose information to other school personnel who have a "legitimate interest" in knowing the information as well as to a school to which a child may be transferring. Other exceptions include health and safety issues and requirements of law.

No Child Left Behind

The most recent piece of legislation to receive considerable attention in the education world is the reauthorization of the Elementary and Secondary Education Act in 2001. This law, which was renamed No Child Left Behind (NCLB), was signed into law in 2002. At the heart of this law is greater accountability by school districts. As mandated by NCLB, students in grades 3 to 8 must take proficiency tests in reading and math annually and at least once in grades 10 to 12. Science testing is to occur at least once in elementary school (grades 3–5), middle school (grades 6–9), and high school (grades 10–12). Schools must show progress on this annual testing. NCLB requires that data from annual testing be reported by race, gender, and disability status. Within each of these groups, at least 95% of the children must participate (although participation rates can be averaged over 3 years). Thus, 95% of children with disabilities must take part in the annual testing. Initially, NCLB regulations stated that 1% of all students could use scores on alternate achievement standards. However, more recently, the U.S. Department of Education has amended this so that districts can allow up to 3% of students to use alternate or modified standards. According to the law, all students must be "proficient" by 2013–2014. Prior to that, each school that receives Title I funding must meet "adequate yearly progress" goals. (Non-Title-I schools are not subject to the same sanctions, but states must have a plan for rewarding and sanctioning these schools.) Schools that fail to make adequate progress for 2 years must offer parents the option to transfer their children to another public school (unless state law prohibits school choice). Schools that fail to make adequate progress 3 years in a row must provide additional instructional services (e.g., tutoring, after-school classes). If adequate progress is not made for 4 consecutive years, corrective measures, such as implementing a new curriculum or replacing staff, are required. If adequate progress is not made for 5 years in a row, then significant changes must be made. These could include a state takeover of the school, conversion to a charter school, or the hiring of a private contract manager. In failing schools, parents may elect to have their children receive additional tutoring services or to use public funds to transport their children to another school. Schools are required to develop report cards showing how their test scores compare with local and state test scores. These report cards must show data for all students as well as subgroups of children, including those with disabilities, children with limited English proficiency, various groups of ethnic minority children, and children from low socioeconomic status (SES) backgrounds.

The law also specifies that all teachers be "highly qualified," generally meaning that they are certified and proficient (as indicated by passing a subject knowledge test) in the subjects they are teaching. This criterion applies to school psychologists, and states that did not previously require testing are now requiring school psychologists to take a pass a test such as the Praxis II.

NCLB also provides individual school districts greater flexibility in spending their federal education monies. School districts can use up to 50% of their federal monies (except those designated for Title I services and excluding IDEIA funds) to support any other educational program as long as student achievement improves.

Although greater accountability by schools sounds positive, the requirements of the NCLB act, particularly those regarding mandatory testing procedures and adequate yearly progress ratings, have generated significant controversy. There are numerous reasons for the controversy, including a lack of adequate funding to implement assessment procedures and concerns regarding the use of test scores for students with disabilities, as well as those not proficient in English, to evaluate the overall performance of a school. Particularly because potential remedial actions for "failing" schools could be severe, schools serving large numbers of students who have limited proficiency in English and/or students with disabilities are concerned about the inclusion of these students in their school performance reports. However, some positive changes may result, including greater exposure to the regular education curriculum for students with disabilities and stronger links between students' IEP goals and the regular education curriculum (Council for Exceptional Children, 2004).

Recently, the Obama administration has issued a blueprint for reform of NCLB (U.S. Department of Education, 2010). The blueprint calls for a continued focus on accountability and improving the performance of all students and calls for states to ensure that their students are college and career ready upon graduation from high school. Additionally, the blueprint calls for the development of quality assessment systems that will assist schools in determining whether students are college and career ready. One of the criticisms of NCLB has been the focus on punitive measures, and the blueprint calls for rewarding teachers and schools that are showing progress and success. In addition, it calls for an increased focus on students' growth rather than simply their meeting a proficiency standard. Congress must now take up the task of the reauthorization of this law. How much of the current law and how much of the blueprint will be included remains to be seen.

Ethical Issues

In addition to legal issues, school psychologists must be aware of ethical principles that guide the practice of school psychology and psychology in general. As indicated early in this chapter, ethical principles differ from legal mandates in that ethical codes are not enforceable by law. They are, however, intended to guide the appropriate practice of psychology, and all psychologists should take these principles just as seriously as they do legal mandates.

Ethical codes provide a model for moral practice and are designed to help protect those whom a professional serves (e.g., children, in the case of school psychologists). In this context, morality involves an evaluation of professional actions based on some broader social or cultural context. Although they are not necessarily enforceable by law, ethical violations are taken seriously by professional organizations and licensing bodies. Individuals may have their memberships in organizations and/or their professional licenses revoked for serious ethical violations (Bersoff, 2008). However, individuals should not follow ethical guidelines simply out of fear of punishment. Individuals should follow ethical guidelines because they help us to best serve and protect our clients and their needs and interests. Both NASP and APA have developed ethical codes to help guide the professional practice of school psychology and psychology in general. However, it should be noted that simple knowledge of these codes is unlikely to be sufficient in helping individuals engage in ethical practice. Many ethical dilemmas faced by school psychologists involve not violations of specific ethical principles but rather ethically challenging situations (Jacob-Timm, 1999). Partly because of this, there has been a focus in ethics education on teaching *ethical decision making* in addition to covering the provisions of the appropriate ethical codes (e.g., Jacob & Hartshorne, 2007; Kenyon, 1999; Welfel, 2006). Although the models used to teach ethical decision making vary in their specific steps, they all involve some similar features, including identification of the ethical dilemma, consideration of ethical guidelines, generation of possible resolutions to the ethical dilemma, evaluation of these possible resolutions and the effects of certain actions on the involved individuals, and making a decision regarding which course of action to follow. As part of this process, consultation with colleagues, reviews of ethics literature and of state laws, and consideration of broad ethical values (e.g., respect for autonomy, fairness) are often taken into account.

As noted, many of the ethical dilemmas faced by school psychologists are not related to specific ethical violations but instead involve ethically problematic situations, thus emphasizing the need for broad ethical problem-solving education. In a survey of school psychologists regarding the ethical dilemmas they have faced, only one-quarter of the respondents indicated that they had not faced an ethical dilemma over the past 2 years (Jacob-Timm, 1999). Of those who had faced ethical dilemmas, the most common incidents involved pressure from administrators to act in a way that was counter to the best interests of the child (e.g., pressure to tailor assessment findings to make or not make a child eligible for special education services or to fit with a certain special education classification; pressure to deliver services in a manner incompatible with ethical principles). Other common ethical problems encountered relate to assessment procedures (e.g., inappropriate use of tests), confidentiality (e.g., struggles with when to report suspected child abuse), and unsound educational practices (e.g., concerns about ineffective programs, discipline methods). Jacob-Timm (1999) argued that these findings support the idea that students must receive training in ethical decision making in addition to being knowledgeable about specific ethical codes. We agree that school psychologists must have knowledge about the content of ethical codes governing practice and that they must also have the ability to engage in problem-solving tactics when faced with an ethical dilemma.

The two primary codes of ethical conduct with which all school psychologists should be familiar are APA's *Ethical Principles of Psychologists and Code of Conduct* (2010a) and NASP's *Principles for Professional Ethics* (2010b). The full text of these ethical codes can be found in Appendices A and B. In addition, NASP also publishes their *Model for Comprehensive and Integrated School Psychological Services* (2010a), which contains NASP's views of best practices in school psychology. It is acknowledged that not all school psychologists will be able to meet every standard in these guidelines, but the document should serve as a guide for the practice of school psychology. The full text of this document is available online at *www.nasponline.org/standards/2010standards/2_PracticeModel.pdf*. Students and practicing school psychologists should read these codes and become very familiar with them. In addition, it is important to note that ethical codes are revised every decade or so, and it is imperative to keep up to date with changes in ethical codes. In fact, APA released amendments to its ethical code in the summer of 2010 specifically dealing with sections related to conflict between the law and the ethical code.

Both the NASP and APA ethical codes have introductory statements that provide some general guidelines and aspirational guidance to practitioners. The introduction to NASP's *Principles for Professional Ethics* states:

> School psychologists are committed to the application of their professional expertise for the purpose of promoting improvement in the quality of life for students, families, and school communities. This objective is pursued in ways that protect the dignity and rights of those involved. School psychologists consider the interests and rights of children and youth to be their highest priority in decision making, and act as advocates for all students. These assumptions necessitate that school psychologists "speak up" for the needs and rights of students even when it may be difficult to do so. (NASP, 2010b, p. 2)

NASP then divides the specific ethical guidelines into four broad categories: (1) Respecting the Dignity and Rights of all Persons; (2) Professional Competencies and Responsibility; (3) Honesty and Integrity in Professional Relationships; and (4) Responsibility to Schools, Families, Communities, the Profession, and Society.

APA's *Ethical Principles* has an Introductory Preamble and General Principles in which psychologists are encouraged, among other things, to "benefit those with whom they work and take care to do no harm" (APA, 2010a, Principle A). Following this, ethical standards in 10 areas are provided: (1) Resolving Ethical Issues, (2) Competence, (3) Human Relations, (4) Privacy and Confidentiality, (5) Advertising and other Public Statements, (6) Record Keeping and Fees, (7) Education and Training, (8) Research and Publication, (9) Assessment, and (10) Therapy.

Although there are some differences between the ethics codes of NASP and APA, there are also many similarities, especially as related to general ethical principles. Because of the number of similarities between the ethical codes, we have chosen to organize the following discussion of ethical principles around major ethical areas, highlighting both NASP's and APA's guidelines on these issues.

Competence

Both the NASP and APA codes state that psychologists should engage in activities for which they are competent and qualified. Psychologists are to seek training, consultation, or supervision as needed to provide competent services. They are also encouraged to make referrals if they are not competent to handle a case. APA's ethical code does state that in an emergency situation psychologists may provide services for which they are not trained to ensure that services are not denied; however, these services are to end as soon as the emergency resolves or more appropriate services are available. Psychologists are also expected to engage in continuing professional development activities to develop and maintain their competence. Psychologists are to refrain from engaging in activities in which they have personal conflicts that would prevent them from providing competent services.

Professional Relationships

Both NASP and APA address psychologists' relationships with others. In NASP's ethical principles, this is addressed under "Honesty and Integrity in Professional Relationships" and in APA's code under "Human Relations" as well as throughout other sections dealing with specific issues. Both codes discuss avoiding dual or multiple relationships. For example, a psychologist who is providing services to a family should not also be engaged in a business relationship with this family. APA's ethical code does state that "multiple relationships that would not reasonably be expected to cause impairment or risk exploitation or harm are not unethical" (§ 3.05). NASP's ethical guidelines state that "school psychologists avoid multiple relationships and conflicts of interest that diminish their professional effectiveness" (Standard III.3.3, p. 10). Both ethical codes specify that psychologists should engage in nondiscriminatory practice and not engage in harassment (including sexual harassment and harassment based on personal characteristics) or in exploitative relationships. Both ethical codes also emphasize working with other professionals to best serve their clients.

Both ethical codes address sexual relationships with clients and relatives of clients. NASP is more absolute in its prohibitions stating that "school psychologists do not engage in sexual relationships with individuals over whom they have evaluation authority, including college students in their classes or program, or any other trainees or supervisees. School psychologists do not engage in sexual relationships with their current or former pupil-clients; the parents, siblings, or other close family members of current pupil-clients; or current consultees" (Standard III.4.3, p. 11). APA's ethical code prohibits sexual relationships with current clients and close relatives of current clients. In addition, psychologists are not to accept into therapy individuals with whom they have had sexual relationships. However, APA does indicate that psychologists could engage in sexual relations with former clients 2 years following termination of the professional relationship, but only under the "most unusual circumstances" (§ 10.08). APA separately discusses sexual relations with students and supervisees and indicates that psychologists are not to engage in sexual relations with "students or supervisees who are in their department, agency, or training center or over whom psychologists have or are likely to have evaluative authority" (§ 7.07).

In addition to general professional relationships, NASP's ethical guidelines address the school psychologist's professional relationships with specific individuals, including the child and family. NASP ethical principles discuss parental participation in services and parental consent for services in some detail (see Standard I), noting when parental consent is required (e.g., consultation about a child is expected to be extensive, administration of screenings for mental health problems) and when it is not (e.g., reviewing educational records, participating in educational screenings that are part of the regular instruction). NASP principles also note that school psychologists should encourage the voluntary participation of minor students in services. However, it is also noted that student assent can be bypassed if the service has a "direct benefit to the student and/or is required by law" (Standard I.1.4, p. 4).

Because school psychologists can practice independently, multiple relationships can exist for school psychologists who work in the schools as well as in private practice. NASP's ethical guidelines include a separate section on professional independent practice that addresses some of the issues faced by school psychologists who are employed by a school district and also have a private practice. In such situations, school psychologists must inform potential clients of no-cost services available through the schools and may not provide services to students of a school or students eligible to attend school where the school psychologists is working. In addition, school psychologists are to conduct their private practice business outside of school hours, and they should not use materials that belong to a public employer unless the employer approves of their use.

APA specifically discusses the issue of informed consent, both in general and in relation to treatment and research. The APA guidelines specify that informed consent be obtained from the individual prior to engaging in research, therapy, assessment, and consulting activities. Assent should also be obtained when an individual is not able to give informed consent. Consent (and assent) must be documented by the psychologist.

Privacy/Confidentiality

Both NASP and APA stress the importance of keeping information confidential. Information should be shared only after receiving informed consent from the client or parent or in situations in which it is required or permitted by law. APA specifies that the sharing of confidential information without consent may include instances in which information needs to be disclosed to "protect the client/patient, psychologist, or others from harm" (§ 4.05). NASP also specifies that confidential information can be shared "in situations in which failure to release information would result in danger to the student or others or where otherwise required by law" (Standard I.2.4, p. 5). Clients should be told about the limits to confidentiality prior to the initiation of services, and the NASP standards note that confidentiality issues may need to be discussed at multiple points. APA specifies that if the clients are being audiotaped or videotaped, permission specifically for these activities must be given by the client (or the parents if the client is a minor). If psychologists are presenting confidential information in a public presentation, they must either take steps to disguise the source of the information or obtain consent from the client for the presentation. APA also specifies that if a psychologist consults with a colleague regarding a case, the psychologist cannot disclose confidential information (unless prior consent has been obtained) and that the psychologist disclose only enough information to meet the purpose of the consultation. The NASP ethical guidelines state that electronic files be protected (e.g., via passwords, encryption) and that parents (or adult students) are notified if records are stored or transmitted electronically. The NASP standards also note that parents should have "appropriate access to the psychological and educational records of their child" (Standard II.4.4., p. 8).

Professional Practice: Intervention and Assessment

The ethical codes of NASP and APA have a number of similarities in their discussion of assessment-related issues. Both codes indicate that psychologists should be knowledgeable about the psychometric properties of instruments they use and should use instruments appropriate to the purpose of the evaluation. NASP also specifically states that school psychologists should use multiple assessment methods when completing an evaluation.

Interpretation of test results is also addressed in the ethical codes of both NASP and APA. APA refers to the use of automated scoring and interpretation programs and indicates that even when such programs are used psychologists must take into account the purpose of the assessment and individual characteristics of the client when interpreting results. The NASP ethical guidelines indicate that school psychologists should adequately interpret information and communicate findings in an understandable manner. With regard to computer-assisted scoring and interpretation programs, NASP guidelines indicate that school psychologists should use programs that meet professional standards and use professional judgment in evaluating the accuracy of the findings.

With regard to engaging in intervention activities, NASP specifies that school psychologists should use a problem-solving process to develop interventions and that preference be given to interventions that have research support. APA states that psychologists must inform their clients if the therapy techniques being used have not been established and the potential risks associated with the treatment.

Research

Both NASP and APA discuss ethical principles as they relate to involvement in research. Both sets of ethical guidelines indicate that institutional approval should be obtained prior to beginning research. The NASP standards indicate that psychologists who are working in an agency without a research review board should have individuals knowledgeable about research and ethics review the research prior to beginning the project and should have the research approved by the school administration. Both ethical codes specify that psychologists do not fabricate data, do not plagiarize, and do not publish the same finding twice. Both codes specify that steps should be taken to correct any errors discovered after publication of data. Both ethical codes indicate that authorship inclusion and order should be based on contributions to the project and that only those who have made substantial contributions should be included as authors. APA ethical codes further specify that, except under unusual circumstances, a student is listed as the first author when the manuscript is based significantly on the student's dissertation. Both ethical codes also specify that reviewers of manuscripts respect the confidentiality of these works.

APA's ethical code goes into more detail than does NASP's code on some of the specifics regarding conducting research. For example, it is specified that deception should not be used unless it is justified given the potential value of the study and the lack of suitable alternative methods. Psychologists are also instructed to not use deception when it is "reasonably expected to cause physical pain or severe emotional distress" (§ 8.07). The APA ethical code also contains a section on ethics when using animals in research.

Training and Supervision

Both sets of ethical guidelines cover issues in training or supervising psychology students, and although the ethical codes are somewhat similar, they address these issues from a slightly different perspective. APA specifies that training programs be designed to provide appropriate knowledge and expertise and that program descriptions be accurate and made available to those interested. APA further specifies that information presented in courses, syllabi, and other training be accurate. Both ethical codes indicate that feedback should be provided to students and others being supervised and that this feedback should be fair. APA specifies that the feedback should be based on "actual performance on relevant and established program requirements" (§ 7.06). The NASP ethical code specifies that school psychologists who supervise trainees or interns are responsible for the professional practice of those they supervise. NASP also specifies that interns and trainees should be clearly identified as such in reports and that supervisors must cosign all reports.

APA addresses disclosure of student personal information and therapy for students. The ethical guidelines state that psychologists cannot require students and others being supervised to disclose personal information, unless (1) the program has clearly identified such information as a requirement of the program in its program materials, (2) the information is necessary to evaluate or obtain assistance for the student if problems could prevent the student from competently completing his or her training duties, or (3) a threat is posed to others. APA specifies that if programs require student involvement in psychotherapy, the program faculty should allow students to select therapists not affiliated with the program. In addition, faculty who are responsible for evaluating the students should not provide the therapy.

Advertising/Media Relations

Both NASP and APA specify that psychologists must provide accurate information in their announcements and advertisements. The APA specifies that psychologists cannot solicit testimonials from former clients and cannot directly solicit clients. The APA also specifies that psychologists do not compensate members of the media in return for publicity in a news item. The APA code contains statements regarding presentations through mass media outlets and cautions psychologists to not indicate that a professional relationship has been established with an individual via this manner.

Record Keeping/Fees

The APA's ethical code has a specific section on record keeping and fees. Likely because these issues are more relevant to psychologists in private practice than to those employed by a school district, the NASP guidelines say little about these issues. As has already been discussed in the confidentiality section, psychologists are expected to keep records confidential, and if information is stored in a database, psychologists should code personal information so that individuals cannot be identified. Psychologists are not allowed to withhold records needed for a client's emergency treatment just because the client has not paid for services. Psychologists are to establish a fee agreement with their clients early in the therapy process. The APA does indicate that psychologists may barter (accept goods, services, and so on in lieu of monetary payment) if this is "not clinically contraindicated" and if the "arrangement is not exploitative" (§ 6.05).

Ethical Decision Making

When ethical principles require a higher standard of conduct than what is set forth in the law, both NASP and APA indicate that ethical principles should be followed. In addition, when ethical behavior conflicts with policy or law, psychologists are expected to state their dilemma and commitment to their ethics and take steps to resolve this conflict. If conflicts exist between ethical practice and the demands of an organization for which a psychologist works, APA's ethical code indicates that the psychologist must attempt to resolve the conflict consistent with the ethical code. Both NASP and APA ethical codes indicate that if a psychologist becomes aware of a possible ethical violation on the part of another professional, an informal resolution should first be attempted by bringing the matter to the attention of the individual. If an informal resolution is not appropriate or, as APA specifies, if the violation is likely to cause substantial harm, the psychologist should contact appropriate organizations (e.g., professional organizations' ethics committees, state licensing boards). The filing of an ethics complaint that is frivolous or made without regard to the facts is itself an ethics violation.

Integrating Ethical Principles and the Law: Limits to Confidentiality

Several of the issues covered in the ethical guidelines of both NASP and APA have also been the subject of case law. In particular, some of the issues related to confidentiality have been the subject of lawsuits that have brought about new laws in some states as well as changes to ethical codes. Although both ethical codes are committed to confidentiality, this confidentiality has limits. The three main limits to confidentiality involve abuse of a minor child, threat of harm to another, and threat of harm to oneself. Where these situations exist, psychologists have an ethical (and often legal) obligation to break confidentiality to ensure the safety of their clients and/or other individuals.

Child Abuse and Neglect

All states have mandatory child abuse reporting laws that require certain individuals (e.g., physicians, mental health workers, teachers) to report suspected child abuse or neglect to the appropriate authorities (generally a state agency such as child protective services). The federal Child Abuse and Prevention Treatment Act as amended by the Keeping Children and Families Safe Act of 2003 (Public Law 108-36) defines child abuse and neglect as "at a minimum any recent act or failure to act on the part of a parent or caregiver, which results in death, serious physical or emotional harm, sexual abuse or exploitation, or an act or failure to act which presents an imminent risk of serious harm." At a minimum, states must use this definition in terms of what they consider to be reportable abuse and neglect. However, states may add to this definition. Reporting laws are generally worded so that an individual does not need to be sure that abuse is occurring but have "reasonable cause" to believe that abuse has occurred.

Duty to Protect

Duty-to-warn or duty-to-protect laws are also common, although not as universal as child abuse reporting laws, and there is no federal statute to guide state laws on this matter. These laws grew out of the *Tarasoff v. Regents of the University of California* rulings in 1974 and 1976. In this case, Prosenjit Poddar had communicated to his psychologist (who was employed by Cowell Memorial Hospital at the University of California at Berkeley) his intention to kill Tatiana Tarasoff. At the psychologist's request, the police detained Poddar, but he was then released. Although the psychologist and two psychiatrists at Cowell agreed that Poddar should be committed, the chief of the Department of Psychiatry disagreed, and no action was taken. Two months later, Poddar murdered Tarasoff. Tarasoff's parents sued, arguing that Poddar should have been confined and that

Tarasoff should have been warned of his threats. The case was initially dismissed, but in 1974 (*Tarasoff I*) the California Supreme Court ruled that therapists have a duty to warn a threatened person. The case was heard again in 1976 (*Tarasoff II*). In this ruling, the police were released from liability, but the court ruled that therapists have a duty to *protect* an intended victim:

> When a therapist determines … that his patient presents a serious danger of violence to another, he incurs an obligation to use reasonable care to protect the intended victim against such danger. This discharge of duty may require the therapist to take one or more of various steps … it may call for him to warn the intended victim or others likely to apprise the victim of the danger, to notify the police, or to take whatever other steps are reasonably necessary under the circumstances.

Thus, based on the second *Tarasoff* ruling, therapists do not simply have a duty to warn an intended victim but must take steps to protect the intended victim.

Although most psychologists are likely familiar with the *Tarasoff* rulings, it should be noted that states differ in terms of their duty-to-protect requirements and that not all states have adopted laws that follow the *Tarasoff* ruling, which covered only the state of California. However, as noted, APA's ethical code indicates that confidential information should be disclosed, where permitted by law, to protect the client or another person. Thus, even if psychologists are not legally required to comply with a duty-to-protect law, they are ethically obligated to break confidentiality when the safety of an individual is in question.

Privileged Communication

Whereas confidentiality is more of an ethical than a legal principle, *privileged communication* is a legal term that prevents the disclosure of information provided in confidence to certain individuals (with exceptions as mandated by law). Attorney–client privilege is the most well-known type of privilege, whereby information transmitted by a client to his or her attorney is considered private and cannot be revealed. In many states, psychologists are also granted privilege. However, school psychologists employed in schools are less commonly granted privilege. If a psychologist has privilege, he or she cannot be compelled to reveal communications with his or her client without the client waiving the right to privilege. If state laws do not consider psychologist–patient communications to be privileged, then the psychologist can likely be compelled to share communications in a court of law. However, even in states in which communication between a therapist and his or her client is considered privileged, the state may allow a judge to waive privilege.

Conclusions

As should be clear from this chapter, legal and ethical issues are complex and multifaceted. They are also not static but rather change over time. Ethics are influenced by legal mandates, and legal mandates can be influenced by ethical principles. For example, prior to the *Tarasoff* rulings, the ethical code of APA stated confidentiality rights in more absolute terms than it does today. Much of what school psychologists do will be guided by both federal legislation and ethical principles. Given this, it is important that school psychologists stay up to date in both areas. Not only should they read texts such as this one, but they should also read professional newsletters and attend to announcements of changes in legislation so that they can receive current information on these important issues.

DISCUSSION QUESTIONS AND ACTIVITIES

1. Search websites such as *Wrightslaw.com* to see what recent court cases have been decided regarding services for children with disabilities. Review these cases in the context of the IDEIA regulations.

2. To school psychologists currently being trained, the requirement that all students (regardless of their disability status) be provided with a FAPE likely seems unquestionable. Research, through readings or talking to educators, parents, or adults with disabilities, what services for children with disabilities were like prior to the passage of Public Law 94-142.

3. IDEIA is detailed in its requirements, but it can be overwhelming for parents to understand. Talk to parents of children with disabilities about their experience with the special education process: Have they understood their rights? Do they know what is in their child's IEP? Have they been satisfied with their child's experience? What suggestions do they have for improving the special education process?

4. Children with disabilities who do not qualify for special education services may be eligible to receive accommodations under Section 504. However, the provision of these services is variable. What is your school district doing to comply with Section 504? How are students in need of accommodations identified? What accommodations are typically offered to these students?

5. Consider an ethical dilemma you have had or have heard about. Examine the NASP and APA ethical codes and list which guidelines apply to your dilemma and what the guidelines suggest in terms of resolving your ethical dilemma.

CHAPTER 7

Facilitating Change
through Data-Driven Problem Solving
A Model for School Psychology Practice

The first six chapters of this volume provided an overview and orientation to the field of school psychology, its historical context, and current trends and issues. In this chapter and those that follow, we shift our focus from a history and current status of the field to mapping a *vision* for the field. In the first edition of this text, we began this chapter by acknowledging that historically school psychology practice has been dominated by traditional refer–test–place models wherein the school psychologist's role is largely that of "diagnostician" (Lentz & Shapiro, 1985) or "sorter" (Fagan, 1995). We then argued that a more promising future for school psychology lies in the data-oriented problem-solving role posited by Susan Gray in 1963 and currently advocated as "best practice" by many leading scholars in the field (e.g., Deno, 2002; Reschly, 2008; Reschly & Ysseldyke, 2002; Shapiro, 2000; Tilly, 2002, 2008). Now, in 2010, our hopeful vision of the field and its future feels less like a wishful description of "what should be" and more of a description of "what is" really taking place in the field *now*. Fueled perhaps by the momentum of the EBP and RTI movements, we see increased attention to and use of approaches consistent with the data-driven problem-solving approach advocated for in the original version of this text. This is not to say, however, that the field has arrived as a coherent profession that fully espouses this approach. Instead, we argue that, unlike our predecessors who pioneered alternative models of school psychology as a problem-solving endeavor (Baer & Bushell, 1981; Gray, 1963; Lentz & Shapiro, 1985) and for decades lamented the disconnects between actual practices and proposed progressive alternatives to traditional refer–test–place models of practice (Deno, 2002; Reschly & Ysseldyke, 2002; Shapiro, 2000; Ysseldyke, 2000), we are beginning to see change occurring (Reshly, 2008; Tilly, 2008). Thus, within this important chapter devoted to a data-driven problem-solving approach, we feel less inclined to devote a great deal of space to issues of past arguments regarding the merits of this approach over more traditional approaches to school psychology. In lieu of rehashing old battles between traditional and alternative approaches to school psychology, we feel compelled to focus a significant amount of our attention on discussing what we see as happening now with an emphasis on how to continue to implement a problem-solving approach within the context of EBP and RTI movements.

This chapter begins with a brief overview of historical roots of this vision of school psychology as a problem-solving endeavor, contrasting the problem-solving approach with more traditional diagnostic approaches to school psychology and acknowledging the contributions of our predecessors, to whom we are grateful for their efforts to bring forth the problem-solving approach to school psychology. Next, we describe how a data-based problem-solving approach is integrally linked with the current EBP and RTI movements. Finally, we describe the approach by detailing its processes and the structures necessary to support its sustained use. In the chapters that follow, we expand on the areas of assessment (Chapter 8), intervention (Chapters 9, 10), systems change (Chapter 11), and research (Chapter 12) within the context of a problem-solving model.

Historical Discussion of Traditional and Alternative Approaches to School Psychology Practice

Historically, arguments in favor of the adoption of a data-based problem-solving approach to school psychology were proposed in light of (1) growing concerns with inadequacies noted in traditional models that dominated school psychology practice; (2) recognition of the critical need for reforms in our practices if we are to address the increasing numbers, complexity, and severity of educational and mental health problems facing our children and youth; and (3) increasing evidence of the utility of alternative approaches in improving educational outcomes for students. As we have noted in earlier chapters, the field of school psychology historically has faced many challenges, one of which has been a general lack of clarity of purpose in our practice roles (Deno, 2002; Reschly, 2008). As discussed in Chapter 4, for example, disparity has existed not only between actual and preferred roles but also often between current and recommended best practices among leading scholars and professional organizations.

We believe that much of the struggle in moving forward and expanding our practice roles from "what is" in our current practice to "what should be" is a result of the difficulties we face as we try to step away from traditional roles that have now become institutionalized. In essence, what has traditionally or historically dominated our practice roles (i.e., traditional diagnostic and refer–test–place tasks) has become our *expected* role. Others (e.g., teachers, administrators, parents), have come to know the school psychologist as one whose primary and most visible function has been the psychoeducational assessment and classification/diagnosis of children to determine their eligibility for special education and/or related services (Fagan, 1995; Lentz & Shapiro, 1985). Despite the fact that alternative models of school psychology as a problem-solving endeavor also have existed for many years (e.g., Baer & Bushell, 1981; Gray, 1963; Lentz & Shapiro, 1985), the more traditional roles seemed to be institutionalized to the extent that others view us as "diagnosticians." Because of these traditional perceptions, policies and regulations have been put into place that in many instances had historically mandated these roles.

It would be easy to continue to do what we have always done and what others have expected us to do, yet leaders in our field have continued to challenge us to critically evaluate our current approaches to practice and, in light of what we find, to consider progressive alternatives (Deno, 2002; Reschly, 2008; Reschly & Ysseldyke, 2002; Shapiro, 2000; Tilly, 2008; Ysseldyke, 2000). In general, we are in agreement with individuals who argued for a fundamental shift away from our traditional practice roles, and we believe that after decades of arguing for such shifts, some movement is finally occurring. For those new to the field, we believe it is important to have some historical awareness and consciousness of our field. In the next few sections, we describe these roots.

Historical Roots of Traditional and Alternative Models of School Psychology

In Chapter 2, we summarized six major historical dichotomies in psychology wherein tension and conflict have manifested in the field of school psychology (pp. 32–35). We now add another, more specific dichotomy to our discussion as we contrast our vision of an alternative approach to school psychology as a data-driven problem-solving endeavor with the more traditional or refer–test–place models of school psychology practice. As aptly noted by Reschly (2008) and Reschly and Ysseldyke (2002), this dichotomy has its historical and philosophical roots in the two approaches that have dominated the broader field of scientific psychology, namely *correlational* and *experimental* psychology. In this section, we describe this dichotomy, place it in its historical context, and illustrate how it has manifested in our notions of traditional and alternative approaches to school psychology practice.

In his 1957 *American Psychologist* article, Cronbach commented that *experimental* psychology and *correlational* psychology were two *disciplines* that characterized the field of scientific psychology. According to Cronbach (1957), the task of a *science* is to "ask questions of nature," and "a *discipline* is a method of asking questions and of testing answers to determine whether they are sound" (p. 671). He noted that psychologists within the correlational discipline were "interested in the already existing variations between individuals, social groups, and species" (p. 671). They measured how these variations related to (correlated with) performance in other domains. With regard to intervention, for example, the correlational psychologist was concerned with predicting performance in treatment conditions based on naturally occurring variations across individuals. One early application of this approach that is relevant to school psychology was the development of the Binet–Simon scales to identify children who were not likely to benefit from the general education curriculum. Performance on these tests was said to positively correlate with school success. Children whose test scores indicated they were not likely to perform well in school settings were placed in alternative settings. Thus, within the correlational discipline, assessments were employed to determine placement based on individual differences, not unlike traditional diagnostic assessment for determining special education eligibility and placement. In contrast, psychologists within the experimental discipline were interested in controlling situational variables to permit "rigorous tests of hypotheses and confident statements about causation" (Cronbach, 1957, p. 672). Within the realm of intervention, the experimental psychologist was concerned with how different treatments resulted in the greatest average effects for individuals (single-subject designs) or groups of individuals (group comparisons). Great emphasis was placed on controlling for situational variations across treatment conditions in order to make valid comparisons of treatment effects. An example of this approach in school psychology is the study of instructional strategies for teaching reading. Within the experimental approach, individuals or groups of individuals would be exposed to different reading interventions to determine which approach resulted in the highest average performance on some reading outcome measure. Thus, whereas experimental psychologists focused on manipulating variables to cause differences (e.g., to determine which treatment condition produced the greatest effect), correlational psychologists focused on studying "what man has not learned to control or can never hope to control" (Cronbach, 1957, p. 672).

After contrasting the experimental and correlational approaches, Cronbach (1957) proposed a merger of these two opposing disciplines when he suggested the aptitude × treatment interaction (ATI) method. He argued that psychologists should consider how aptitudes (naturally occurring or existing variations between individuals, social groups, and species) might interact with certain aspects of treatment to attenuate effects. The idea was that we should design treatments to fit individuals or groups of individuals with certain aptitudes or aptitude patterns. In this approach, what is meant by *aptitude* is "any characteristic of the person that affects his response to treatment" (Cronbach, 1975, p. 116). Some major assumptions behind ATI were as follows: "A person learns more easily from one method than another, and this best method differs from person to person, and that such between-treatments differences are correlated with tests of ability and personality" (Cronbach, 1957, p. 681).

This idea had intuitive appeal and was the focus of much attention in research and practice in psychology in the decades following Cronbach's proposal. Tests were developed to assess and classify students according to their preferred learning modalities or underlying processes (e.g., perceptual–motor, visual, auditory). In the field of special education, and learning disabilities (LDs) in particular, many researchers set out to design instruction in accord with assessed patterns of modality strengths and weaknesses (e.g., Kirk, McCarthy, & Kirk, 1968). Despite the fact that research on the ATI model was in its infancy and evidence confirming its utility still pending, this approach enjoyed enormous attention from scholars who advocated its use:

> In some children information is absorbed more easily through auditory pathways; in others, learning is facilitated primarily by using visual channels.... We feel that exploration of modality strengths and weaknesses is of more than theoretical interest and should largely determine teaching methods. (deHirsch, Jansky, & Langford, 1966, pp. 80–83)

> The visual dyslexic rarely is able to learn by an ideo-visual approach since he cannot associate words with their meanings. He cannot retain the visual image of a whole word and consequently needs a more phonetic or elemental approach to reading. (Johnson & Myklebust, 1967, p. 156)

The school psychologists' role in this process was the careful assessment of processing and modality issues. With its intuitive appeal and widespread dissemination from educational leaders (e.g., Barbe & Milone, 1980; Dunn, 1979), this approach also pervaded special education practice. In one survey, for example, the overwhelming majority (i.e., 99%) of special education teachers reported that they believed a child's modality strengths and weaknesses should be a major instructional planning consideration (Arter & Jenkins, 1977). Although it is not surprising that this occurred, because we know that educational practice is not always driven by research (Carnine, 1997), the widespread adoption of ATI becomes problematic in light of mounting empirical evidence that failed to support the efficacy of this model.

During the decades following Cronbach's 1957 proposal of ATI, empirical investigations on the efficacy of this approach abounded. Contrary to the conventional wisdom that endorsed ATI, research syntheses did not substantiate its efficacy (e.g., Arter & Jenkins, 1979; Cronbach & Snow, 1977; Kampwirth & Bates, 1980; Kavale & Forness, 1987; Tarver & Dawson, 1978). In 1975, Cronbach reconsidered ATI in another *American Psychologist* article. This time he addressed ATI in light of its empirical evidence, commenting that as "important as ATIs are proving to be, the line of investigation I advocated in 1957 no longer seem sufficient" (Cronbach, 1975, p. 116). Cronbach was concerned with the inconsistency of findings across relatively similar studies (e.g., studies investigating the same treatment variables but finding different outcome-on-aptitude slopes), because only a fraction of these inconsistencies were due to statistical sampling error. He argued that these inconsistencies were evidence of unidentified, complex interactions with other variables such as sex, ability, skill level, prior knowledge in the domain of interest, and so forth. In proposing the ATI model, Cronbach overlooked the possibility that the interactions he was interested in studying (i.e., ATI) might be moderated by other factors he had not considered. His original hypotheses were as follows: (1) When ATIs are present, generalizations about treatment effects are problematic because the effect will come and go (interact) across the kinds of individuals who are treated; and (2) when ATIs are present, general predictions about treatment effects from aptitudes is uncertain because effects will vary depending on the selected treatment. After studying ATI, Cronbach realized the importance of other unforeseen interactions, noting that "interactions are not confined to the first order; the dimensions of the situation and of the person enter into complex interactions" (Cronbach, 1975, p. 116). He emphasized that "once we attend to interactions, we enter a hall of mirrors that extends to infinity" (p. 119) and "when we give proper weight to local conditions, any generalization is a working hypothesis, not a conclusion" (p. 125).

In light of the evidence derived from ATI research, Cronbach (1975) argued the need for applied psychology to embrace short-run empiricism and evaluation of interventions within local contexts. According to Cronbach (1975, p. 126), "Short-run empiricism is 'response sensitive' ... one monitors responses to the treatment and adjusts it, instead of prescribing a fixed treatment on the basis of a generalization from prior experience with other persons or in other locales." Later, Reschly (2008) and Reschly and Ysseldyke (2002) drew parallels between Cronbach's suggested *short-run empiricism* and an alternative or *problem-solving approach* to school psychology practice. They commented that the majority of school psychology's practice (past and current) has been more consistent with the correlational and ATI approaches, as they urged us to consider the lack of evidence for traditional models and challenged us to consider the adoption of a problem-solving model of school psychology (Reschly, 2008; Reschly & Ysseldyke, 2002). We also encourage school psychologists and school psychologists in training to consider the adoption of a data-driven problem-solving approach to school psychology. We ask them to do so in light of the history we have presented thus far and with consideration of other factors that we present in the next sections.

Rationale for Adopting a Problem-Solving Approach

As we have noted in the preceding section, the philosophical assumptions driving traditional practice have not been substantiated empirically. Despite this fact, these approaches monopolized the majority of school psychologists' professional practices for decades and, in some places, still do. Why would school psychologists and educators in general continue to engage in practices that have been deemed questionable? One plausible explanation can be found in commentaries positing that education (Carnine, 1999) and, within education, school psychology (Tilly, 2002, 2008) are relatively immature professions that do not necessarily rely on the scientific method to determine the efficacy of their respective practices. According to Carnine (1999, p. 2), "An immature profession is characterized by (a) expertise based on the subjective judgments of the individual professional, (b) trust based on personal contact rather than on quantification, and (c) autonomy allowed by reliance on perceived expertise and trust that staves off standardized procedures based on experimental research findings." He commented that the field of education fits these criteria. Similarly, Tilly (2002, 2008) argued that school psychology is currently evolving, as do all sciences, from a philosophically based system to a scientifically based system. In a philosophically based system, reasoning occurs "from premise to conclusions: *If this is true, then that would be true*" (Tilly, 2002, p. 21). Within school psychology, for example, this logic is seen in traditional diagnostic work. The premise that assessment based on form and structure of symptoms leads to diagnosis, and that, in turn, *diagnosis informs treatment*, is presumed to be "true." Thus, the focus of practice becomes systematic assessment (e.g., diagnostic testing) to determine the presence of a disability (diagnosis). And the practice of diagnostic assessment is deemed an important endeavor because it presumably leads to a diagnosis that will inform treatment. Within this model, which is predicated on the medical model, problems are conceptualized as residing primarily within patients (students), and the role of the therapist (school psychologist) was to treat the illness (disability) and to maximize adjustment (learning; see Tilly, 2008). Thus, problems were dealt with in a reactive fashion (i.e., diagnosis and intervention took place after a problem was apparent), and the approach focused on remediating problems for individuals in a child-by-child fashion (Tilly, 2008).

As professions mature, however, they reach "a point in their development where philosophical reasoning, assumptions, and practice no longer sufficiently addressed problems at hand" (Tilly, 2002, p. 21). When faced with sufficient practice "failures," practitioners begin to question the premises and conclusions of their current practices. At this point, reasoning begins to shift and becomes more scientifically based, by which observation leads to a tentative hypothesis that is subsequently evaluated. Carnine (1999, p. 2) claims that maturation of a profession is triggered by "pressures from groups that are adversely affected by the poor quality of service provided by a profession." When this occurs, there is "(a) a shift from judgments of individual experts to judgments constrained by quantified data that can be inspected by a broad audience, (b) less emphasis on personal trust and more emphasis on objectivity, and (c) diminished autonomy by experts and a greater role for standardized measures and procedures informed by scientific investigation" (Carnine, 1999, p. 3). Tilly (2002) states that school psychologists and educators in general have amassed a significant enough number of "failures" resulting from current assumptions and practices to warrant movement from a philosophically based system to a scientifically based system. Further, Tilly (2008) and Reschly (2008) argue that, with legal mandates for accountability in schools, we are currently experiencing further movement toward science-based practices, and that we ultimately have both moral and ethical reasons for continuing to evolve our profession toward adopting science into our applied practices. Reschly (2008) comments that embedded within the implementation of a problem-solving and RTI approach to school psychology, there is a self-correcting process that occurs from the frequent monitoring of progress that informs decision making surrounding the implementation of prevention and intervention strategies. This self-corrective process is akin to Cronbach's notion of "short-run" empiricism.

Individuals who are currently practicing, in training for, or simply considering a career in school psychology will no doubt encounter differing opinions and controversy regarding traditional and alternative professional practice roles. We are hopeful that, as they are faced with choices regarding how they approach their professional practice, they do so in a very conscious and informed manner. Further, and in keeping with the problem-solving approach we are advocating, we hope that school psychologists carefully evaluate the practices they choose and make adjustments as necessary.

In this section, we provide a rationale for why selection of the data-oriented problem-solving approach to school psychology practice over a traditional approach has been advocated, namely (1) evidence that traditional systems have many problems, despite improvements in theory and methods of cognitive assessment; (2) information suggesting the urgency of the need for a change; and (3) continued evidence supportive of the problem-solving approach to professional school psychology practice.

Evidence That Traditional Systems Have Many Problems

Foundational assumptions underlying much of the traditional refer–test–place approaches to school psychology practice have been challenged for decades. For example, extensive efforts to document the efficacy of assessing processing strengths or learning modalities and matching these to instructional strategies to capitalize on strengths have failed to produce intended results (e.g., Kavale & Forness, 1987; Vaughn & Linan-Thompson, 2003). In her early critique of this approach as it applies to reading, Snider (1992) eloquently illustrated the logical fallacy behind this approach as she considered the application of modality instruction or learning styles interventions to the nonacademic skill of basketball. She supposed that a physical education teacher gives a learning styles inventory to her class and discovers that her students were auditory/analytical learners who had weaknesses in tactile/kinesthetic areas. She imagined further that the teacher attempts to match basketball instruction to the students' learning styles through auditory means (e.g., having them listen to tapes) and analytic means (e.g., analyze plays, engage in group discussions). Snider asked, "Why do some educators reject the notion that students can learn to play basketball by only thinking and talking about it, but embrace the idea that students can learn to read by only global and visual or tactile/kinesthetic methods?" (p. 15). Further, she wondered why this approach to instruction considers *who* and *how* to teach but ignores *what* is to be learned. The "what" of beginning reading involves certain analytical and phonological skills, whereas the "what" of basketball requires certain tactile and kinesthetic skills. She cautioned the use of any process that disregards this part of the teaching equation.

In addition to criticisms of the theoretical basis for our current practices, the methodological soundness (i.e., reliability and validity) of diagnostic approaches, particularly with regard to LDs, has been questioned. Historically, a diagnosis of an LD involved assessment of a discrepancy between a child's ability (via IQ tests) and achievement (via norm-referenced achievement tests). Alarmingly, evidence indicated that practitioners do not diagnose LD consistently across students or districts (Epps, Ysseldyke, & McGue, 1984; Ysseldyke, Algozzine, & Epps, 1983). In addition to problems noted in the reliability of the assessment process across practitioners, other methodological issues surround traditional assessment processes (Francis et al., 2005; Hoskyn & Swanson, 2000; Stuebing et al., 2002). The ability–achievement discrepancy model that dominated early assessment approaches, for example, was "fraught with measurement error," yet significant decisions were made on the basis of a few ability–achievement discrepancy points (Reschly & Ysseldyke, 2002, p. 9). Further, when the model was applied to students with low reading performance, results did not support the validity of differential diagnosis based on an ability–achievement discrepancy compared with assessment based simply on low achievement in reading (Fletcher et al., 1994). In light of the evidence regarding problems with ability–achievement discrepancy approaches to diagnosis of LDs, a consensus statement was released following the LD summit, noting that that this IQ–achievement discrepancy was "neither necessary nor sufficient for identifying individuals with LD" (Bradley, Danielson, & Hallhan, 2002, p. 796). Finally, concerns have been raised about delays in service delivery that result when children who are initially referred for reading problems in the early grades and do not qualify for services (i.e., do not meet the ability–achievement discrepancy) are referred again in later grades, when their achievement levels fall far enough behind to qualify for the ability–achievement discrepancy (Fletcher et al., 1998). This practice is quite concerning when evidence suggests that there is a critical and short period in which we can alter reading trajectories (Simmons & Kame'enui, 1998).

Within the traditional system, one assumed benefit is that diagnosis leads to treatment via access to special education placement and/or related services and, more important, that special education and related services benefit students. Given the amount of time and resources devoted to diagnostic and classification activities, some researchers have attempted to evaluate the degree to which diagnostic assessments actually inform treatments as well as the degree to which students who are diagnosed and receiving services actually benefit from those services. Early studies failed to demonstrate the efficacy of special education placement (e.g., Carlberg & Kavale, 1980; Glass, 1983; see Reschly, 2008) for students with high-incidence disabilities such as specific learning disabilities (SLD), speech–language impairments, emotional/behavioral disorders, mild intellectual disabilities, and other health impairments (OHI). For students with high-incidence disabilities, meta-analyses regarding the overall effects of special education identification and placement (e.g., Kavale, 2005) have been equivocal (see also Reschly, 2008). Further, some studies indicated that students identified through the assessment process were not necessarily receiving instruction that differed from instruction provided to their peers without disabilities, thus calling into question the differential service delivery assumption behind diagnostic assessments (e.g., Thurlow & Ysseldyke, 1982) and special education placements (e.g., Ysseldyke, Christenson, Thurlow, & Bakewell, 1989; Ysseldyke & Thurlow, 1984). Because students with and without disabilities are not randomly assigned to various educational services, one cannot conduct true experimental studies in this area, so studies must rely on outcomes for individual students. This is also a difficult process because students with disabilities have often been exempted from state- and district-level assessments. With recent movements toward accountability within systems, these data are becoming more available, yet the evidence does not systematically demonstrate benefits for students with disabilities. In fact, "when performance over time is tracked, the gap in performance of students in general and special education gets wider every year, with a continual decline in the performance of the group of students assigned to special education" (Reschly & Ysseldyke, 2002, p. 7). Clearly, more research is needed in this area, because preliminary evaluations have failed to demonstrate the effectiveness or efficiency of special education placement alone as an intervention (Reschly, 2008; Reschly & Ysseldyke, 2002).

Criticisms of the traditional role of the school psychologist have been long-standing:

> The school psychologist is not a well man. His malady, while not particularly acute, is nonetheless a chronic one, endemic to his profession. The patient often presents such symptoms as distention of the referral ... rupture of the arteries of communication ... atrophied recommendations ... and accumulation of jargon deposits in the report.... The syndrome might best be described as a "paralysis of the analysis." (Forness, 1970, p. 96, as cited in Ninness & Glenn, 1988, p. 6)

Despite early awareness of the potential shortcomings of our practices, educational systems have tended to be deficit focused, wherein the school psychologists' role in that system is to respond after problems are apparent and to search for pathology (e.g., Alessi, 1988). This practice is troublesome when one considers the stigma associated with many diagnostic or categorical labels, their typical lack of treatment utility, and the need for a preventive focus to comprehensively address student needs and to consider *all* students, not just those who are experiencing difficulties or who are eligible for special services (e.g., Hoagwood & Johnson, 2003; Hunter, 2003; Power, 2003; Shapiro, 2000; Strein, Hoagwood, & Cohn, 2003). "The search for pathology dominates eligibility evaluations and confers an overall, often implicit, obsession with deficits that deflects attention from effective treatment and the explicit pursuit of goals related to adult social roles" (Reschly & Ysseldyke, 2002, p. 7).

Within the current literature, scholars who advocate for practices more in line with traditional approaches continue to defend the use of such approaches and also question the utility of alternatives that are consistent with an RTI process (e.g., Hale, Fiorello, Kavanagh, Holdnack, & Aloe, 2007; Kavale, Kauffman, Bachmeier, & LeFever, 2008; Kavale & Spaulding, 2008; Reynolds & Shaywitz, 2009; Learning Disabilities Association of America, 2010). Specifically, critics argue that (1) the use of RTI is "premature" and "lacks a trustworthy evidence-base" (Reynolds & Shaywitz, 2009); (2) comprehensive psychometric assessments are required to achieve reliable and valid diagnosis of SLD under IDEA (Kavale et al., 2008; Kavale & Spaulding, 2008); and (3) idiographic interpretation of intellectual measures for children will inform intervention (Hale et al., 2007). Such commentary is in large part fueled by reactions to new provisions in the 2004 reauthorization of IDEA with respect to identification of students with SLD that (1) no longer require consideration of IQ–achievement discrepancy and (2) allow for the use of an RTI process as part of the diagnostic evaluation of SLD. Within the United States, SLD accounts for approximately 46% of the school-age population and represents the largest category, slightly less than 50%, of all students with identified disabilities (U.S. Department of Education, 2009). Thus, the advocacy surrounding this group of students is strong, and fears regarding the potential outcomes of policy changes regarding the identification/diagnosis process may be driving some of the current conflict surrounding what might seem to others as progress. According to the 2010 white papers written by the Learning Disabilities Association of America, for example, concern was raised that in the published regulations for IDEA eligibility criteria emphasized the identification of students who were not achieving adequate progress for the child's age or attainment of state-approved grade-level standards, not cognitive abilities. The papers noted specifically "the new criteria virtually eliminated a great many students with SLD, including some who have high academic achievement in some areas, but markedly low achievement in other areas" (Learning Disabilities Association of America, 2010). In contrast, scholars who advocate in favor of these alternative and RTI approaches have responded to arguments for the continued use of more traditional approaches (e.g., Fletcher & Vaughn, 2009a, 2009b; Fuchs & Fuchs, 2009; Torgeson, 2009), stating that such traditional views are "outdated and unsupported by research" (Fletcher & Vaughn, 2009b, p. 48). For psychologists new to the field or in training, we believe the task of navigating through the arguments between noted scholars of the field and emerging with some clear sense of where the evidence falls is difficult. Both sides argue that their position is grounded in evidence and that the "other side" is on shaky ground. So, who is right? Or is this question relevant? What approach would be in the best interest of the children and families we serve?

In the companion publication to this introductory text (*Practical Handbook of School Psychology*), we argued that school psychologists, who are successful problem solvers, likely adopt a set of beliefs, including the following (Ervin, Gimpel Peacock, & Merrell, 2010):

- Are open, flexible, and responsive to new information or changing circum-stances.
- Are willing to recognize when they fail (i.e., when their initial hypotheses or assumptions are incorrect).
- Are committed to EBP.

We ask you to think about these as you consider arguments among scholars as well as practitioners within the field. Given these assumptions, when we contemplated the inclusion of chapters relevant to a practical handbook of school psychology, we wanted to present a balanced assessment of current advances in psychoeducational assessment practices more in keeping with traditional approaches to school psychology. Thus, we asked a colleague well versed in the literature on cognitive assessment to provide us with an assessment of the current state of the literature on this topic in light of noted advances in theories of cognitive abilities as well as improvements in the tests themselves. Our goal for this chapter was to provide a current appraisal of the state of the field on cognitive assessment and its utility in aiding school psychologists in applying a problem-solving model to improve meaningful outcomes for students with whom we work. We encourage those new to the field to read this chapter carefully (see Floyd, 2010).

In considering the use of such tests, Floyd (2010) notes that advancements in cognitive assessment theories and tests have not overcome such issues as difficulties associated with their use in identifying problems (e.g., lack of alignment with curriculum, problems with error associated with measurement taken at one point in time in contrast to serial measurement, relative time and cost-effectiveness) as well as with analyzing problems (e.g., substantial inference associated with the use of these measures, recognition that these approaches have a tendency to focus on narrow aspects of within-child variables). Further, despite notable efforts to address issues of treatment utility, Floyd (2010, p. 59) comments that "at present, there is no sizable body of evidence revealing that scores from tests measuring cognitive abilities distal to achievement provide direct links to effective academic interventions." In contrast, he states that, irrespective of the source of evidence from which intervention selection is informed, it is likely that "interventions that are based on principles of learning and that have solid empirical support will most likely be the most effective" (Floyd, 2010, p. 60). And with respect to arguments for the use of cognitive abilities by school psychologists in the identification of aptitudes, he concludes that results have not typically supported the practices of differentiated instruction based on assessment of cognitive ability aptitudes. Further, the "taxonomy of CHC [Cattell–Horn–Carroll] theory (with 10 or so broad abilities and 70 or so narrow abilities) may only complicate the selection of cognitive ability aptitudes" (Floyd, 2010,

p. 60), and this may be compounded by the notion that generalization of ATIs from basic research will not necessarily generalize to applied settings (such as classrooms) and that generalizations of ATIs from applied settings such as classrooms may not generalize to other applied settings such as different classrooms or schools. This is not to say that it is not possible that, at some point in the future, advances in understanding cognitive ability aptitudes (based on CHC theory) or aptitude complexes could yield results more supportive of such differentiated instruction; however, "at present, consideration of ATIs based on most cognitive ability aptitudes does not appear fruitful for those engaged in problem-solving" (Floyd, 2010, p. 61). In his review of the current state of the research, Floyd concludes:

> Finally, after more than a year of consideration of the content of this chapter and several revisions, I ask myself with humility, If my daughter begins struggling with reading, mathematics, or writing when she begins first grade in 2009, what questions would I want for a school psychologist to ask about her? Would I like for him or her to be focused primarily on cognitive abilities and cognitive processes and to ask, What is her IQ? What does her profile of CHC broad cognitive ability strengths and weaknesses look like? Does she have discrepancies between IQ and achievement? Where does she rank compared with age-based peers on a measure of Comprehension-Knowledge and Fluid Reasoning? Does she have auditory processing problems or visual processing problems? Does she have weak working memory? Or would I prefer that the school psychologist determine the existence of a perceived problem, complete an ecologically minded assessment and develop low-inference hypotheses to explain the reason for the problem, draw on empirically based interventions to remedy the problem, and collect data to determine whether the interventions led to reductions in the problem? There is no doubt that I would prefer the second option, which represents the problem-solving process. I expect that, in the near future, the passion for cognitive ability tests felt by many school psychologists in the past will be transferred to a passion for the problem-solving model applied to academic problems. (2010, pp. 62–63)

In light of current evidence, we are in agreement with Floyd's conclusion, and we also remain committed to being open, flexible, and responsive to new information or changing circumstances, including recognition that we might be wrong at times when information suggests that our initial hypotheses or assumptions are incorrect, based on the evidence. As new information becomes available, it is important that school psychologists consider the evidence and allow their assumptions to be modified in light of evidence that may be contrary to current practices.

Urgency of the Need for Change

As we noted in Chapters 2 and 3, schools are currently faced with many challenges, such as rising numbers and diversity of students; complexity and severity of student behavior and learning needs; the need to prepare students for the ever-changing workforce; and increasing accountability requirements. Further, educators are often expected to address these issues in the face of decreasing resources or support, particularly in light of current economic challenges facing much of the world. According to Carnine (1999, p. 3), "Because educational performance determines economic well-being for individuals and society as a whole, widespread underachievement is detrimental and unacceptable to the public as well as to government and to business." He argues that when conditions become unacceptable to the public, this serves as a catalyst for systemic changes in practice. For some time now in education, we have been facing such a crisis. For some students, for example, learning or behavior problems are often chronic and associated with significant later-life difficulties that are quite costly to society (Adams, 1990; Walker, Colvin, & Ramsey, 1995). To efficiently address these growing concerns, research indicates that schools need to adopt a systemic approach with a focus on preventive and early intervention (e.g., Hoagwood & Johnson, 2003; Hunter, 2003; Strein et al., 2003). For example, some pivotal skills such as reading present a critical and short period in which we can alter developmental trajectories (Simmons & Kame'enui, 1998). Similarly, research suggests the importance of prevention and early intervention if the development of severe behavior problems is to be curtailed (Biglan, Mrazek, Carnine, & Flay, 2003). In the face of these concerns, scholars in school psychology have urged us to consider the "big picture" and to solve the "big instructional problems" that our schools are facing (Shapiro, 2000; Ysseldyke, 2000). Further, they continue to argue that our traditional approaches are insufficient in doing so.

Continued Evidence Supportive of a Problem-Solving Approach

Within the literature, support for the data-oriented problem-solving approach to school psychology is growing. Some developments in this area have their history embedded in the problem-solving approach posited by Susan Gray in 1963, and others developed in response to frustrations with traditional approaches. A few noteworthy examples include the development of assessment tools for direct measurement of academic and behavioral outcomes, advances in problem-solving approaches for linking assessment to intervention, expanding knowledge on effective instruction and interventions, improved methods for data-based decision making, and the development of alternative service delivery systems that are noncategorical in nature.

Tools for direct measurement of academic learning outcomes have been developed and show great promise in assessing student progress in the curriculum. Curriculum-based assessment (CBA; e.g., Shapiro, 1996, 2004), curriculum-based measurement (CBM; e.g., Deno, 1985; Shinn, 1989, 1998), curriculum-based evaluation (e.g., Howell & Nolet, 2000), and Dynamic Indicators of Basic Early Literacy Skills (DIBELS; e.g., Good, Gruba, & Kaminski, 2002) are examples of assessment methods that focus on assessing learning outcomes rather than learning modalities or processes. These tools have demonstrated efficacy for direct assessment and monitoring of student academic performance within the curriculum in the domains of reading (see Marcotte & Hintze, 2010), mathematics (see Burns & Klingbeil, 2010), and written expression (see Gansle & Noell, 2010). They provide an alternative to traditional norm-referenced assessment practices and have the advantages of being more closely tied to the curriculum, of shorter duration, sensitive to incremental changes, and they can be used repeatedly to monitor growth formatively. Further, these tools have been embedded within school psychology practice and are considered acceptable by practitioners (e.g., Eckert, Shapiro, & Lutz, 1995; Shapiro & Eckert, 1993, 1994). Advances in this area have led scholars to argue for the use of these tools in tackling screening and monitoring of student progress to identify students at risk for school failure and to promote early intervention and prevention efforts (e.g., Good et al., 2002; Shapiro, 2000; Simmons, Kuykendall, King, Cornachione, & Kame'enui, 2000).

In addition to assessment tools that lend themselves to direct measurement of student progress, school-based technologies for linking assessment to intervention have proven useful for problem solving in school settings (e.g., Gresham & Noell, 1999; Jones

& Wickstrom, 2010; O'Neill et al., 1997; Witt, Daly, & Noell, 2000). Functional behavioral assessment (FBA) is a process that focuses on collecting information pertaining to relations between *behaviors* (e.g., aggression, work completion), their *antecedents* (i.e., environmental factors that tend to precede and possibly predict them, such as a teacher prompt to begin reading), *consequences* (i.e., environmental factors that tend to follow and possibly maintain them, such as escape from a task, access to a preferred object or activity, or social attention), relevant *setting events* (i.e., distal antecedents, such as an argument with a parent or sibling before school, that may play a role in exacerbating problem behavior) and *establishing operations* (i.e., conditions of satiation or deprivation, such as hunger, that tend to alter the reinforcing value of certain stimuli, such as preference for food). Information on behavior–environment relations is then considered in the development of interventions. For example, if data suggest that a student's disruptive behavior (e.g., calling out in class) is *functionally* related to access to teacher attention, then an intervention is built around this hypothesis (e.g., the student could be taught to use a different and more appropriate means of accessing teacher attention, such as raising his or her hand; or the teacher could provide attention only when the student is not being disruptive). Alternatively, if data suggest that a student's disruptive behavior is functionally related to escape from task (e.g., reading group), a quite different intervention strategy might be used. Thus, functional assessment helps the problem solver to consider not just the "what" (i.e., form or structure) of behavior but also the "why" or "what for" of behavior (i.e., function). Empirical evidence indicates that functional assessment has shown promise in school settings and is an integral part of a movement toward a more data-driven, problem-solving orientation to the field (e.g., Gresham & Noell, 1999; Jones & Wickstrom, 2010; McIntosh, Reinke, & Herman, 2010). Currently, methods and procedures have been developed that are useful for schoolwide analysis of data for social behavior problems (see McIntosh, Reinke, & Herman, 2010).

Advances in instructional and intervention technologies and data-based decision-making methods have helped to enhance the utility of curriculum-based and functional assessment tools. We have accumulated a wealth of information regarding effective intervention strategies for a wide range of presenting problems (e.g., Eyberg, Nelson, & Boggs, 2008; Shinn & Walker, 2010). *Evidence-based practice* (EBP) is a term that has received a great deal of attention in recent literature. This term has been used to refer to "a body of scientific knowledge defined usually by reference to research methods or designs, about a range of service practices (e.g., referral, assessment, case management, therapies, or support services)" (Hoagwood & Johnson, 2003, p. 5) but more recently has come to encompass a model of practice that integrates research evidence for treatments with clinical expertise and patient characteristics (APA Presidential Task Force on Evidence-Based Practice, 2006). With respect to the literature on instructional strategies, the evidence base is quite large and has been around for several decades despite the fact that proposed school reform ideas might ignore such evidence (for further discussion, see Kaufman, 2010). With respect to interventions for social–emotional and mental health concerns, our evidence base is growing (see Kazdin, 2008a). Strategies for evaluating and selecting interventions also are being articulated within the field of psychology more broadly (e.g., APA Presidential Task Force on Evidence-Based Practice, 2006) and within school psychology (e.g., Kratochwill, 2007; Stoiber & DeSmet, 2010). These efforts are promising, because evidence-based interventions (EBIs) offer a useful place to start when selecting interventions. Equally important, however, is the need to carefully evaluate EBIs, because we cannot assume that interventions with demonstrated efficacy in one setting or with one population will result in similar effects with a different population or in different contexts (Campbell, 1988; Cronbach, 1975). Thus, improvements in intervention technologies are useful when paired with concomitant advances in alternative assessment tools (e.g., CBA/CBM, FBA) and careful attention to monitoring and evaluation of learning outcomes.

In addition to evidence suggesting the utility of practices related to a data-driven problem-solving orientation to school psychology, efforts have been made to develop and implement administrative and policy alternatives to traditional categorical service delivery systems (e.g., Reschly, Tilly, & Grimes, 1999). Unlike many current systems that search for pathology and produce labels that may be stigmatizing, "non-categorical approaches facilitate placing more emphasis on gathering assessment information related to designing interventions that enhance competencies" and are permitted under U.S. federal law (Reschly & Ysseldyke, 2002, p. 7). The noncategorical approach to special education eligibility assessment has been used successfully for several years now in certain area education agencies in the state of Iowa and in other educational systems as well. This approach is consistent with a problem-solving approach and is in keeping with the RTI movement discussed in the next section. We believe that the emerging noncategorical approach movement is an interesting and worthwhile endeavor and that the idea has several positive aspects.

Whether these systems offer a worthwhile alternative to current categorically based systems remains an empirical question worthy of further investigation (see Floyd, 2010). From a problem-solving standpoint, we believe these systems are worth our exploration and careful evaluation prior to wholesale endorsement. It is likely that school psychologists who are just entering the field will encounter one or more of these alternative service delivery systems in their practice.

A Context for Change: EBP and RTI

In addition to advancements in tools and procedures relevant to applications of a problem-solving model of school psychology, two current movements in the field of education, namely, the EBP and RTI movements, are relevant to school psychology practice. The EBP movement emphasizes the identification, dissemination, promotion, and adoption of practices (e.g., assessment, intervention) that have demonstrated research support, and this movement has been viewed as having the potential to significantly improve the quality of school psychology services (Kratochwill, 2007). The EBP movement, described briefly in an earlier section, is linked to response to intervention (RTI), a movement that has grown out of special education but has potential for much broader applications (Glover & Vaughn, 2010). RTI involves the integration of assessment and intervention within a multilevel/multi-tiered problem-solving approach to address learning and social–behavioral needs of *all* students (see Glover & Vaughn, 2010). The RTI and EBP movements are compatible and have gained significant momentum in the field of education. They are of particular relevance to the applications of a problem-solving approach to school psychology practice. Essentially, within the context of a problem-solving approach (described in the next section), taken together, the RTI and EBP movements suggest that practitioners consider and utilize the best available practices (of intervention and assessment) to address and prevent problems for *all* students by providing services across a continuum. RTI provides a framework from within which educators work together to address learning and social–behavioral needs of students. Key components of this approach include (1) coordination of service delivery efforts via involvement of key stakeholders; (2) multilevel/multi-tiered service delivery; (3) collection and use of data for screening and progress monitoring purposes within a data-based decision-making process; and (4) provision of evidence-based instruction and prevention/intervention services (Glover & Vaughn, 2010). These components are in keeping with the problem-solving process advocated for in this text and described in the next section.

Overview of the Data-Driven Problem-Solving Model

According to Deno (2002), the purpose of schooling is to foster the cognitive, affective, social, and physical developmental outcomes of students. Viewed in this light, Deno argues that school itself is an intervention that we as a society have deemed important to implement on a universal level. In other words, *all* children who participate in schooling are part of this widespread intervention designed to alter their development from its "natural" (i.e., unschooled) course. Within this context, it follows that the purpose of problem solving is to "eliminate the difference between 'what is' and 'what should be' with respect to student development" (Deno, 2002, p. 38). Thus, at a universal or school-wide level, the problem-solving process begins with determination of the discrepancy between where students are with regard to their skill levels in various developmental domains when they enter school and where we would like them to be when they graduate. Schools establish a general scope and sequence of competencies that students should master along the way (i.e., benchmarks or indices of progress), and instruction is focused on moving students forward through the various curricula toward the desired goal at graduation.

Movement along this continuum of curricular materials and mastery of desired skills and outcomes do not occur at the same pace for all students or evenly across domains for individual students (Deno, 2002). Within a second-grade classroom, for example, the range of skills in the domain of reading may vary widely across students, with some reading at or above targeted benchmarks and others reading slightly or significantly behind desired levels. Teachers must employ a problem-solving process and adapt instruction to address the varying instructional needs of all students within a particular instructional domain (e.g., reading). Similarly, at the individual student level, teachers will need to address varying student needs across domains. For example, an individual child may be viewed as not making adequate progress in a particular domain, such as reading, when his or her level of performance is not at the level expected along the continuum set by the school; yet the same student may be viewed as on target across other domains of functioning (e.g., social, mathematics, writing). Thus, even for children who are making adequate progress within the general education curriculum, problem solving is needed to address various instructional needs as they move along all the continua of development.

The problem-solving model so construed is *outcome focused* and *context specific*. Emphasis is placed on measuring discrepancies between current and expected performance on important domains of functioning, and problem solving focuses on the development of interventions to reduce this discrepancy (outcome). All of this (assessment of the discrepancy, intervention development, and evaluation) occurs within the context (setting and activity) in which the problem occurs. This focus directs the problem-solving agent (e.g., the school psychologist) toward solutions (e.g., instructional modifications) that fit the problem context (e.g., independent seat work during math class). When school problems are viewed from this perspective, one might argue that "failure to profit from general education is relatively common and results to some extent from idiosyncratic, inappropriately arranged environmental events" (Lentz & Shapiro, 1985, p. 199). Further, school psychology within a problem-solving system might be viewed as "a system of service provision designed to help remediate school-based problems of children [that is] preventative [and] incorporates explicit efforts to resolve problems before child placement in special education is required" (Baer & Bushell, 1981, p. 192). This perspective, although not new, is very different from the reactive focus of traditional diagnostic assessment, described earlier, that has traditionally dominated school psychology practice. The problem-solving model is focused on gathering information about the problem (i.e., quantifying discrepancies) and the problem context to develop working hypotheses about why problems are occurring and what solutions might work. These hypotheses are then evaluated within the natural context. In contrast, the traditional model is focused on gathering information about presumed underlying learning processes and individual differences that might lead to diagnoses with the assumption that the diagnosis will inform treatment. *Thus, the problem-solving model uses the scientific method to determine what works, whereas the traditional model is more likely to produce recommendations based on diagnosis.*

Problems that present themselves in school settings can vary on many dimensions (e.g., intensity, frequency, duration, severity, magnitude, complexity, resistance to intervention). Thus, the intensity of problem solving exists along a continuum and can be varied to match the presenting problem. For example, for some students, the discrepancy between actual and desired performance may be quite small, and problem resolution may be achieved with relatively minor adjustments (e.g., increased practice, corrective feedback, prompting) to instruction that could be managed by the classroom teacher within the general education curriculum. Other students, whose presenting problems are of a higher level of intensity, severity, or complexity, may require additional problem-solving efforts (e.g., consultation between the teacher and a special education teacher or school psychologist) and perhaps more intensive instructional supports to resolve their presenting concerns and to curtail the development of more significant problems. For a smaller percentage of students, current functioning in some domains may occur at levels that are severely discrepant from expected levels or that are extremely complex, intense, or resistant to intervention. These students might require ongoing problem solving to systematically address their needs and prevent exacerbation of existing problems. Finally, when a child's problem becomes pronounced (e.g., the discrepancy between a child's current rate of acquisition and retention occurs at a level that is significantly behind his or her peers), it may be necessary to provide instructional supports beyond what would typically be delivered in general education.

As noted, the problem-solving approach can be applied along the continuum of student needs to address the wide range of problems presented by students within school settings. At each level of intensity, problem solving also may vary in intensity, yet it will always follow a consistent process (i.e., series of steps). Many models of problem-solving appear within the literature (e.g., Bergan & Kratochwill, 1990; Kratochwill & Bergan, 1990; Witt et al., 2000). Across these models, Tilly (2002, 2008) notes that "four thematic questions guide practitioner thinking: What is the problem? Why is it occurring? What should be done about it? Did it work?" (p. 27). This same line of questioning is used not only to guide problem solving along the continuum of student needs but also to address problems at small-group and schoolwide levels. In this next section, we summarize the line of questioning and the steps involved in the problem-solving process

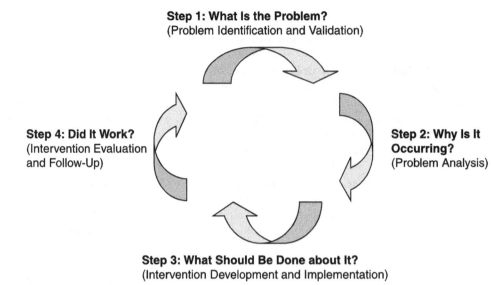

Step 1: What Is the Problem?
(Problem Identification and Validation)

Step 4: Did It Work?
(Intervention Evaluation
and Follow-Up)

**Step 2: Why Is It
Occurring?**
(Problem Analysis)

Step 3: What Should Be Done about It?
(Intervention Development and Implementation)

FIGURE 7.1. Questions and steps involved in a data-driven problem-solving process.

(see Figure 7.1). We end with a description of how this process might be embedded and sustained within the school context to address the needs of *all* students from a preventive stance consistent with current RTI and EBP movements.

Step 1: What Is the Problem? (Problem Identification and Validation)

The initial step in solving any presenting problem is, first, recognizing and confirming its existence as a problem and, second, determining that it is, in fact, a problem worth solving. As we noted earlier in this chapter, in a data-oriented problem-solving model, problems are defined as discrepancies between "what is" (current performance/outcome) and "what should be" (expected/desired performance) on some domain of functioning (e.g., reading). For example, when there is a discrepancy between a student's *current* and *expected* reading performance, in some circumstances this discrepancy may be viewed as a *problem*. In order for this step to occur, someone (e.g., a teacher or parent) must first notice the problem (i.e., discrepancy). This recognition requires some monitoring of or experience with the student's current reading performance, as well as experience and/or information pertaining to expected reading performance (e.g., relative to same-age peers or some other criterion). Further, in order to gain a clear understanding of the problem, it is important to use objective means to measure the discrepancy and confirm its existence.

Selecting standards for comparison to determine expected levels of performance (e.g., professional experience, teacher preference, parental expectations, developmental norms, medical standards, template matching, curriculum standards, local norms, national norms, and classroom peer performance) is not always an easy task. It requires professional judgment and some understanding of measurement issues. In Chapter 8, we discuss a variety of assessment tools that are used in school psychology practice, and in Chapter 12 we cover important measurement issues relevant to this process (see also

Daly, Barnett, Kupzyk, Hofstadter, & Barkley, 2010; Daly, Hofstadter, Martinez, & Andersen, 2010; Hawkins, Barnett, Morrison, & Musti-Rao, 2010; Hintze & Marcotte, 2010). Within a problem-solving framework, it is important that selected assessment tools and measurement techniques help to clearly define the problem in objective, observable, and measurable terms. In addition, we need to consider direct measurement of problems within the context in which they occur. Precision is extremely important at this stage of the problem-solving process, and quantifying the problem as a "discrepancy or difference score causes problem solvers to be objective about the problem" (Tilly, 2002, p. 29). The question becomes, How wide is the gap between actual and desired performance in this particular domain of functioning? To quantify discrepancies, it is important to think in terms of measurement categories (e.g., frequency, duration, latency, magnitude).

This careful measurement process helps to formalize goals for students (i.e., a reduction in the discrepancy). When the discrepancy is large, it is sometimes necessary to consider short- and long-term goals. For example, a student who is reading at a level that is significantly below that of his or her peers (e.g., a discrepancy of three grade levels) is not likely to catch up in a short period (e.g., 1 year). Instead, a more reasonable goal might be set and progress monitored along the way (formative assessment). Direct and frequent measurement is helpful in identifying problems, promoting agreement across stakeholders (e.g., parents, administrators, and teachers) about what the problem is, and, once an intervention is in place, determining whether or not it is improving. Further, with discrepancy scores, one can discern magnitude or problem severity in an objective fashion, and this can be helpful when prioritizing problems within and across students. Of course, there are certain practical constraints to measuring discrepancies in applied settings (e.g., time, resources, and skills). Thus, skillful practitioners will need to consider the precision, objectivity, practicality, and social validity of various measurement options when engaging in this first step of the problem-solving process. The problem identification phase of the problem-solving process does not end until the problem is defined and validated as a quantifiable discrepancy between current and desired performance.

Step 2: Why Is It Occurring? (Problem Analysis)

Once we have established that a problem exists and is worth our time and effort to solve, we move to the next stage in the problem-solving process. In this stage, we gather information about the problem and ask the question, Why is this problem occurring? In a problem-solving approach to school psychology, emphasis is placed on linking assessment to treatment and evaluation (Lentz & Shapiro, 1985). In this stage of the process, "instead of measuring student performance to find disabilities, our purpose is to diagnose the conditions under which students' learning is *enabled*" (Tilly, 2002, p. 29). To do this, we need to conduct an analysis of the problem context and function (see also Jones & Wickstrom, 2010). One important question to answer in this phase of the process is whether the problem is a *skill* (can't do) or *performance* (won't do) problem (for more information on this process, see Witt et al., 2000). More specifically, if the issue is a behavioral deficit (i.e., the student's actual performance level is less than what is expected), is the reason for this deficit that (1) the student does not want to perform the task or activity, (2) the student gets something (e.g., attention, access to a preferred activity or object, sensory stimulation) as a result of not performing the task, (3) the work is being presented at a level that is too difficult for the student, (4) the student has not been provided enough assistance to acquire the skill, (5) the student has not been given suf-ficient time or practice with the skills to do it fluently, or (6) the work is being presented in a way that is different from the way the student has usually done the work?

This phase of the problem-solving process is focused on gathering information to answer questions such as those just posed in order to gain an understanding of why the problem exists and to use this information to generate hypotheses about what might be done differently to enable learning to occur. For example, if we suspect that the student's reading problem is related to the fact that he or she has not been provided enough assistance to acquire the skill (i.e., the student has an acquisition problem), then our hypothesized intervention strategy might focus on providing instructional assistance directed toward skill development in reading (e.g., cueing, prompting, corrective feed-back). Alternatively, if we suspect that the student's reading problem is due to the fact that the student has not had enough time to practice the skill (i.e., a fluency issue), then our hypothesized intervention strategy might focus on increasing opportunities to read (e.g., paired reading, reading at home). If we are concerned that the student's reading problem is not related to a skill deficit but is instead a performance (won't do) prob-lem—a way of escaping the task—then our hypothesized intervention strategy will focus on addressing this problem. For example, we might make the task less aversive (e.g., considering the use of interesting reading materials or choice of materials), teach the student a different and more appropriate way to let us know that the task is aversive (e.g., asking for a break), and/or allow escape from the task contingent on some criterion of performance (e.g., allowing brief breaks from reading for appropriate performance for a certain number of minutes). In each of these scenarios, the problem is the same (i.e., a discrepancy between actual and desired reading performance), but the solutions are very different.

During the problem analysis phase, information may be gathered from a variety of sources (e.g., student, teacher, parent, peers, administrator) via a variety of assess-ment tools (e.g., formal and informal direct observational methods, semistructured and unstructured interviews, anecdotal reports, rating scales, review of records, CBA of skills) to answer the preceding questions. The purpose is to understand why (under what conditions) problems are more pronounced and to identify patterns and factors that contribute to the problem. We focus on directly measuring when, where, with whom, and during which activities the problem is more or less likely to occur or become exacer-bated. Given the assumption that many, if not most, student problems are a result of inap-propriately arranged classroom and instructional events, attempts are made to examine potential contributing factors (e.g., materials, instructional strategies) that can be easily altered. Of course, factors that are outside of the school's control (e.g., allergies, illness, divorce) may play a role in the development or maintenance of the presenting problem. Yet when developing interventions it is important to focus on what we can change to enable learning and reduce the discrepancy. For example, knowing that a student has a significant visual impairment is important for instructional planning, but it is unlikely that the cause of the visual impairment will be the focus of the intervention for school personnel. Instead, it is likely that the school will consider instructional accommodations (e.g., modified materials, vocal cues) to enable the student to benefit from instruction, despite the visual impairment. This phase of the process ends with the development of hypotheses regarding why the problem is occurring (e.g., under what conditions) and, based on this information, of hypotheses about what intervention strategies are likely to be effective.

Step 3: What Should Be Done About It? (Intervention Development and Implementation)

When we conceptualize problems as discrepancies between "what is" and "what should be," we are driven by the need to identify a solution that will reduce this discrepancy. It is at this stage of the problem-solving process that we use the information gathered thus far and decide what should be done about the problem. In addition to developing hypotheses about why the problem is occurring and linking this information to the selection of intervention strategies (contextual fit), one should consider interventions that have demonstrated empirical validity (see Chapters 9 and 10 for more discussion; see also Chapters 12 to 28 from our companion text, Gimpel Peacock et al., 2010). Thus, in a problem-solving approach, an intervention strategy is selected based on its functional relevance to the problem, contextual fit, and likelihood of success. After identifying an appropriate intervention strategy, it is important to specify the intervention tactics that will be used. For example, when deciding what we should do about a problem, we need to clarify the intervention steps, roles, and responsibilities as well as monitoring and evaluation techniques. In addition, it is important to determine the adequacy of existing resources and the need for additional resources in plan development. Further, time lines for implementing objectives and achieving desired goals should be specified. A clearly delineated intervention plan is the outcome of this phase in the process.

Step 4: Did It Work? (Intervention Evaluation and Follow-Up)

As indicated previously, the goal of the problem-solving process is to resolve the discrepancy between "what is" and "what should be." Thus, the process does not simply end with a thorough description or analysis of the problem. Nor does it end with a careful description of a potential solution or solutions to the problem. In order for the process to be completed, the problem should be resolved. Collecting ongoing information regarding the discrepancy between desired and actual performance is the best way to determine whether or not the intervention is effective. Thus, continuous monitoring and evaluation are essential parts of an effective problem-solving process.

At this stage, objective evidence should be gathered to determine whether plans are effective (i.e., change behavior in the direction of the goal), practical (i.e., relatively easy to implement with integrity), and acceptable. To ensure that the intervention and not some other factor was responsible for problem resolution, it is important to compare the extent of a problem (discrepancy) during intervention and its extent when the intervention was not in place. Single-subject design methods (discussed in Chapter 12) are useful for evaluating the effects of treatments for individual students (see also Daly, Barnett, et al., 2010). Information gathered during this phase of the process is analyzed, and, if necessary, intervention plans are revised and/or goals adjusted accordingly.

Summary of the Critical Features of a Data-Driven Problem-Solving Model

The data-driven problem-solving model is *outcome focused, data driven*, integrally *linked to intervention*, and *context specific*. One of the most important features of this approach is the emphasis on measurement to guide decision making throughout each phase of the process. In fact, if we were asked to identify the most important feature of this process, it would be *its focus on data*. Consistent with an empirically or scientifically based approach to practice, this model depends less on subjective judgment than on quantifiable feed-back provided from the information collected throughout the process. An important feature of the type of information used in this process is that it is objective, observable, and measurable. The focus is on learning outcomes and alignment of student skills with curriculum and instruction rather than internal processes alone. In addition, data collection emphasizes direct over indirect methods as well as methods that are repeatable and lend themselves to formative assessment of learning outcomes. At all stages of the process, attempts are made to use tools and procedures that do not require significant levels of inference (Tilly, 2002). Similarly, the problem-solving process is context specific, and disabilities are viewed as problems only if they result in a functional impairment within a particular context. This viewpoint keeps the focus on aspects of the problem situation that are modifiable (i.e., what we can change) and reduces the interpretive leap necessary to move to intervention.

Systems to Support Sustained Use of Problem Solving

As with any shift in practice, one must consider how new practices fit within the existing school context in order to ensure their sustained use. As we noted in Chapters 2 and 3, school contexts are quite complex systems. They serve a diverse student population with a continuum of learning and social–behavioral needs. Concern with ever-increasing numbers, diversity, and severity of student needs urges us to examine our practices and, in light of evidence suggesting that what we are currently doing is not working, to explore alternatives. Further, recognized leaders in school psychology have promoted the adoption of an EBP data-oriented problem solving model (e.g., Reschly, 2008; Tilly, 2008; Ysseldyke et al., 2006). Despite advocacy for this approach and despite advances in alternative assessment techniques, problem-solving methodologies, and interventions, schools do not readily adopt EBIs (e.g., Abbott, Walton, Tapia, & Greenwood, 1999; Carnine, 1997, 1999; Forness, 2003a; Friedman, 2003; Gersten, Vaughn, Deshler, & Schiller, 1997; Hunter, 2003). When external supports are provided to schools to facilitate the adoption of evidence-based, problem-solving approaches, these endeavors have demonstrated improved outcomes for students, yet schools fail to sustain these practices when external supports are subsequently removed (e.g., Fuchs, Fuchs, Harris, & Roberts, 1996; McDougal, Clonan, & Martens, 2000). These failures have led researchers to consider that an important but often neglected aspect of translating research into effective school-based practices is the careful consideration of the "fit between empirically validated interventions and organizational structures" (Hoagwood & Johnson, 2003, p. 5). In order to facilitate lasting change, we need to consider systems and organization structures of school systems and to work directly with stakeholders and policymakers (e.g., Curtis & Stollar, 2002; Grimes & Tilly, 1996).

   In recent years, efforts to promote adoption of evidence-based, problem-solving approaches to addressing literacy (e.g., Simmons et al., 2000, 2002) and behavior (e.g., Sugai & Horner, 2002a, 2002b; Sugai, Horner, et al., 2000) have emphasized the need to address organizational issues and contextual fit to promote successful adoption and sustained use of data-based decision making. On a larger scale, the state of Iowa has focused on combining many aspects of general and special education services to meet the needs of all students through the adoption of a "problem-solving orientation to assessment, intervention design, data-based decision making, and outcome orientation" (Grimes & Tilly, 1996, p. 466). Many of these efforts have focused on schoolwide, districtwide, and/or statewide applications of data-driven problem solving and EBPs to address the needs of *all* students in the system in a proactive and preventive manner. Systems-level challenges that arise when attempting to build capacity for schools to adopt such approaches are discussed in detail in Chapter 11, but it is important to note here that consideration of these issues is paramount to successful adoption of a data-oriented problem-solving approach to school psychology.

A Focus on Prevention

In addition to organizational and systems issues, in order for the data-driven problem-solving model to successfully address the learning, social, and behavioral needs facing today's youth, a prevention focus is critical. The following quote aptly illustrates this point:

> Communities cannot afford, and I mean this in hard economic terms as well as in humanitarian terms, to invest only in repair services.... To illustrate the point there is a fable concerning three people who were having a picnic beside the river. As they were enjoying their lunch in the sunshine, one looked up to see a child floating down the river. Immediately he leaped in and brought the child ashore. As he did so, his companions saw two more children helplessly bobbing in the water. Upon diving in to bring them out, they were dismayed to find still three more children in the river. Very quickly, they realized that the river was alive with struggling children in need of rescue. As they frantically worked to save as many as possible, one of the three suddenly left the water and began to run upstream along the bank. Seeing this, the others shouted after him in alarm, "Where are you going? Come back, we must help these children!" Continuing to run, he yelled, "You do the best you can there, I'm going up the river to try to stop them from falling in!" (Kisler, 1967, as cited in Drum & Figler, 1973, p. 13)

To date, school psychologists have invested much in "repair services." The children we typically serve are referred to us because they are already experiencing difficulties of some sort. Using the preceding analogy, one could argue that school psychologists spend a great deal of their time attempting to "pull kids from the river" or, if we are unable to pull them out, throwing them supports so they can stay afloat. Within the mental health literature, the work that we do falls into the category of *tertiary prevention* (Walker et al., 1996). In tertiary prevention, emphasis is placed on reducing the intensity, severity, and complications of chronic cases. This is accomplished through the delivery of specialized and individual interventions. Whether this occurs through traditional diagnostic approaches or through a problem-solving orientation, the focus is on addressing student needs on a case-by-case basis (i.e., one child at a time) in a reactive manner (i.e., after problems are noted). Problems are noticed, students are referred to us, we assess the issue using traditional or alternative means, and from this information interventions are determined, implemented, and, it is hoped, evaluated. Given the ever-increasing number of students in need of such services, tertiary prevention efforts are essential.

Unfortunately, and as the preceding parable indicates, a focus on repair services alone takes great effort and still may not be successful because of the increasing number, severity, and complexity of problems that we face. We know, for example, that by late elementary school learning and behavior disorders are often chronic, resistant to intervention, and associated with negative long-term outcomes and costs to the individual and to society (e.g., Adams, 1990; Biglan et al., 2003; Hunter, 2003; Walker, Colvin, & Ramsey, 1995). Without early intervention services, the stability of learning and behavior problems is alarming. In contrast, with proactive services, prevention, and early intervention, prognosis is much more promising (e.g., Biglan et al., 2003; Simmons & Kame'enui, 1998). Further, comprehensive prevention and intervention efforts that focus on building competencies and resiliency characteristics on a schoolwide level seem to be the most promising from a public health standpoint (e.g., Biglan et al., 2003; Hunter, 2003; Shapiro, 2000).

Several scholars in school psychology have argued for the adoption of a public health model of school psychology (e.g., Hoagwood & Johnson, 2003; Power, 2003; Strein et al., 2003). We agree with this perspective. As Figure 7.2 illustrates (OSEP Center on Positive Behavioral Interventions and Supports, 2000; Walker et al., 1996), public health models focus on comprehensive service delivery at three levels of prevention for:

1. Students who currently are not experiencing learning and/or social–behavioral difficulties (primary prevention).
2. Students determined to be at risk for the development of learning and/or social–behavioral difficulties (secondary prevention).
3. Students who currently are experiencing significant learning and/or social–behavioral difficulties (tertiary prevention).

The triangle in Figure 7.2 represents all students within a school setting, the majority of whom are not experiencing difficulties (i.e., the bottom portion of the triangle), some of whom are at risk to develop significant problems (i.e., the middle portion), and an even smaller percentage who are currently experiencing significant difficulties (i.e., the top portion). Using the river analogy, children who are already "in the river" are like

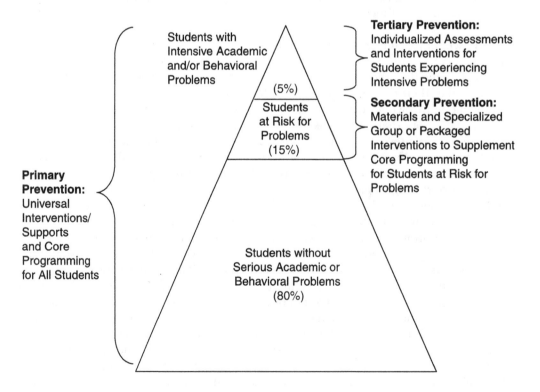

FIGURE 7.2. Triangle of support for the prevention of academic and behavioral problems.

those at the top of the triangle who are currently experiencing learning and/or social–behavioral difficulties. School psychologists currently spend the majority of their time and effort providing tertiary prevention (i.e., individualized assessment and intervention services) to these students on a case-by-case basis. These students make up the smallest percentage of the school population, but because of the significance of their problems, they often require the majority of time and resources from school personnel (Walker et al., 1996).

Shifting to a prevention model requires that we take a step back and look at the "big picture" by considering the needs of *all* students, not just those who are referred to us because they are experiencing difficulties (Shapiro, 2000). The foundation of a prevention approach is the use of universal interventions (i.e., *primary prevention*) designed to enhance the delivery of effective instruction and improved school climate designed to promote the academic, social, and behavioral resilience of *all* students in the school. The idea is that we send some folks "up river" to attend to students by implementing practices that are likely to enable them to remain on safe ground. More specifically, *primary prevention* for students who are not currently experiencing learning and/or social–behavioral difficulties is accomplished through schoolwide reform that involves the consistent use of research-based effective teaching and behavior management practices, ongoing monitoring of these practices and student outcomes, staff training and professional development, and systems-level decision making. The goal of primary prevention is to create school and classroom environments that promote student learning and decrease the number of students at risk for learning and/or social–behavioral problems.

We also know, however, that not all students respond similarly to prevention and intervention efforts. Thus it is important to monitor student progress and to assess whether students are at risk (i.e., in need of secondary prevention efforts) or experiencing significant learning and/or social–behavioral difficulties (i.e., are in need of tertiary prevention efforts). In other words, the people who are working to keep students on safe ground should monitor students to determine those who are at risk for falling in the river. Identifying students at risk of learning and/or social–behavioral difficulties is an important aspect of comprehensive prevention efforts. For students identified as at risk and in need of *secondary prevention* efforts, the focus is on the delivery of specialized interventions (often at a small-group level) to prevent the exacerbation of problems and the development of more significant concerns. In contrast to traditional diagnostic approaches, wherein students may actually "wait" to meet criteria for a disability prior to receiving services, in a prevention model, efforts are made to identify at-risk students early and to provide immediate services. The focus on early identification and early intervention is important. With regard to reading problems, for example, current evidence suggests that there is a critical and short period in which we can alter reading trajectories (Simmons & Kame'enui, 1998). In addition, if low-achieving students can be brought up to grade level within the first 3 years of school, their reading performance tends to stay at grade level (Adams, 1990). Thus, if we focus on early prevention and intervention services, our impact is likely to be greater.

The School Psychologist's Role

With a data-oriented problem-solving approach, we believe the school psychologist can make significant contributions at all levels of prevention noted in the triangle in Figure 7.2. The same problem-solving process (i.e., What is the problem? Why is it occurring? What can be done about it? Is it working?) can be applied at the school, classroom, and individual levels. One key to success in this model is the use of quantifiable, objective data to guide decision making. Thus, school psychologists are in a unique position to make significant contributions to prevention and intervention efforts given their knowledge and skills in the use of alternative assessment tools (CBA/CBM, FBA) for frequent and formative monitoring of student progress along expected continua of development, of proactive screening of students at risk, and of intervention evaluation purposes. Overall, we believe the school psychologist of the future has much to offer in a preventive data-oriented problem-solving system.

DISCUSSION QUESTIONS AND ACTIVITIES

1. Visit the library and consult the early issues (i.e., prior to 1980) of *School Psychology Review*. See if you can find at least one example of an article that espouses a traditional (i.e., correlational or ATI) approach and one example of an article that espouses a problem-solving (i.e., experimental) approach. Now, read Floyd (2010) and examine the more recent literature (i.e., post-2000) and see if you can find a more current article that is consistent with a traditional approach (i.e., correlational or ATI) and one that is more consistent with a problem-solving (i.e., experimental) approach. Discuss whether the issues raised regarding the utility of ATI have been resolved.

2. Interview parents, teachers, administrators, and school psychologists regarding their perceptions of the current role and their ideal/preferred role of the school psychologist. If differences between current role and ideal/preferred roles are expressed, ask what barriers the individual thinks are getting in the way of the ideal/preferred role. Were there differences between perceptions of current and ideal/preferred roles? Were perceptions of the school psychologist's *current* role more consistent with a traditional (diagnostic) or an alternative (problem-solving) approach? What about perceptions of the ideal/preferred role?

3. Despite evidence that was unsupportive of the ATI approach (i.e., Cronbach, 1975), in a 1977 teacher survey, the overwhelming majority of special education teachers reported that they believed a child's modality strengths and weaknesses should be a major instructional planning consideration. Interview 10 special education teachers and 10 school psychologists to discover whether this view is still held today.

4. Interview a school psychologist about the typical process (steps) she or he follows when working with an individual referral. Is the process more consistent with a traditional approach or with a problem-solving approach? Do they define problems as discrepancies? Is measurement an integral part of the process? What type of information is collected to inform treatment? Is evaluation of the treatment part of the process, or does this process end with assessment and recommendations?

5. Search the literature for problem-solving formats that were developed for use in school settings. From the information you collect, examine the forms and create your own version of a line of questioning that helps guide the process.

CHAPTER 8

The School Psychologist's Role in Assessment

Models, Methods, and Trends in Gathering, Organizing, and Analyzing Data

Assessment is one of the more controversial topics in school psychology. If one were to interview 10 school psychologists on their views of assessment and what constitutes an appropriate evaluation, there would likely be significant disagreement. Historically, school psychologists have been very tied to assessment in terms of their job function (as discussed in Chapters 2 and 5). However, more recently many school psychologists have attempted to move away from the evaluator/diagnostician role, at least as their primary role. As should be clear from earlier chapters, we do not endorse the diagnostician role as one to which school psychologists should be primarily tied. However, we do believe that assessment is critical in identifying children who may benefit from additional services as well as tracking the progress of these students over time. Historically in school psychology, assessment has been thought of as standardized testing, particularly using standardized measures of intellectual ability and achievement for the purpose of determining diagnosis and/or eligibility for special education services. However, when assessment is viewed in the context of the problem-solving process (as outlined in Chapter 7), it should be clear that the traditional view is very limited. Further, assessment is a critical component in the problem-solving/data-driven process. Although the view of school psychologists as problem solvers was gaining momentum when we wrote the first edition of this book, the past several years have seen a dramatic increase in the discussion of assessment as part of a problem-solving process, most notably in the context of the RTI paradigm. Although much has changed since we wrote the first edition, what has not changed is that assessment and the use of assessment in critical decision making remains an important, controversial, and highly debated topic within the field of school psychology, as we briefly note in Chapter 7.

A helpful distinction between assessment practices that have historically been used by school psychologists and problem-solving assessment is made by Howell and Nolet (2000), who differentiate between evaluations conducted for purposes outside the classroom and those conducted for purposes inside the classroom. Evaluations conducted for outside purposes include those typically conducted by school psychologists to determine whether a child meets criteria for a certain disability category. Evaluations conducted for inside purposes are those intended to obtain data to identify students who need specific skills, to inform intervention decisions, and to monitor implemented interventions. At a broader program evaluation level, inside assessments may be conducted to determine whether educational programs are having the intended positive effect. Evaluations with an inside purpose facilitate the problem-solving process in which information is gathered to help answer the questions that guide the process (i.e., What is the problem? Why is it occurring? What can we do about it? Did it work?) in an objective manner. This type of assessment is formative in nature; it is conducted in an ongoing fashion to guide decision making at all levels of problem solving (e.g., individual child, classroom, school, district).

Although trends are changing, many school psychologists have historically engaged primarily in assessment focused on outside purposes with significantly less attention paid to inside, intervention-focused assessment. With the increased focused on accountability and RTI, however, we are seeing an increase in the use of inside assessment.

We acknowledge that standardized norm-referenced assessment practices may be useful for some evaluation purposes (e.g., comparisons of performance across schools, comparison of a student's performance with that of a large normative sample). We also are aware that most, if not all, school psychologists in training are still expected to learn certain standardized assessment measures and procedures – and that these measures will continue to be used in the schools, although likely at a lower rate than they have been used in the past. The purpose of this chapter is to present an overview of different assessment methods and techniques. We outline some of the common assessment techniques utilized in school psychology practice. We include assessments that are used for a variety of evaluation purposes and give an overview of standardized, norm-referenced measures as well as alternative methods of assessment. We conclude this chapter with an integrated view of assessment and the problem-solving process.

Assessment Standards and Psychometric Properties

Before discussing specific assessment techniques, it is important to provide some background regarding assessment standards and psychometric issues. Understanding the reliability and validity of instruments is a key part of evaluating the usefulness and appropriateness of assessment measures and systems. Although a complete overview of these important psychometric properties is beyond the scope of this chapter, we briefly review these concepts and urge readers to familiarize themselves with these issues.

Assessment Standards

Most ethical codes address assessment standards in some manner. For example, as noted in Chapter 6, the ethical codes of both NASP and APA require that psychologists be knowledgeable about the psychometric properties of instruments and use instruments appropriate to the purpose of the evaluation. In addition to the assessment standards mentioned in specific ethical codes, the *Standards for Educational and Psychological Testing* were published in a joint effort of the American Educational Research Association, the American Psychological Association, and the National Council on Measurement in Education (1999). As stated in the introduction to these standards, their purpose is to "promote the sound and ethical use of tests and to provide a basis for evaluating the quality of testing practices" (p. 1). These standards are divided into three parts: test construction, evaluation, and documentation (including standards related to reliability and validity); fairness in testing; and testing applications. These standards are quite numerous and lengthy, covering everything from the importance of using reliable and valid measures to best practices in assessing individuals of diverse linguistic backgrounds to standards relating to the use of tests in specific applied settings (e.g., educational testing, employment). Related specifically to assessment in educational settings, the Joint Committee on Testing Practices has published the *Code of Fair Testing Practices in Education* (2004; available online at *www.apa.org/science/programs/testing/fair-testing.pdf*), which provides guidance for both test developers and test users in four different areas: developing and selecting appropriate tests, administering and scoring tests, reporting and interpreting test results, and informing test takers. These guidelines are intended to help professionals develop and use tests that are fair to all individuals. Readers are encouraged to familiarize themselves with these various standards and general best practices in assessment.

Reliability

The reliability of a measure refers to the *extent to which the measure is consistent*. This consistency can be shown across the items within the measure (internal consistency reliability), over time (test–retest reliability), across respondents or raters (interrater reliability), and across different forms of the same measure (alternate-form reliability). Reliability coefficients are expressed as correlation coefficients ranging from .00 (no association, meaning no reliability) to 1.00 (perfect reliability). An important related concept is the *standard error of measurement*, which is the amount of error associated with a score. The lower the reliability of a measure, the larger the standard error of measurement associated with the measure. The standard error of measurement can then be used to form confidence intervals, or ranges of scores that are likely to contain an individual's "true" score (Sattler, 2008). It is important to note that not all forms of reliability should be expected to be high. For example, interrater reliability between parents and teachers on behavior rating scales is typically quite low. This does not necessarily indicate that the test is unreliable, but instead may reflect that parents and teachers often observe different behaviors in different settings.

Validity

Validity is a somewhat more complex concept than reliability. Validity refers to *the extent to which a test measures what it is intended to measure*. Given this, validity must be considered in the context of the purpose of the test. Although validity is generally viewed as a unitary construct, there are various ways of determining validity. Traditionally, the three main forms of validity are *content, criterion*, and *construct*. Content validity refers to whether the items on the test are representative of the domain they are intended to evaluate (e.g., do items on a depression inventory actually measure depression, or do they represent another, perhaps related, construct, such as anxiety?). Criterion validity has to do with the relationship between the score on the measure and an outcome, such as a classification. There are two types of criterion validity: concurrent validity (which examines the test score as it relates to some currently available outcome) and predictive validity (which examines the test score as it relates to future performance). Construct validity is considered to be the overarching or superordinate form of validity. This notion refers to whether the test measures the particular construct it is intended to measure. When evaluating construct validity, both convergent validity (whether the test correlates with other, similar measures) and discriminant validity (whether the test does not correlate with measures of unlike constructs) are evaluated (Sattler, 2008).

Although validity is often thought of as relating specifically to the technical adequacy of a measure, Messick (1995) argues that one must also consider the "social consequences of test interpretation and use" (p. 744). As such, Messick refers to both evidential bases of validity (the psychometric/technical adequacy of a measure) and consequential bases of validity (the appropriateness of a test's use in terms of social consequences). The consequential basis of validity is an "appraisal of the value implications of score meaning" (p. 748), which relate to labels and actions generated as a result of testing. Thus, Messick argues that we should evaluate tests based not only on their psychometric grounds but also on their ethical grounds.

Clearly, both reliability and validity are important in helping us evaluate whether we should use a certain test for a given purpose. Although test developers should attend to these issues when developing new assessment instruments, it is imperative that test users also attend to these issues, especially those related to validity because the documentation of a test's validity tends to be an ongoing process and not limited to studies conducted prior to a test's publication.

Intellectual Assessment

As discussed in Chapter 5, school psychologists spend much of their time in assessment-related activities. In terms of actual assessment measures administered, standardized measures of intellectual ability (IQ tests) are some of the most commonly used, with the Wechsler intelligence scales (Wechsler, 2002, 2003, 2008) consistently being the most widely used. Wilson and Reschly (1996) surveyed school psychologists in 1991–1992 and compared school psychologists' use of certain assessment instruments in that year with their use in 1986. The Wechsler scales were the most commonly administered measures at both times (although observation was the most commonly used assessment method in 1991–1992). Almost all school psychologists in 1991–1992 reported that they used the Wechsler scales, with the average use being about nine times per month. Other measures of intelligence were used, but their use was reported by less than half of the school psychologists. In a more recent survey, school psychologists reported that intellectual measures, behavior rating scales, and projective measures were the most commonly used assessment techniques (Hosp & Reschly, 2002). School psychologists in this survey reported giving an average of 15 intellectual measures a month (these were not broken down by specific measures). Although data on the use of intellectual measures since the passage of IDEIA-2004 could not be found, Machek and Nelson (2010) did survey school psychologists regarding the assessment of reading disabilities, including their perceived usefulness of IQ measures. In general, more than half of the respondents indicated that they believed IQ measures could be useful in understanding a child's disability, and 86% indicated that IQ measures should be used to rule out intellectual disabilities when working within an RTI context. Thus, although this study did not ask about actual use of IQ measures, results imply that many school psychologists see utility in their use and, therefore, are likely to continue to use them at a relatively high rate.

Although measures of intellectual ability are commonly used, they are certainly not without controversy. A complete discussion of the controversy surrounding IQ instruments is well beyond the scope of this chapter, but numerous other books, chapters, journal articles, and scholarly talks are available for this purpose. We attempt to outline briefly some of the main issues involved in this controversy, but we encourage readers to seek additional information from these other sources. Although a significant focus of past debates regarding IQ tests centered on whether these measures are biased against certain populations (e.g., students from ethnic minority backgrounds), more recently the debate has been focused on the utility of these measures, although it should be noted that the issue of potential bias has not been resolved. In addition, as RTI methods have grown in popularity, the controversies regarding the use of IQ measures, particularly within the context of *identifying* LDs – has expanded.

The question of what is being assessed via IQ measures is theoretically complex. A number of different theories of intelligence have been developed over the years. In general, these theories can be placed into two different categories: (1) those that focus on intelligence involving a *general factor* (generally referred to as *g*) and (2) those that subscribe to the notion that intelligence has *multiple factors*. Even most professionals who subscribe to the notion of a general factor of intelligence agree that there are a variety of specific skills that contribute to a person's overall level of intelligence. However, those who subscribe to a multiple-factor theory of intelligence believe that these different facets of intelligence are distinct and cannot be simply combined to obtain one general intelligence factor (Sattler, 2008). One of the most well-formed and well-researched theories of intelligence is the Cattell–Horn–Carroll (CHC) theory. This theory consists of three levels of abilities: Stratum I, which consists of a large number of narrow abilities; Stratum II, which are clustered broader ability categories; and Stratum III, which is an overall or general ability factor (Floyd, 2010; McGrew, 2009). Just as there are many theories of intelligence, there are many definitions of intelligence. In reviewing these definitions, Sattler (2008) noted that many definitions include "the ability to adjust or adapt to the environment, the ability to learn, or the ability to perform abstract thinking" (p. 224).

The issue of whether IQ measures have treatment validity has received greater attention in school psychology as researchers and practitioners are increasingly advocating for a more direct link between assessment and intervention. If the goal of assessment is to guide treatment planning, how do results from traditional IQ tests fit in with this goal? It is clear that IQ measures do have moderate predictive validity; children with higher scores are more likely to perform well in school than those with lower scores, with the correlation between IQ scores and grades being about .50 (Neisser et al., 1996). However, as Reschly (1997) noted, IQ measures "are rarely used as predictors of how well children will perform in an academic setting. Rather such tests are used *after* children have performed poorly" (p. 238). Reschly further stated that the concerns for these children have more to do with identifying "goals and instructional methodologies that will result in improve academic performance" (p. 238) than with identifying whether there is a difference between a referred child's current abilities and those of his or her peers.

Historically, the use of intellectual measures has been necessary in schools to help determine whether a child qualified for special education services. Prior to IDEIA-2004, SLDs were required to involve a "severe discrepancy between achievement and intellectual ability." The definition of *intellectual disabilities* also references intellectual abilities (i.e., "significantly subaverage intellectual functioning, existing concurrently with deficits in adaptive behavior") (34 C.F.R. § 300.8); however, the identification of children within this category has produced far less controversy in recent years. Given that the procedures for identifying these disabilities have been directly tied to intellectual measures, it has been difficult for school psychologists to get away from performing IQ tests, even if such assessments do not seem to be necessary to develop an appropriate treatment plan for a child. However, given the changes to the definition of a SLD in IDEIA-2004 (discussed in Chapter 6) that eliminate the requirement that students have a severe discrepancy between their intellectual and achievement abilities to be classified as having a SLD, the issues of what constitutes a SLD and how best to identify a SLD have created significant discussion within the school psychology and special education communities. Although IDEIA-2004 provides that the RTI approach *can* be used in the identification of SLDs, research on how this approach would be used is lacking, because RTI procedures have historically been used more to identify children who may benefit from preventive services (e.g., increased academic instruction in reading) and to rule out inadequate instruction as a potential cause for problems rather than to classify children. Debate about the usefulness of RTI procedures, particularly in the identification of SLDs (e.g., Fletcher & Vaughn, 2009a; Reynolds & Shaywitz, 2009), is likely to continue for some time.

We assume that, even as RTI becomes more common, the use of IQ tests will not disappear from the practice of school psychology. For intellectual measures to be used responsibly, it is important that users understand what these measures are and what they are not. IQ measures provide an estimate of *current* intellectual functioning. Although IQ scores are relatively stable in most individuals by the early elementary school years, variation in scores may occur across testing times, and it is important to understand that there may be changes in an individual's IQ score across time as a result of changes in environment or circumstances (Sattler, 2008). It is important that users and consumers of IQ measures understand that these measures do not assess only some "innate" intellectual ability. Although genetics and biology obviously play an important role in the development of intellectual ability, environmental factors, such as early exposure to reading and quality of environment in the infancy and preschool years, are also important (Neisser et al., 1996). We also need to understand that the scores obtained from IQ measures are *estimates* of a person's true abilities. Confidence intervals are important in interpreting the limits or realistic ranges of test scores. The inclusion of confidence intervals when reporting results helps demonstrate that the obtained IQ score is not the specific IQ but rather our best estimate of a person's current intellectual ability.

Before deciding to use an IQ measure, it is important to determine whether it is needed and justified for the decision that is to be made. Using a measure just because it is typically what is administered or because "that's just the way it is done" is not good practice and has likely contributed to some of the negative perceptions of IQ measures. It is also important to choose a measure that will provide valid information. School psychologists must remember that although an instrument may have adequate psychometric properties, it is not necessarily valid for the purpose or the populations for which it is being used. For example, an IQ measure may be a valid measure of current intellectual functioning, but it is not a valid measure of whether a child has impairments in reading. An intelligence test normed on an American, English-speaking population may be a valid measure of current intellectual functioning for a child who is a U.S. citizen and a native English speaker. It is likely not a valid measure of current intellectual functioning for a child who recently emigrated from Mexico and speaks little English. When interpreting results, it is also important to remember that no decisions should be made on the basis of one data point (e.g., one test score) alone. Results from the assessment must be interpreted within the context of other information. For example, how the child approached the task is important to consider: Did the child rush through items and complain about being there, or was the child focused and on task? Are there other pieces of information that may argue against a certain conclusion? For example, perhaps a child scored poorly on an IQ measure but has always obtained adequate grades in school and complained of receiving little sleep the night before the test. In this case, it seems likely that the results from the IQ measure may underestimate the child's true abilities— perhaps because of his or her extreme fatigue.

Historically, school psychologists have had little choice when selecting an IQ measure, but an increasing number of such measures are being developed, and many of the newer tests bear little resemblance to the traditional IQ measures. Even with the increasing availability of measures, the Wechsler Intelligence Scale for Children, now in its fourth edition (WISC-IV; Wechsler, 2003), remains the measure with which most clinicians are familiar. Parallel measures for young children (Wechsler Preschool and Primary Scales of Intelligence—Third Edition; Wechsler, 2002) and adults (Wechsler Adult Intelligence Scale—Fourth Edition; Wechsler, 2008) are also commonly used, although less so in schools because of the age of the school clientele. The WISC-IV has undergone some significant revisions from its earlier versions in terms of its factor structure. On the current version of the WISC, a Full Scale IQ score is obtained as well as index scores in four areas: Verbal Comprehension, Perceptual Reasoning, Working Memory, and Processing Speed. The WISC-IV contains 15 individual subtests, 10 of which contribute to the overall or Full Scale IQ score. The WISC-IV is considered to have excellent reliability and strong validity (Sattler, 2008). As reported in the manual and by Sattler, factor analyses support the general factors on the WISC-IV.

Another IQ measure with a long history is the Stanford–Binet, currently in its fifth version (SB-V; Roid, 2003). Like the WISC-IV, the Stanford–Binet has a Full Scale IQ score as well as a several composite scores (Fluid Reasoning, Knowledge, Quantitative Reasoning, Visual Spatial Processing, and Working Memory). Verbal and nonverbal IQ scores can also be obtained. However, Sattler (2008) notes that although factor-analytic studies have found support for a general factor on the SB-V, neither a two-factor nor a five-factor model has been supported at all ages.

The Kaufman Assessment Battery for Children (K-ABC-II; Kaufman & Kaufman, 2004a) provides users with two theoretical models (the Luria neuropsychological model and CHC theory) that can be used to interpret the results of this measure. The K-ABC-II is purported by the authors to be more culturally fair than other traditional measures of IQ; it attempts to achieve this fairness by limiting verbal instructions and responses as well as using items with limited cultural content. Sattler (2008) reports that the K-ABC-II has satisfactory reliability and validity, with factor analyses supporting a general factor as well as specific factors.

The Woodcock–Johnson Tests of Cognitive Abilities (WJ-III-Cog; Woodcock, McGrew, & Mather, 2001b) was co-normed with the Woodcock–Johnson Tests of Achievement (Woodcock, McGrew, & Mather, 2001a). The WJ-III-Cog is based on the CHC theory of intelligence, with subtests designed to target factors of intelligence as outlined in this theory (McGrew & Woodcock, 2001). As noted by Sattler (2008), reliability and validity of this measure are strong, with factor-analytic support for the WJ-III-COG supporting the CHC model. Based on anecdotal data from individuals employed in school districts, the WJ-III-Cog seems to be increasing in use.

The Differential Ability Scales (DAS-II; Elliot, 2007) is another standardized measure of intellectual ability that is used with some frequency. Sattler (2008) reports that the measure has excellent reliability and strong validity. However, he notes that factor-analytic studies do not consistently replicate all DAS-II factors.

In addition to these more traditional measures of IQ, which tend to have a significant verbal component to them, are newer, "nonverbal" measures of intelligence designed to rely less heavily on verbal skills. Some of these measures include the Wechsler Nonverbal Scale of Ability (Wechsler & Naglieri, 2006); the Universal Nonverbal Intelligence Test (Bracken & McCallum, 1998), the Leiter International Performance Scale—Revised (Roid & Miller, 1997), and the Comprehensive Test of Nonverbal Intelligence (Hammill, Pearson, & Weiderholt, 2009). These nonverbal tests have gained in popularity as school populations have become more diverse, with larger non-English-speaking populations. Nonverbal tests can also be helpful when evaluating children with limited language abilities resulting from disabilities. Although nonverbal measures of intelligence correlate substantially with more traditional measures of intelligence and thus appear to be still measuring the theoretical construct of general intelligence, significant variability still exists in the psychometric properties of nonverbal measures. Users should be cautious when selecting nonverbal tests and ensure that the test they choose has been adequately standardized and normed and has strong psychometric properties (Bracken & Naglieri, 2003).

Assessment of Academic Skills

In contrast to the assessment of intellectual abilities, relatively less controversy surrounds achievement testing. This situation likely occurs in part because achievement tests are considered to have more "face validity" than IQ measures. They are intended to measure current academic performance, and the subtests on these measures clearly involve basic academic skills such as reading, math, and writing. However, as noted, in recent years, discussion of how best to evaluate LDs, and therefore also how to evaluate academic skills, has grown. Traditionally, academic skills were evaluated via standardized, norm-referenced measures of achievement. Increasingly, though, alternative methods of assessment such as curriculum-based assessment (CBA) and curriculum-based measurement (CBM), a specific type of CBA procedures (as discussed further later) have been growing in popularity, and as the RTI movement has become more mainstream in schools, we expect the use of CBA procedures to increase over time.

It is interesting to note that although texts such as the most recent editions of *Best Practices in School Psychology* (Thomas & Grimes, 2008) and *Handbook of School Psychology* (Reynolds & Gutkin, 2009) include specific chapters on intellectual assessment, they contain no specific general chapters on the assessment of academic skills, only chapters on the use of CBM (and the *Handbook* briefly covers academic achievement testing within the same chapter as assessment of intelligence). Although historically standardized achievement tests have been widely used, the use of CBA methods is increasing. School psychologists who responded to Wilson and Reschly's (1996) survey indicated that they were using standardized achievement tests much more frequently than they were using CBA/CBM methods. In this survey, the three most commonly used achievement measures were used, on average, approximately eight times per month, and CBA/CBM methods were used only once per month. In a more recent survey, school psychologists also reported using standardized achievement tests more often than CBA methods (Chafouleas, Riley-Tillman, & Eckert, 2003). However, Shapiro, Angello, and Eckert (2004) indicated that more school psychologists reported using curriculum-based methods in

2000 (54%) than in 1990 (46%). In addition, school psychologists who had recently completed their graduate training were much more likely to have received training in CBA methods than were those who had been in the workforce for some time. Shapiro et al. (2004) reported that, of school psychologists who have been working 1 to 3 years, 90% had received training in CBA during their graduate education, whereas less than 20% of those in the workforce 13 years or longer had received training in CBA in their graduate programs. Training in CBA and the use of CBA methods have been noted to be significantly correlated, and school psychologists do rate CBA methods as acceptable; in fact, these methods have been rated as more acceptable than norm-referenced measures of achievement (Chafouleas et al., 2003). Given that school psychologists seem open to the use of CBA methods and that they are increasingly receiving training in these methods, and that RTI models (which make use of CBA methods) are increasing in schools, it seems likely that CBA methods will continue to increase in use over time.

In the following sections, we discuss the use of both standardized, norm-referenced measures of academic skills and CBA. Although school psychologists should be familiar with these assessment techniques, it should be noted that in many school districts it is not the school psychologist who is responsible for assessing a child's academic achievement but rather the special education teacher or an educational diagnostician. However, even in such districts, school psychologists will need to be familiar with these measures to aid in interpretation and intervention planning.

Standardized, Norm-Referenced Achievement Tests

As noted, although CBA methods appear to be gaining in use, standardized, norm-referenced achievement tests are still frequently used to evaluate academic skills. Some of the more common measures include the Woodcock–Johnson Tests of Achievement—Third Edition (WJ-III; Woodcock et al., 2001a), the Wechsler Individual Achievement Test–Third Edition (WIAT-III; Wechsler, 2009), the Wide Range Achievement Test—Fourth Edition (WRAT-4; Wilkinson & Robertson, 2006), the Peabody Individual Achievement Test—Revised (PIAT-R; Markwardt, 1989, 1997), and the Kaufman Test of Educational Achievement—Second Edition (K-TEA-II; Kaufman & Kaufman, 2004b). These measures all include subtests intended to assess a variety of achievement abilities (e.g., reading, math, written language, oral language). In addition to these broad measures of academic achievement are measures that assess academic ability in one specific area. Examples of such instruments include KeyMath—3 (Connolly, 2007), Woodcock Reading Mastery Tests—Revised (Woodcock, 1987, 1998), and the Gray Oral Reading Test—Fourth Edition (Wiederholt & Bryant, 2001). These single-subject tests are used less frequently than the multiple-subject tests and are typically used to follow up on problems noted when using a comprehensive achievement measure. Obviously, the advantage to using a comprehensive test is that one can obtain information on a student's abilities in a variety of academic areas with the use of a single assessment instrument. However, a single-subject test might be used when the referral question relates directly to a specific problem or when more in-depth information is needed in a certain area (Stetson, Stetson, & Sattler, 2001).

Two trends in the development of comprehensive achievement tests have become evident over the past several years. One is that achievement tests are increasingly being developed to match specific IDEIA categories of learning disabilities (oral expression, listening comprehension, written expression, basic reading skills, reading comprehension, mathematics calculation, and mathematics reasoning). The other trend is that achievement tests are increasingly being co-normed with parallel IQ tests, theoretically for a more accurate comparison of whether there is a significant discrepancy between a student's intellectual ability and achievement performance. For example, the K-TEA-II, WJ-III, and WIAT-III all have subtests that match the seven areas of learning disabilities identified in IDEIA. Each of these tests is also linked to an IQ test, either through co-norming (as was done with the K-TEA-II and K-ABC-II and the WJ-III tests of achievement and cognitive ability) or via administering intelligence tests to a subset of those in the achievement test sample (as was done with the WIAT-III and associated Wechsler intelligence scales). Both the PIAT-R and WRAT-4 are more limited in scope than these newer measures of academic achievement. Most notably, neither has a subtest that assesses oral language. The WRAT-4, for example, contains only four subtests measuring comprehension, reading, spelling, and arithmetic.

A complete review of the available tests of achievement is beyond the scope of this chapter. However, it should be noted that each of the comprehensive multiple-subject tests of achievement described here has adequate psychometric properties. Which of these measures one ends up using (if a standardized, norm-referenced test is being used at all) may depend in part on personal preference. School psychologists should also make sure they stay updated on the literature regarding psychometric properties of the achievement measures they may use to ensure they are selecting those that are most psychometrically sound.

Curriculum-Based Assessment/Measurement

As noted, CBA/CBM (a type of CBA with emphasis placed on progress monitoring) methods are rapidly gaining in use as alternatives to standardized, norm-referenced achievement testing. CBM involves a set of specific procedures that are technically adequate, that include standardized measurement tasks, and that have specific administration and scoring guidelines (Deno, 2003). CBM methods are intended to be time efficient and generally consist of probes that last a maximum of several minutes.

As outlined in Shinn (2008, pp. 245–246), some of the common CBM measures include:

1. Reading: The child reads aloud from a text for 1 minute. The total number of words read correctly is calculated.
2. Math: The child completes math problems during a 2- to 4-minute timing. The number of digits correct is calculated.
3. Spelling: The child writes dictated words for 2 minutes. The number of correct words and correct letter sequences are calculated.
4. Written expression: The child is provided with a story-starter and then asked to write for 3 minutes. The number of words written and spelled correctly as well as the number of correct word sequences can be calculated.

For more details on specific CBM methods, readers may want to consult Hosp, Hosp, and Howell (2007).

Although school psychologists often are not involved in the administration of CBM probes (teachers are), they must understand the data obtained from such probes and understand how to use these data in making decisions regarding services for children within the school context. As Shinn (2008) notes, CBM techniques are increasingly being used in the schools and are an integral part of the RTI approach to identifying children who are struggling and may benefit from additional services. They are also an important part of monitoring students' progress when more intensive interventions are implemented.

Within the RTI/problem-solving model, CBM techniques are seen as an integral part of identifying children who may benefit from additional or specialized instruction as well as tracking the progress of students over time to ensure that the instruction they are receiving is beneficial to them. Increasingly, schools are adopting programs in which all students are screened via CBM probes. For children who do poorly on these screenings, additional supports are put in place. As Shinn (2008) discusses, CBM may be used within a three-tiered model as follows:

- Tier 1: benchmark assessment three to four times per year to help identify students at risk; monitoring of student progress across the year.
- Tier 2: strategic monitoring on a monthly basis.
- Tier 3: frequent (e.g., weekly) progress monitoring on individualized goals.

One example of a specific CBM system that is widely used in the schools is the Dynamic Indicators of Basic Early Literacy Skills (DIBELS) system developed by researchers at the University of Oregon (for more information, see the DIBELS homepage: *dibels.uoregon. edu*). DIBELS is intended to be used to assess several of the "big ideas" in basic literacy skills, including phonological awareness (the ability to hear and manipulate sounds into words), alphabetic principle (the ability to link letters to sounds and to form words), and fluency with connected text (the ability to effortlessly read words in context). The DIBELS system includes brief measures that address each of these areas. The measures are standardized and can be used over time to help monitor the reading progress of students (Kaminski, Cummings, Powell-Smith, & Good, 2008; see DIBELS homepage). Five main measures are used in the DIBELS system. These include two that measure phonological awareness: Initial Sounds Fluency (in which the child is asked to identify out of four pictures one that begins with a certain letter) and Phoneme Segmentation Fluency (in which the student is asked to verbally break words into their individual phonemes). Nonsense Word Fluency is a measure of alphabetic principle and requires students to read nonsense words presented on paper or to verbally produce the letter sounds in the nonsense word. Oral Reading Fluency is a measure of fluency with connected text in which students are required to read passages aloud. Letter Naming Fluency, in which students are asked to name letters presented on paper, is intended to provide a measure of risk for early literacy problems (see DIBELS homepage). The DIBELS system is intended to be used with children in kindergarten through sixth grade. The system contains benchmark goals for the beginning, middle, and end of the year to help determine whether students are achieving at an adequate level. Students considered to be at risk would be provided with instructional support to attempt to increase their literacy skills (Kaminski et al., 2008; see DIBELS homepage).

Given the significant research regarding CBM procedures over the past quarter-century, the strong advocates for the use of CBM procedures in the evaluation of student performance, and the link to academic interventions, it seems likely that this momentum will continue and that CBM will increasingly be used as a means of assessing academic achievement and, more important, of students' responses to intervention. This method, which is viewed as highly acceptable by most school psychologists, more clearly ties assessment to intervention than do most other methods of assessing academic skills.

Brief Experimental Analysis

Although functional assessment methods have historically been tied more to behavior problems than to academic problems, this methodology has also been used to address academic issues. Daly, Witt, Martens, and Dool (1997) describe a functional approach to understanding academic failure as one that relates "academic performance to aspects of the classroom instruction that precede and follow student performance" (p. 555). They argue that because aspects of the classroom are external to the child, viewing academic difficulties from this perspective allows one to identify areas for instructional intervention. Daly et al. (1997) discuss five "reasonable hypotheses" about why students perform poorly from a functional perspective: (1) The student does not want to do the work, (2) the student has not spent enough time on the work, (3) the student has not had enough help to successfully complete the work, (4) the student has not previously had to do the work in the requested manner, and (5) the work is too hard for the student. If the function of the difficulty is identified, interventions can be developed that match (e.g., if the student does not want or is not motivated to do the work, provide incentives for completion of the work).

When using a functional approach, hypotheses regarding the function of the academic problem are formed and are then evaluated using mini-experiments in a brief experimental analysis procedure (Jones, Wickstrom, & Daly, 2008). CBA techniques are integral to this process, because the evaluator must be able to make quick, repeated assessments of a child's performance under different conditions. For example, a student's reading level may be assessed under several different academic interventions, each tied to a functional hypothesis (e.g., with a reinforcer for completing work; with repeated practice with correction). After the student's performance is assessed under these different conditions, the one that produces the most benefit is chosen to implement in an ongoing manner. CBM probes continue to be used to monitor the effectiveness of the chosen intervention.

Assessment of Social–Emotional and Behavioral Functioning

The assessment of social–emotional and behavioral problems has typically not generated as much controversy and discussion within the field of school psychology as has the assessment of intellectual ability and academic achievement. Likely this gap has to do with the fewer number of children being served under the IDEIA-2004 category of emotional disturbance (7.9% of all children in special education in fall 2004; U.S. Department of Education, 2009) compared with the number of children being served under the category of LDs (46.4% of all children in special education in fall 2004; U.S. Department of Education, 2009). However, there are signs that attention to this topic is picking up. This trend is likely due to several factors, including an increased recognition that school psychologists have expertise in mental health issues as well as academic issues. In addition, the number of children identified as having attention-deficit/hyperactivity disorder (ADHD), a disorder that requires an assessment of behavior, is increasing. Although there are no exact numbers on school-based evaluations for ADHD, many children with ADHD who are eligible for special education services receive them under the "other health impaired" (OHI) category, and the number of children being served in this category has risen significantly over time, with 8.4% of all students in special education now classified under OHI (U.S. Department of Education, 2009). In fact, only the

OHI and autism categories have seen a significant increase over time in the percentage of children served under these categories (from 1995 to 2004 the percentage of all students receiving service as OHI increased from 0.2 to 0.8 and the percentage of students receiving services in the autism category increased from 0.1 to 0.3; U.S. Department of Education, 2009).

As with the other areas of assessment, some controversy exists regarding the utility of certain measures in this area. Much of the controversy centers on the use of projective assessment techniques (which almost always have significant problems with test–retest reliability and construct validity; see Merrell, 2008, for a discussion) versus the use of other techniques considered by many to be reliable and valid measures of emotional and behavioral functioning (e.g., observations, rating scales, functional assessment methods). Although earlier surveys of school psychologists' assessment practices indicated that behavioral rating scales were used less frequently than projective measures (e.g., Wilson & Reschly, 1996), this trend seems to be reversing. Hosp and Reschly (2002) reported that school psychologists administer slightly more behavior rating scales per month (17.2) than projective measures (15.2), and Shapiro and Heick (2004) reported that behavior rating scales were the most common assessment method used in cases involving a referral for emotional or behavioral problems.

In addition to behavior rating scales and projective measures, numerous other procedures can be used in the assessment of emotional and behavioral problems. These include interviews (with parents, teachers, and the child), observations (which may be either informal or formal), and self-report measures. In addition, functional assessment methods have been gaining in popularity over the past 5 to 10 years and are currently seen as key in linking assessment to intervention in the area of emotional and behavioral problems. Each of these methods is described briefly here. However, as with the discussion of intellectual and achievement measures, this discussion is not intended to be a comprehensive overview of these methods but instead an introduction. School psychologists should consult other sources (e.g., Merrell, 2008; Shapiro & Kratochwill, 2000, 2002) for more detailed information.

Projective Techniques

We discuss projective assessment techniques first because they have the longest history in the assessment of emotional and behavioral problems. Their use dates back to at least the early 1920s, and, by some accounts, projective drawing techniques were used as long ago as the 1890s (Merrell, 2008). Projective techniques include drawing techniques (e.g., Draw-a-Person, House–Tree–Person, Kinetic Family Drawing), thematic techniques (e.g., Children's Apperception Test [Bellak & Bellak, 1949]; Roberts Apperception Test for Children [McArthur & Roberts, 1982]), and sentence completion techniques. These methods are all based on the assumption that, when presented with ambiguous stimuli, children will "project" their own feelings, thoughts, and emotional conflicts onto these stimuli. As noted, the use of projective techniques by school psychologists has historically been very common. In Wilson and Reschly's (1996) survey, the Draw-a-Person test was the fourth most commonly used measure overall (not just for evaluating children referred for emotional and behavioral problems); House–Tree–Person was sixth; and Kinetic Family Drawing was eighth. In a more recent survey (Hosp & Reschly, 2002), projective methods were the second most common assessment procedures used overall, just behind rating scales and ahead of IQ measures. Shapiro and Heick (2004) indicate that about one-third of school psychologists regularly use projective methods for children referred for emotional and behavioral problems, and that about one-third never use projective methods. In another recent survey of NASP members (Hojnoski, Morrison, Brown, & Matthews, 2006), on average, school psychologists reported using projective measures in only 10.6% of their social–emotional assessments. Sixty-two percent of the respondents reported never using projective measures in social–emotional assessments, leaving 38% who indicated some use of the measures for social–emotional assessments. In addition, 61% of respondents reported using sentence completion tasks in assessments in general.

Although projective methods continue to be commonly used by many school psychology practitioners, they are certainly not without controversy. In fact, other than IQ measures, projective measures have likely created the most controversy within the field of psychology (although, unlike with IQ measures, there has been a lack of controversy regarding the use of these methods among non-psychologists). The controversy regarding these methods stems from questions regarding the validity of these techniques: Do they really measure what they say they measure? Most projective measures lack adequate psychometric properties, and many professionals argue that such measures do not reflect internalized feelings but are simply a sample of overt behavior. Others argue that at least some of the projective techniques have changed considerably over time (the Rorschach with its more objective scoring system being the prime example) and that one should not dismiss all projective measures simply because the measures as a group lack adequate data to support their use (Prevatt, 1999). However, given the poor validity of many projective measures and the wide availability of other measures with superior psychometric properties, we do not believe that projective measures should be routinely used in the schools. They provide little useful information in terms of either diagnostic decision making or treatment planning. They may be helpful in building rapport with a child (they are typically nonthreatening to a student and are sometimes perceived as fun) and may help generate hypotheses for further evaluation with measures with adequate psychometric properties. However, when used in this fashion, these measures cease to be truly assessment measures. Therefore, in our opinion, the use of projective measures is outdated, and they provide little to no useful information, either in terms of identifying problem areas or linking assessment to intervention.

Behavior Rating Scales

Although behavior rating scales have become increasingly popular (and psychometrically sound) over the past several decades, their use also dates back to at least the early part of the 1900s. Wickman (1928) discussed behavior problems as rated by children's teachers and divided problems into "attacking" traits and "withdrawing" traits, which are similar to our conceptualization of externalizing and internalizing problems today. However, it was not until much more recently that behavior rating scales became the well-standardized and normed tests that they are today. In 1973 Spivak and Swift reviewed the available behavior rating scales and found that, although there were 19 such measures, only three had norms and reliability information. Today there are numerous behavior rating scales that are well normed, are based on large standardization samples, and have extensive reliability and validity information.

Behavior rating scales are generally divided into two categories: broad band and narrow band. Broad-band measures, such as the Child Behavior Checklist (CBCL) and Teacher's Report Form (TRF) that are part of the Achenbach System of Empirically Based Assessment (Achenbach & Rescorla, 2001) and Behavioral Assessment System for Children (BASC; Reynolds & Kamphaus, 2004), measure behaviors in a variety of domains and include subscales that evaluate both externalizing (e.g., aggression) and internalizing (e.g., anxiety, depression) problems. Narrow-band measures assess functioning in just one domain (e.g., ADHD, autism). Broad-band measures are particularly useful in gathering a significant amount of information in a relatively short period of time. However, because broad-band scales do not provide detailed information on specific areas, narrow-band scales are typically used to obtain more information on problems noted on broad-band scales.

Rating scales are considered to be objective measures, given that the assessor does not interpret responses to individual items nor insert his or her potential bias in the rating process. However, it should be noted that rating scales provide the point of view of the person completing the scale, and that different informants often do not agree on the severity (or even the presence) of behaviors. Thus, although it is an advantage that rating scales can be used to gather information from multiple sources and that many rating scales have parallel parent and teacher versions, it is up to the evaluator to integrate the findings from the scales.

As noted, behavior rating scales are the most common assessment method that school psychologists currently report using for children referred for emotional and behavioral problems (Shapiro & Heick, 2004). This finding is encouraging given the positive qualities that behavior rating scales have. However, school psychologists must ensure that they are using measures with adequate psychometric properties and that are germane to the referral question. In addition, it is all too easy with behavior rating scales to say "Levi scored high on measures of ADHD so he must have ADHD." School psychologists must remember that scores do not dictate diagnoses. Scores on behavior rating scales provide data that can help in the diagnostic process, but these scores must be considered in the larger context (e.g., Are the symptoms impairing? Have they been present for a significant amount of time and since early childhood? Can the symptoms be better accounted for by something other than ADHD?). In addition, behavior rating scales do not provide information that is directly linked to interventions. Behavior rating scales are more helpful in assessing the severity of a problem (e.g., Does Levi have more symptoms of ADHD than his peers?) but are less useful in providing direction on what to do about those problems.

Interviews

Interviews are a commonly used method of obtaining information related to a child's social–emotional functioning, with informal clinical interviews being the most common method. Clinical interviews involve the practitioner asking the interviewee (e.g., child, parent, teacher) a series of questions regarding symptom presentation and background information in order both to obtain more information on the referral problem and to put this information in a broader context. In addition to the commonly used clinical interviews, there are also structured and semistructured interviews. Structured interviews are highly scripted and typically involve the interviewer asking a series of yes–no questions regarding the presence of symptoms. Although such interviews are relatively common in research, they are rarely used in clinical practice. Semistructured interviews allow the interviewer slightly more leeway in questioning and typically consist of open-ended as well as structured questions (Merrell, 2008).

Clinical interviews are useful for several reasons. They allow the clinician to obtain a large amount of information on a wide variety of topics at one time in a flexible format.

The flexible format of the clinical interview allows the clinician to build rapport with the interviewee. This is one reason interviews are typically conducted as the first step in the assessment process. Interviews can also be used to obtain information from different sources and to informally compare the perceptions of the problems as well as to clarify issues. As is discussed in more detail later in this chapter, interviews can also be used to help conduct a functional assessment by asking questions about antecedents and consequences of behaviors. Although interviews have numerous advantages, as with all assessment methods, they also have disadvantages. Clearly, with informal clinical interviews, there is no way to evaluate their psychometric properties, and it is likely that different interviewers will obtain somewhat different information from the same respondent because of differences in questioning style, rapport built, and so forth. It is also possible that interviewers will have some biases that will color their interpretation of the information presented. For example, if the interviewer has already formed an impression about the child, he or she may ask questions that are geared toward supporting this impression. With young children in particular, interviews can be difficult. Children may have difficulties verbalizing thoughts and feelings, and young children can easily become confused regarding temporal aspects of events. It is very important when interviewing not to ask leading questions but instead to make questions open ended (e.g., instead of saying "You like school, don't you?" say "Tell me what you think about school"; Hughes & Baker, 1990).

Although interviews are standard practice when conducting evaluations in clinical settings and are used frequently by school psychologists, we believe they are underutilized in school psychology. Shapiro and Heick (2004) indicated that only about one-third of school psychologists regularly use interviews with parents and teachers for children referred for emotional and behavioral problems, and that about 20% do not use interviews at all. Involving parents and teachers in the assessment process is critically important, and interviews are an easy method to solicit this involvement as well as to obtain significant background information on the child. In fact, given the many assessment advantages of interviewing, we believe that the use of this method among school psychologists should be standard practice.

Observations

Observations are another commonly used assessment procedure. Shapiro and Heick (2004) reported that school psychologists complete observations on most of the students they evaluate for emotional and behavioral problems. Observations are typically done in a child's classroom and often involve the assessment of several key behaviors of concern. Observations provide the assessor with a direct picture of a child's problems (as well as positive behaviors). In addition, the observer is able to see the child's behaviors in the context in which they naturally occur. This ecological–contextual information may be particularly helpful when conducting a functional assessment. The observer can obtain information on the child's behavior as well as the context in which the behavior occurs and the antecedents and consequences of the behavior.

Although observations have clear advantages and we believe they are an important part of the assessment process, they are also relatively time consuming and can require extensive training. It is impossible to obtain data on many behaviors at once with observational techniques, as can be done with interviews and behavior rating scales. In addition, although theoretically observations are objective (the observer directly sees the behavior), the observer can bias the observation results by focusing on negative (or positive) behaviors. It is generally best to observe several behaviors and to include at least one positive behavior. It is also important to observe comparison peers to help determine whether the observed behavior of the child is unusual in the context of the child's classroom and peers (Merrell, 2008).

Self-Report Measures

Self-report measures include both rating scale-type measures (e.g., the Youth Self-Report [Achenbach & Rescorla, 2001], which is the parallel self-report measure to the CBCL), as well as measures of "personality." The rating scale-type measures are similar to those completed by parents and teachers, and most broad-band parent–teacher rating scales have parallel self-report forms. It is also common to assess internalizing constructs such as anxiety and depression with narrow-band scales (e.g., Children's Depression Inventory [Kovacs, 1992]; Multidimensional Anxiety Scale for Children [March, 1997]). The most common self-report personality measure for adolescents is the Minnesota Multiphasic Personality Inventory—Adolescent (MMPI-A; Butcher et al., 1992). Although this instrument is used extensively in clinical practice, its use in the field of school psychology is still relatively limited for several reasons, including a lack of emphasis on this measure in training programs, the focus of this tool on pathology, the length of time it takes for a child to complete the measure (about 90 minutes), and the relatively limited age range of children evaluated in the schools (it is generally recommended that this test not be given to children younger than 14). In Shapiro and Heick's (2004) study, school psychologists reported commonly using self-report rating scales but uncommonly using measures of personality assessment such as the MMPI-A. In fact, 70% of school psychologists reported that they had not used such measures at all in their previous 10 evaluations.

Self-report measures are advantageous because they allow clinicians to assess children's perceptions of the problems. Self-report measures may be particularly helpful when evaluating internalizing symptoms, because these symptoms are ones that frequently cannot be observed by others. Children do have to have adequate reading abilities to complete self-report measures, and for this reason most self-report measures cannot be administered to children younger than 8. Although self-report measures are helpful in providing the child's perspective on issues, self-report ratings typically do not correlate highly with ratings from parent and teacher measures. Thus, the clinician is left to make sense of these differences and attempt to determine the "true" presence of symptoms. As with informant-based rating scales, self-report measures are more useful in assessing the severity of a child's problem compared with his or her peers than in identifying specific behaviors of concern for the child that might be targeted in an intervention.

Functional Behavioral Assessment

In much the same way that the use of CBA methods has been increasing for evaluating academic problems, FBA methods are increasingly being used to link assessment to intervention for emotional and behavioral problems. However, according to Shapiro and Heick's (2004) survey, such methods are by no means commonplace. One-quarter of school psychologists reported not using such methods at all in their previous 10 evaluations of children suspected of having emotional and behavioral problems, and only 14% reported using these methods in almost all of their last 10 evaluations.

Functional assessment procedures are a broad group of procedures that are based on the concept of identifying the behavioral function, or purpose, of a behavior. In functional assessment, the antecedents and consequences of the behavior are identi-fied, with the goal being to understand the environmental conditions that maintain the behavior in question. Through a better understanding of the relationship between the behavior of the individual and the contextual factors that precipitate and reinforce the behavior, interventions can be implemented that attempt to change the behavior by addressing the function (Steege & Watson, 2009). For example, if a student is disruptive in class (e.g., talks to other students, is out of his seat) and consistently receives attention (in the form of teacher reprimands) for this behavior but no positive feedback for appro-priate classroom behaviors, we might hypothesize that the function of the behavior is to obtain attention. Our intervention recommendations would follow from this hypoth-esis and include the suggestion to cease providing attention for the disruptive behavior. Instead, this behavior should be ignored and attention should be provided to more posi-tive behaviors (e.g., raising his hand to speak).

Steege and Watson (2009) outlined three forms of FBA: *indirect, direct descriptive,* and *functional behavioral analysis.* With indirect FBA, interviews as well as rating scales and records reviews are used to identify and describe the behavior of concern and to generate hypotheses regarding the function of the behavior. As described by Gresham, Watson, and Skinner (2001, p. 161), functional assessment interviews have four main purposes: (1) to identify and define the behavior of concern; (2) to identify anteced-ents of the target behavior; (3) to obtain initial information on the possible function of the target behavior; and (4) to identify behaviors that can be substituted for the target behavior. These purposes are accomplished by asking questions about what the behav-ior looks like as well as the context and setting in which the behavior occurs. Although indirect FBA can provide valuable information, direct descriptive FBA, in which obser-vations are conducted, should be used to help better identify functional relationships between the behaviors of concern and environmental factors. Observations allow the school psychologist to directly observe the behavior and to see the antecedents and con-sequences associated with the behavior in the context in which the behavior occurs. However, even observations do not allow one to confirm that a certain function is main-taining the behavior. In order to confirm hypotheses regarding behavioral function, a functional analysis would need to be conducted. This involves mini-experiments in which the behavior of concern is observed under different conditions (e.g., providing attention to the behavior, allowing escape from a task following the behavior). Although true functional analysis procedures are relatively common in inpatient clinical settings in which functional methods are employed, these procedures are less common in school settings.

The FBA framework encompasses three functions of behavior. These include obtaining attention or access to desired activities or tangibles for engaging in a certain behavior, escaping or avoiding an aversive task, and sensory stimulation (Steege & Wat-son, 2009). It is important to remember that attention can be both positive (e.g., get-ting peers to laugh at a joke) or negative (e.g., teacher reprimands) in content and still positively reinforce the behavior in question. As long as the consequence (in this case, attention) increases the likelihood that the behavior will occur again, the consequence is considered to be positively reinforcing.

The information obtained from the functional assessment is used to develop a plan for intervention that addresses the function of the behavior. For example, as noted, if it is hypothesized that a student's disruptive behavior during class is reinforced by attention from his or her teacher, we would provide attention to positive, on-task behaviors and remove attention from disruptive behaviors. Because functional assessment techniques lead directly to interventions, they have significantly more treatment utility than many other methods of assessment. Functional assessment methods are particularly useful with behaviors that are externalized (e.g., oppositional behaviors) but are less useful with internalized behaviors (e.g., depression) that are not clearly tied to environmental contingencies. Although functional assessment methods were initially developed with children with severe behavior problems who were institutionalized, they have been adequately adapted to the school setting, and we expect that their use will continue to increase as more training programs emphasize these methods and more clinicians experience the utility of such methods in tying assessment to intervention.

Diagnosis and Classification in the Schools

As with other assessment issues discussed thus far in this chapter, a lack of agreement exists in the field of school psychology on the usefulness of providing diagnostic and/or classification labels for children. By way of definition, *classification* is the term typically used in the schools when assigning special education labels (e.g., LD, emotional disturbance), whereas *diagnosis* is typically used in clinical practice when assigning *Diagnostic and Statistical Manual of Mental Disorders* (fourth ed., text rev. [DSM-IV-TR] American Psychiatric Association, 2000) labels (e.g., ADHD, separation anxiety disorder). However, these terms are often used interchangeably, and they have in common the assignment of a label to a child.

One concern regarding the use of diagnostic and classification systems is that they may lead to "self-fulfilling prophecies." For example, a child labeled as having an LD may cease to try as hard and his or her parents and teachers may cease to expect as much, leading to a decline in academic performance. Concerns have also been expressed that the process of diagnosing or classifying children artificially places them in categories that are not reliable. In addition, because diagnostic systems typically used require categorical decisions to be made (i.e., either the child has the problem or does not), individuals with the same label can display different behaviors and varying levels of behavior severity, and children with "subclinical" problems (who may benefit from treatment) may not receive a classification because a certain threshold of symptoms is not met. One of the most commonly leveled criticisms against diagnostic systems in the field of school psychology is that they are not directly linked to intervention (Dowdy, Mays, Kamphaus, & Reynolds, 2009; Merrell, 2008). Although we acknowledge that there are significant problems with classification systems, we do believe that they serve a purpose. In many systems, classifications are required for individuals to access and/or be reimbursed for services. For example, although states can provide noncategorical services under IDEIA, most states use the categories provided in the federal guidelines. This situation means that, for a student to receive special education services, he or she *must* be assigned to a certain special education category (although it should also be noted that there may be a variety of services available to children that do not require special education classification). In the private practice sector, almost all insurance companies require a DSM-IV diagnosis for insurance reimbursement. Although these issues of access to services are very practical and many would argue that we should work toward changing these system requirements, it seems unlikely that significant change will occur any time in the near future.

Practical issues aside, there are other, more theoretically based arguments for the use of diagnostic systems. Such systems do allow for better communication between professionals (Dowdy et al., 2009; Merrell, 2008). For example, if a school psychologist is talking with the pediatrician of a child who has been diagnosed with ADHD, both can use this term and know they are referring to generally the same set of symptoms and that the symptoms are not better accounted for by another disorder (such as depression). Although there is variability in the specific behaviors exhibited by children with ADHD, the use of this term nevertheless provides some common understanding. Of course, this enhanced communication does assume that the diagnosis was correctly made. If the diagnosis was made in error, the communication ceases to be helpful and meaningful. In addition, although we acknowledge that classification systems do not directly lead to interventions, we believe they can help guide the selection of appropriate intervention techniques. As noted in Chapter 7, increasing emphasis is being placed on EBP and "empirically supported interventions" (i.e., those that have well-conducted research to support their use) in the psychology literature. The participants in the studies that support these interventions are typically labeled in some manner, either with specific DSM-IV labels (e.g., children with separation anxiety disorder) or with general categories (e.g., children with anxiety). Thus, by classifying a child, we can know in general what treatments might be effective for that child. Our job is then to implement the treatment in a manner that is compatible with the child's specific symptom presentation and the context in which these symptoms are being exhibited. This may involve conducting additional assessments to better understand the function of the child's behavior in the context in which the behavior is occurring. It is important to remember that just because most children within a certain diagnostic category respond to a certain treatment (e.g., the majority of children with anxiety respond positively to cognitive-behavioral interventions) does not mean that all children with a certain label will respond to a certain treatment. Thus, it is still important to take into account individual differences and to continuously evaluate the effectiveness of an intervention with the individual child.

Although the purpose of an assessment is not always to provide a label for the difficulties a child is experiencing, frequently in schools at least part of the purpose of an evaluation is to determine whether a child meets criteria for a certain special education category. Because of this, school psychologists are often faced with making decisions (as a member of a multidisciplinary team) about the appropriate classification for a child. Thus, regardless of a school psychologist's philosophy on the use of labels, all school psychologists will need to be knowledgeable about classification systems. However, even though assessment may lead to a determination of which, if any, diagnostic labels fit the child's symptom presentation, assessment should also, and more importantly, lead to intervention recommendations. Although it may appear that this state of events would naturally follow (especially given our point that classifications can help lead to intervention selection), this is certainly not always the case. For example, if a child is diagnosed as having ADHD, we know from the research that behavioral interventions are likely to reduce ADHD-related behaviors in the classroom setting. However, we do not know what specific behaviors we should target. Does the child engage in significant out-of-seat behavior? Does the child have difficulty following instructions? Does the child have peer relationship problems because he or she is always acting impulsively? In addition, we do not know the function of these behaviors through the diagnostic process. Is the child engaging in out-of-seat behavior for attention, to escape an aversive task, or as a self-stimulatory behavior? These types of questions must also be answered as part of the assessment process so that, in addition to providing a diagnostic label for a child, we can provide parents and teachers with recommendations about what can be done to help reduce the child's problem behaviors and to increase positive behaviors. Currently, we contend that school psychologists should view the assignment of a classification or diagnosis as one part of the assessment process in many cases, while at the same time realizing that a label by itself is likely to be of minimal benefit to the child and those who interact with the child.

Assessment as a Problem-Solving Process

Much has been written about assessment as a problem-solving process and, as discussed earlier in this chapter as well as in Chapter 7, as RTI procedures have been implemented more broadly, the discussion of assessment within a problem-solving paradigm has increased dramatically. Within this approach, assessment information is collected to guide decision making throughout each of the steps. We strongly believe that this approach to school psychology is the most useful one for effectively addressing the academic and behavioral problems facing today's children and youth. As discussed in Chapter 7, when using the problem-solving model, one seeks to identify the discrepancy between a child's current academic and/or behavioral performance and the desired performance for the child. Given this model, the goal of an evaluation should not simply be to provide numerical values regarding the child's functioning and to choose a category that best fits the child. Rather, the goal is to identify conditions that will enable a child to learn most effectively (Tilly, 2008). Assessment as part of the problem-solving process is directly linked to intervention. This is in contrast to more traditional assessment activities in which assessment is not directly linked to intervention and the goal is typically to make a diagnostic decision. We stress that the traditional approach to assessment is not inherently bad; it just serves a different purpose than the problem-solving approach. In addition, traditional assessment requires a higher degree of inference to generate intervention strategies than does assessment under the problem-solving method, which obtains a direct measure of a student's skills in the context in which they occur. Higher inference is a problem in that the greater the inference, the less confidence we can have that the intervention will be effective in remediating the student's problem (Tilly, 2008).

Next, we outline the problem-solving process of assessment and use a hypothetical example to help illustrate this process. We also provide a graphic representation of this process in Figure 8.1.

Identification of the Problem: The Referral and Clarification

An assessment begins with a referral. Typically, the referral is from a child's teacher or parent. The referral contains some information on the problems of concern but typically does not provide detailed information. For example, the referral issue might be, "Tony is having difficulty learning and attending in class." After receiving the referral, the school psychologist should clarify the nature of the problem with the referring source via an interview. The goal of this interview is to obtain more information on the behaviors of concern, the context in which these behaviors occur, and the desired level of performance. Information should be obtained on the following: specific behaviors of concern, expectancies for the behavior, opportunities for the expected behaviors to occur, how long the problem behaviors have been occurring, situations in which the behaviors occur, situations in which the behaviors do not occur, any changes that have occurred in the child's life, and positive aspects of the child's behaviors. This initial interview can also be used to help clarify the discrepancy between the actual performance of the child and the desired performance.

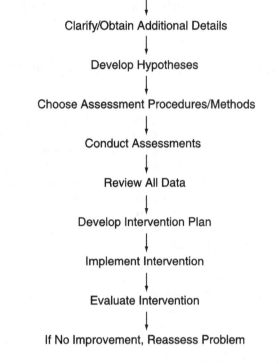

FIGURE 8.1. Problem-solving process in assessment.

In addition to clarifying details regarding the referral problem, the school psychologist should obtain additional background information on the student to help put the behaviors in context and rule out other potentially contributing factors, for example: Does the child have any major health problems? Did the child meet developmental milestones on time? Is the child currently on any medications? This information is most likely obtained via an interview with the child's parents.

Observations of the child may also be conducted by the school psychologist. These observations may help clarify the nature of the problem as well as identify potential antecedents and consequences surrounding the problem.

Analysis of the Problem: Development of Hypotheses and Collection of Assessment Data

Once the referral question has been clarified, the psychologist should develop hypotheses that will guide additional assessment. In our example referral problem, let's assume that there have been no significant changes in Tony's life, that he has no medical problems, and that he has reached major development milestones as expected. He is now in the third grade but has struggled with school since beginning kindergarten. He is currently behind his peers in reading, according to this classroom teacher. In addition, his parents report that he has always been a bit on the active side, and that they have had difficulties getting him to attend to and follow their instructions. His teacher reports many of the same problems. His parents and his teacher agree that they would like to see Tony reading on grade level, being more attentive to academic work, and being more compliant with their requests.

At this point, we conclude that there is a discrepancy between Tony's actual current performance and his desired performance in reading. In a traditional approach to assessment, it is likely that Tony would be administered standardized measures of intellectual ability (e.g., WISC-IV) and achievement (e.g., WJ-III) to determine whether he meets criteria for a learning disability. However, in the problem-solving model, our primary goal is to identify interventions that may help improve Tony's reading skills and decrease his problematic behaviors in the context of his current classroom setting. As discussed earlier in this chapter as well as in Chapter 7, there are a variety of reasons why Tony may not be performing well, including that he does not want to complete his reading assignments, he has not spent enough time on his assignments, he has not had enough help to complete assignments, he has not had to do the tasks in that manner before, or the reading material is too difficult for him. Following the functional approach outlined by Daly et al. (1997), we administer Tony a variety of curriculum-based reading probes under different conditions (e.g., incentives for reading at a certain rate, repeated reading practices), alternating with a baseline probe with no modifications. We ascertain that Tony is reading at the frustrational level in third-grade material but is at the instructional level when reading first-grade material. In addition, Tony's performance improves when he is provided with a reinforcer for improving his performance.

Regarding assessment of Tony's behavioral and attention problems, if our goal was to decide whether Tony's behaviors were symptomatic of ADHD, we would likely have Tony's parents and teachers complete norm-based behavior rating scales. However, as noted earlier, in the problem-solving model, diagnosis is not the focus of our assessment. Thus, to help us learn more about conditions in which Tony exhibits inattentiveness and conditions in which he is on task, we conduct a more detailed classroom observation to obtain additional data on the times when Tony is inattentive and on the antecedents and consequences of this behavior. We note that Tony is frequently off task and inattentive during reading and that the consequence for his behavior is typically to be sent away from the class group, either into the "quiet corner" in the classroom or to an isolated seat in the back of the classroom where the teacher cannot see what he is working on. In an interview with Tony's parents, they reported that they have difficulties getting Tony to do his homework; he often jumps up from the table, attempts to engage his parents in conversations, and doodles on his homework papers. They also noted that he is often noncompliant with their requests in general. They noted that they had tired of repeating their commands and that once they asked him several times to do something, they dropped the request, even if he did not follow through.

Review of Data

Once we have completed our assessments, we compile all the data (including our initial interview data) and attempt to draw some conclusions about the problems present as well as what interventions may be effective in remediating these problems. As noted, Tony read more words per minute when provided with a reinforcer than with no reinforcer and is also finding grade-level reading to be too difficult. Thus, it seems likely that Tony's difficulties with reading are a combination of issues: The reading he is currently assigned is too difficult for him and he is not motivated to complete reading assignments. Observations of Tony in class, as well as interview data from his parents, indicate that he is most likely to be inattentive and off task when engaged in tasks he finds aversive. Typically, the consequences of his behavior are removing him or allowing him to remove himself from the setting. Based on these data, it seems likely that the function of Tony's behavior is to escape from aversive tasks (e.g., reading time, homework time).

Intervention Development

Once the data have been reviewed (and additional data collected if necessary to follow up on issues not initially presented as concerns), we are ready to make intervention recommendations. In Tony's case, based on our assessment of his reading skills and attention problems, we recommend that he be provided with frequent reinforcement for completing reading assignments. For example, Tony might earn points toward a larger reward or might be given the option to choose from a menu of reinforcers after completing a reading assignment at home or at school. In addition, we recommend that Tony be given reading assignments within his current instructional level. With regard to Tony's difficulties with inattentiveness and off-task behavior, we noted that Tony's teacher provides him little feedback in the classroom and that she allows him to escape from reading activities by separating him from the rest of the class. We recommend attending to Tony when he is on task and providing mild consequences for off-task behavior, but not allowing him to choose not to engage in reading. At home, we recommend that Tony's parents be consistent in their requirements and that they not allow Tony to escape an aversive situation by simply not complying with parental requests. We further recommend that Tony's homework time be broken into small chunks, with frequent reinforcement provided for completing assignments.

Evaluation of the Intervention

To determine whether an intervention is successful, we must evaluate it in an ongoing manner. Observations can be repeated, CBM probes administered, and feedback obtained from parents and teachers. If an intervention is not having the desired effect, we must evaluate why it is not. Have we targeted the wrong problem? Did we target the right problem but not use an effective method? The evaluation process must be continuous so that we know when we must rethink our intervention plans to make them produce the desired results.

Final Thoughts

We encourage school psychologists not to approach assessments with dread and not to think of assessment as a purely psychometric exercise. Let's face it: With some minimal training, almost anyone can administer the measures mentioned in this chapter. If all there were to assessment was administering and scoring a standardized measure or two, assessment would indeed be a tedious activity. However, we must learn to look beyond the numbers and beyond traditional assessment techniques. We must learn to *think* about the child who has been referred to us and the context in which the child interacts (school, home, community). We must remember that the goal of an evaluation is not simply to decide on an appropriate classification for a child but to improve the child's educational and/or social–emotional functioning. To do that, we must approach evaluations from a problem-solving model. Assessment done right should be interesting—all children are unique, and our assessment practices should reflect that.

DISCUSSION QUESTIONS AND ACTIVITIES

1. Compare two of the recently revised measures of intellectual ability (e.g., WISC-IV, SB-V, WJ-III). What theory of intelligence are the tests based on? What was the norming process for the tests? Are the test(s) psychometric properties adequate?

2. Interview school psychologists from different school districts regarding their opinions of the need for the achievement–ability discrepancy in identifying children with learning disabilities. Have their practices changed since the implementation of IDEIA-2004? If so, how?

3. Search for existing FBA interview and observation forms. Compare and contrast these and use them to create a form you can use when conducting functional assessments in the schools.

4. Interview parents and teachers for their opinions about requiring children to be classified as having a certain disability to receive special education services. Would they prefer a noncategorical system? Why or why not?

5. Talk with current school psychologists about their approach to conducting assessments. Are they using a problem-solving approach/RTI approach? If so, what makes their approach a problem-solving one? If not, how could they change their approach to more directly reflect the problem-solving approach?

CHAPTER 9

The School Psychologist's Role in Prevention and Intervention

Part 1. Academic Skills

It has been our experience that one of the main reasons why individuals enter the field of school psychology is to "help" others, to assist children and youth who experience learning and/or behavioral difficulties. The development of knowledge and skills in prevention and intervention services is an integral part of school psychology training programs, deemed important by professional organizations and leaders in the field and valued by practitioners. Preference for this role is matched with evidence indicating the need for prevention and intervention services if we are to address pressing issues facing our children and youth (e.g., Carnine, 1999; Forness, 2003a, 2003b; Friedman, 2003; Hunter, 2003; Power, 2003; Reschly, 2008; Shapiro, 2000; Strein & Koehler, 2008; Tilly, 2008; Ysseldyke, 2000). Despite the overwhelming consensus regarding the importance of this aspect of school psychology service provision and the evidence indicating its urgency, practicing school psychologists tend to spend a minimal portion of their time in this role (see Chapter 5). This apparent lack of attention to evidence-based prevention and intervention practices in school settings is not limited to the field of school psychology. For quite some time now, scholars have recognized gaps between our existing knowledge of effective prevention and intervention practices and actual adoption of those practices in educational settings (e.g., Abbott et al., 1999; Carnine, 1997, 1999; Forness, 2003a; Friedman, 2003; Gersten et al., 1997; Hunter, 2003; Reschly, 2008). Recognition of this gap has led researchers to carefully consider issues essential to the promotion of EBP in school settings (Kratochwill, 2007).

In this chapter and in Chapter 10, we discuss prevention and intervention issues in school psychology. We describe how a data-driven problem-solving approach is helpful in facilitating the provision of effective prevention and intervention services for addressing learning (this chapter) as well as social–emotional or mental health (Chapter 10) needs of children and youth. In addition, we summarize the key areas of knowledge and skills that school psychologists will need in order to embark on this endeavor. We include a discussion of the literature on resiliency, which provides a wealth of information regarding important risk and protective factors that influence development. Knowledge in this area is helpful as a starting point for prevention and intervention because it provides information regarding who should be the focus of intervention, what domains of functioning we should target, and when certain domains should be targeted. We also provide a brief overview of some of the effective prevention and intervention strategies that are supported in literature. Knowledge in this area is useful in guiding the problem-solving process toward intervention strategies that are likely to be effective. We end each chapter with a description of the process for using this information to inform treatment planning at each level of prevention (i.e., primary, secondary, and tertiary) in school settings. Throughout our discussion, emphasis is placed on the use of evidence (from the literature as well as from the immediate problem-solving context) to inform the decision-making process as it relates to intervention selection, implementation, and evaluation.

Prevention and Intervention as Part of a Data-Driven Problem-Solving Process

When we view the entire process of schooling as an "intervention" that alters development (cognitive, affective, social, and physical) from its natural (i.e., unschooled) course (Deno, 2002), it is easy to see how prevention and intervention services are an essential part of education. As we discussed in Chapter 7, within domains of functioning important to schooling (e.g., reading), children learn and develop at different rates. Similarly, within individuals, developmental progress varies over time and across domains. We also know that individuals respond differently to various interventions. Taking these natural variations into account, it is clear that education and mental health professionals must monitor outcomes and be responsive by adapting intervention techniques to meet the individual needs of the students they serve.

Advancements in our knowledge regarding effective instructional strategies and intervention techniques can help build our capacity for improving educational services and creating school environments that promote positive outcomes and reduce the risk of learning and mental health problems. Despite these advances, we must still acknowledge that our ability to predict a priori how our knowledge from research studies will generalize beyond the research contexts and into real-world settings is limited. In light of this limitation, we advocate the use of an *experimenting society* approach to solving problems in school settings (e.g., Campbell, 1988; Cronbach, 1975). This approach relies on the scientific method to determine the efficacy of prevention and intervention strategies within the contexts in which they are used. Thus, as we discussed in Chapter 7, it is necessary to view prevention and intervention efforts as being embedded in a data-driven problem-solving process that focuses on the contexts in which problems occur.

Our current empirical knowledge base can inform and guide certain aspects of the decision-making process, but ongoing evaluation and feedback are necessary for ensuring effective outcomes. The problem-solving process does not provide us with a crystal ball so that we can predict in an *absolute* manner how successful various prevention and intervention efforts will be for different students, but it can help to facilitate the selection of strategies with a *higher probability* of being successful. Further, it incorporates measurement and evaluation methods so that we can at least answer the question, Did our prevention or intervention efforts work? As noted, we cannot assume that an intervention that has been effective in one setting with one individual or group of individuals will work with the same individual or group of individuals for a different problem or problem context or for a different individual within the same context. This uncertainty does not mean that group-level research is not useful in informing the decision-making process. We have neither the time nor the resources to haphazardly implement interventions on a trial-and-error basis. Thus, we must find a balance between our current knowledge base (i.e., existing research on empirically sound prevention and intervention practices) and information we collect about the problem and its context. From this information, we can derive working hypotheses regarding what prevention and intervention strategies are *likely* to facilitate problem resolution. Then we need to test these hypotheses.

To illustrate the preceding points, consider the important domain of reading. Here it is easy to see how research can inform our decision-making process regarding prevention and intervention efforts. First, information from the research literature can help us determine *who to target* and *in what important domains of functioning*. Studies indicate that more than one in six children in the United States will have problems learning how to read in their first 3 years of school (National Reading Panel, 2000), and national data collected in 2009 indicated that 33% of grade 4 students and 25% of grade 8 students are reading below basic levels (National Center for Education Statistics, 2009). These data are alarming when we consider the fact that reading is a pivotal and enabling skill that translates into meaningful personal, social, and economic outcomes for individuals (Joseph, 2008; Simmons & Kame'enui, 1998). More specifically, children who develop poor reading skills are more likely to experience learning and behavioral difficulties in school and are at risk for later-life problems (e.g., dropout, unemployment, adjudication). Alternatively, those who develop strong reading skills are more likely to experience academic success and positive outcomes in later life. Further, children with special needs and those living in poverty are at an extremely high risk for the development of poor reading skills. Thus, the research literature indicates that reading is an important skill and that some children are at higher risk for the development of reading problems, making them potential targets for prevention and intervention efforts.

Research literature can also inform the problem-solving process by indicating *when* we need to intervene (i.e., critical periods of development), and sometimes it helps inform *how* we should intervene (i.e., what intervention strategies are likely to work for particular problems, contexts, or populations). For example, some longitudinal research indicates that when children develop early reading difficulties, these problems tend to persist. According to a seminal study by Juel (1988), the probability of being a poor reader in fourth grade for those who were poor readers in first grade was 88%. Similarly, students with poor reading skills at the end of third grade failed to significantly improve their skills by the end of eighth grade (Felton & Pepper, 1995). Further, when we consider research examining the natural course of reading development for students with and without early reading problems, data indicate that a critical time exists in which we should focus on altering reading trajectories. Longitudinal research illustrates this point, demonstrating how the discrepancy in reading performance between groups of poor readers and strong readers becomes more pronounced as children progress through the early school grades (Good, Simmons, & Smith, 1998). Persistence of reading problems has been explained as emanating from early foundational skill deficits and being exacerbated by reduced exposure to print and eventual reductions in motivation and their desire to read (Stanovich, 1986, 2000). By the time students with poor reading skills enter the third and fourth grades, they are performing well below their same-age peers, and, at this point in time, it is too late to simply modify initial reading instruction to facilitate the acquisition of beginning reading skills (Kaminski et al., 2008; Hosp & MacConnell, 2008).

As we just noted, a critical, short period exists in which we can alter reading trajectories (Hosp & MacConnell, 2008; Simmons & Kame'enui, 1998). Further, the evidence indicates that proficiency in foundational skills in beginning reading is causally linked to the development of reading competence (National Reading Panel, 2000; National Research Council, 1998). Development of these foundational skills differentiates successful from less successful readers (Hosp & MacConnell, 2008; Kame'enui & Carnine, 2001; Simmons & Kame'enui, 1998). These foundational skills include "(a) phonemic awareness or the ability to hear and manipulate the individual sounds in words, (b) alphabetic principle or the mapping of print (letters) to speech (individual sounds) and the blending of these letter sounds into words, (c) accuracy and fluency with connected text, (d) vocabulary and oral language including the ability to understand and use words orally and in writing, and (e) comprehension" (Kaminski et al., 2008, p. 1182). According to Pressley (2006), the majority of students with reading difficulties experience problems attending to the sounds in words (phonemic awareness) and learning to decode (alphabetic principle). The good news is that, through instruction, these important skills are teachable (Carnine, Silbert, Kame'enui, & Tarver, 2004; Coyne, Zipoli, & Ruby, 2006). In particular, explicit phonics instruction (synthetic phonics), wherein children are taught to convert letters into sounds or phonemes and to blend the sounds to form words, has been associated with the greatest overall gains in decoding, comprehension, and collateral skills (e.g., spelling; National Reading Panel, 2000; Pullen & Lloyd, 2008). Furthermore, intervention research demonstrates that if low-achieving students can be brought up to grade level within the first 3 years of school, their reading performance tends to stay at grade level (Adams, 1990; Adams & Carnine, 2003). In addition, when a systematic, multi-tiered approach is employed, wherein reading instruction is differentiated depending on student need and responsiveness to instruction, preliminary research demonstrates that the majority of students can be brought up to grade-level expectations when secondary interventions (additional focused reading instruction to smaller homogeneous groups) are implemented (see Linan-Thompson & Vaughn, 2010, for a review of this work and an overview of the multi-tiered intervention process in reading). Taking all of this into account, reading scholars have suggested that "what is needed for prevention of reading failure is to begin early and assess dynamically" (Good et al., 2002, p. 699).

From our rather brief review of the literature on the development of reading skills and reading intervention research, it is possible to surmise how knowledge in this area would be helpful in addressing the needs of students who are referred for reading problems. It tells us that reading is an important and pivotal skill that affects success in school and later-life outcomes. In addition, it tells us that many students experience reading problems, and that some (e.g., students who are economically disadvantaged or have special needs) are more at risk for the development of reading difficulties than others. It also indicates that we should intervene early and focus on teaching foundational reading skills as a means of primary prevention. The research literature on reading instruction also tells us that most, though not all, students can reach grade-level expectations with the addition of secondary-level reading supports provided outside of core reading instruction (see Linan-Thompson & Vaughn, 2010). Still, this wealth of empirical knowledge does not tell us the whole story regarding specifically how we should address Joey Smith's reading problems within the context of Sunshine Elementary School. In order to address Joey's reading concerns, we need to answer the questions in the problem-solving process as they relate to his particular situation (What is the problem? Why is it occurring? What can we do about it? Did it work?). It is our belief that effective problem solvers *integrate* knowledge of the factors that influence important developmental outcomes, knowledge of empirically supported treatments, and the information they collect about the problem and its context. Thus, school psychologists who are involved in prevention and intervention of reading problems at an individual, small-group, or schoolwide level should be cognizant of the empirical literature on reading difficulties and should employ a data-oriented problem-solving approach to addressing such issues. Further, these problem-solving efforts should be conducted within a multi-tiered, RTI framework, wherein resources are utilized to address a continuum of learning and social behavioral needs of all students (Ervin et al., 2010; Reschly, 2008; Tilly, 2008).

Factors That Influence Development

Research on child development, including risk and resiliency factors, has much to contribute to our understanding of effective prevention and intervention services in schools. Psychologists who study the natural course of development for typically and atypically (e.g., children with autism) developing children and youth have provided us with mapped trajectories of important developmental outcomes across various domains of functioning. This information helps inform the problem-solving process because it helps us to know when students typically meet various levels of performance across developmental domains. This information thus contributes to our definitions of "expected levels of functioning" as we try to determine discrepancies between current and desired levels of performance. In addition, knowing when we can expect students to achieve certain skills helps us to match our instructional techniques to a child's developmental level. Friman and Blum (2002) provided a clear example that shows how a mismatch can occur between our expectations and a child's developmental readiness Their example does not address a specific academic skill per se but does clearly and eloquently illustrate how learning can be affected by such mismatches. Specifically, Friman and Blum (2002) argued that mismatches between parental expectations or assumptions about their child's knowledge and what children actually understand are central to problems of child compliance. One example is Jean Piaget's work on the development of a child's ability to understand abstractions and abstract relations. Piaget's work on *conservation* (i.e., the capacity to conserve and apply certain qualities of an object or event to another object or event) is helpful in understanding how children develop the concept of "sameness." Friman and Blum (2002) suggested that parents often assume that a child has the capacity to understand similarities across behavioral episodes even when that capacity may not be well developed. Parents may get frustrated when their child, who has just been disciplined in one situation, seemingly does the "same thing" again. Parents might comment, "That's the same thing I told you not to do yesterday" or "Didn't I warn you not to do that again?" When young children have underdeveloped capacities for understanding abstractions such as "sameness," it is very difficult for them to see how what they did yesterday in the living room at Aunt Michelle's house is in any way similar to what they did today at home in the kitchen. Similarly, mismatches between a child's capacity for understanding instructions and parental delivery of commands can lead to significant issues of noncompliance.

As Friman and Blum (2002) noted, when working with children to teach them new skills, it is helpful to know something about how children learn and develop the capacity for understanding language. Similarly, problems may occur in classroom settings when there is a mismatch between a student's level of understanding and a teacher's instructional cues. Psychologists who are interested in prevention and intervention services in the school or in other settings must have some understanding of the natural course of development, as their focus may be on detecting progress along a particular domain (e.g., reading, capacity to understand language and abstractions) and intervening to alter trajectories when they detect a gap between actual and expected rates of progress.

Risk Factors

In addition to knowing the natural course of development, psychologists interested in prevention and intervention services should be familiar with research regarding the factors that tend to influence development and subsequent later-life outcomes. An extensive amount of research has demonstrated that children who are raised under certain conditions (e.g., poverty, abuse, family dysfunction) are at significantly higher risk for problems in their adult lives (e.g., marital discord, unemployment). This line of research has focused on the identification of *risk factors* that are predictive of later-life dysfunction. Research consistently indicates that poverty is the most powerful risk factor that predicts adult dysfunction. Poverty, or a lack of resources, can result in certain adverse living situations, such as economic dependence, overcrowding, and disorganization within the family system (Doll & Lyon, 1998; Gutman, McLoyd, & Tokoyawa, 2005; Tornquist, Mastropieri, Scruggs, Berry, & Halloran, 2009). For example, poverty can place children at risk of learning problems as a result of risks associated with health, nutrition, and adequate health care (e.g., lower birthweights resulting from inadequate prenatal care, continued poor nutrition, and lack of proper health care) as well as from risks associated with low educational achievement of parents and the ways in which poverty can impede access to educational materials (e.g., books, computers) and activities (e.g., travel experiences). Another powerful predictor of negative adult outcomes is an ineffective or uncaring parenting environment. The importance of warm, caring, consistent parental environment to the development and general well-being of children has been well documented (see Masten & Coatsworth, 1998; Taylor, 2010). The occurrence of physical or emotional maltreatment in childhood is a third predictor of negative adult outcomes, particularly the development of adult psychopathology. A fourth factor predicting adult problems is marital discord and/or family dysfunction. Children raised in conditions of chronic family conflict tend to end up in similarly dysfunctional family conditions in adulthood. All four factors (poverty, uncaring parental environments, abuse or maltreatment, and family conflict) have been linked to negative later-life outcomes. Further, evidence suggests that "factors tend to be chronic life conditions rather than acute hazards" and that "the rate and intensity of undesirable outcomes appears to increase geometrically with exposure to each successive risk factor" (Doll & Lyon, 1998, p. 356). This information tells us that children with prolonged exposure to multiple risk factors are at the greatest risk of developing problems and are, therefore, in great need of support services. They also, however, are likely to be the most difficult to treat (i.e., they fall at the "top of the prevention triangle").

Protective Factors

In addition to risk factors, some research has examined factors associated with the development of competence in spite of adversity (i.e., *protective factors*). The concept of resilience refers to "manifested competence in the context of significant challenges to adaptation or development" (Masten & Coatsworth, 1998, p. 206). Researchers who study resilience are often interested in the questions, Why do some children succeed amidst a sea of adversity? Is there something special or unique about these children? In a recent review of this literature, Masten and Coatsworth (1998) reported that "converging evidence suggests that the same powerful adaptive systems protect development in both favorable and unfavorable environments" (p. 205). These include (1) quality parent–child relationships (i.e., warm, caring, competent relationships with a parent or surrogate caregiver figure); (2) good cognitive development; and (3) self-regulation of attention, emotion, and behavior. Further, research indicates that early prevention and intervention to foster the development of competence and prevent problems is critical to successful later-life outcomes.

Our knowledge base of protective and risk factors is increasing. In this section we provide a very cursory overview of the risk and resiliency literature, the major findings of this work, and its implications. "Development is biased towards competence, but there is no such thing as an invulnerable child" (Masten & Coatsworth, 1998, p. 216). Thus, it is important for prevention and intervention efforts to focus on ameliorating risk factors and enhancing protective factors for children in school settings. We encourage school psychologists to advance their knowledge of this literature and to keep abreast of new findings, because these will have important implications for our prevention and intervention work (e.g., Cohn, Fredrickson, Brown, Mikels, & Conway, 2009; Luthar & Cicchetti, 2000; Taylor, 2010).

Evidence-Based Instruction and Intervention Strategies

Equally important to our understanding of the natural course of child development and of important risk and protective factors that influence this development is our knowledge of empirically supported instructional techniques and intervention strategies. This literature is enormous, and sifting through it can be overwhelming. Thus, we highlight some of the major findings in the effective teaching and intervention literature. As we do so, we caution readers to keep in mind that when selecting intervention practices one should consider practices with demonstrated (1) trustworthiness and effectiveness, (2) relevance to the current problem and its context, and (3) efficiency. One should also keep in mind the following limitations to EBIs: (1) Research findings may not generalize to the problem situation that you are working with; (2) when empirical findings indicate that the intervention was effective for a group of students, individual differences in response to the intervention are also likely to be noted; (3) intervention strategies found to be *efficacious* (i.e., to produce desired outcomes in controlled research) may not be *effective* (i.e., efficient, practical, acceptable, feasible in practice contexts); and (4) we cannot know whether a prevention or intervention strategy works with the problem we are addressing until we evaluate it.

Literature on Effective Instruction

As Shapiro (2004) aptly notes, "A substantial literature has demonstrated that a child's academic failure may reside in the instructional environment rather than in the child's inadequate mastery of skills" (p. 30). Over the past few decades, researchers have examined how effective teachers structure their classrooms and utilize strategies to create instructional environments conducive to learning (e.g., Good & Brophy, 1994; Good &

Brophy, 2007). The literature on effective teaching indicates that quality of instruction is influenced by what effective teachers *think* about teaching and learning as well as what they *do*. What teachers think about how children learn influences what the teachers do in the classroom. Research indicates that teacher expectations about learning characteristics of particular students can have a profound impact on the manner in which they interact with those students. Further, students are more likely to learn when teachers hold high expectations and less likely to learn when they hold low expectations.

With regard to classroom management, it is interesting to note that effective teachers generally use the same kinds of consequences for misbehavior as ineffective teachers. How they tend to differ from ineffective teachers is in the manner in which they manage problem situations before they arise (Kounin, 1970). Effective teachers prevent problems by establishing classroom environments in which students are engaged in functional, interesting, worthwhile materials and activities so that participation in classroom activities is meaningful, a focus is placed on group aspects of classroom management, and there are fewer incentives to misbehave (Bear, 2008; Gettinger & Ball, 2008; Wolery, Bailey, & Sugai, 1989).

When learning problems arise, effective teachers tend to be *active problem solvers* and to focus on *alterable variables* (i.e., what they can change) when deciding what to do to improve outcomes for students (Howell & Nolet, 2000). Moreover, "effective teachers know *when* and *how* to make changes to meet the needs of students who are not progressing" (Howell & Nolet, 2000, p. 10). Teaching requires knowledge of the *content* of instruction as well as the *structure* or *format* of instructional delivery. Lesson preview, explanation, demonstration, guided practice, correction, and independent practice are a few examples of the structure or formats that effective teachers use in the classroom. What teachers do or the instructional practices they use is only one part of the equation for effective teaching. In order for learning to occur, there needs to be consideration of the interaction between and alignment of three important factors (Howell & Nolet, 2000; Howell & Schumann, 2010): (1) *students* (i.e., who is being taught or what the learner brings to the instructional context), (2) *curriculum* (what is being taught or the set of learning outcomes and expectations), and (3) *instruction* (how things are taught or what the teacher does). "The interactive nature of learning points out the truism that evaluations designed to guide instruction must focus on the learning interaction, not on individual components of the interaction" (Howell & Nolet, 2000, p. 19). As we have noted in earlier chapters, one limitation of traditional approaches to assessment is the focus on child factors to the exclusion of the learning context. The effective teaching literature suggests that decisions about interventions should be determined by consideration of the interaction of student, curriculum, instruction, and educational environment factors. Further, the focus should be on *alterable* (i.e., those amenable to change) characteristics of these factors.

The Student (Who Is Being Taught?)

What the learner brings to the instructional context is one aspect of the learning equation. For example, as Howell and Nolet (2000) note, one important alterable variable that a student brings to the learning context is his or her *prior knowledge* (i.e., skills, strategies, perceptions, expectations, and beliefs). When a student does not have adequate prior knowledge or skill in a particular area, tasks become difficult. Tasks that have missing information or ambiguous cues or that lack predictability are considered difficult. Of course, whether or not a task is difficult varies for individuals with different prior knowledge bases and skills (e.g., novices vs. experts). Thus, task difficulty has more to do with the interaction of the task and the learner's prior knowledge than with the task itself. Unfortunately, "many people attribute difficulty in school to deficits in a student's fixed capacity to learn—not missing prior knowledge" (Howell & Nolet, 2000, p. 21). In addition to task-specific knowledge (i.e., content knowledge and skills in the subject matter being taught), students need to have sufficient task-related knowledge (i.e., skills required to learn). Task-related knowledge is learned and, therefore, alterable. It includes such things as attention, motivation, and problem-solving skills. Students who are effective learners, for example, are able to analyze task demands and, from this information, select strategies for task completion. They are good at *solving problems* (Carnine, 1989; Howell & Nolet, 2000; Pressley, 1996), and they are able to *self-regulate* and *self-monitor* their behavior and their learning with respect to awareness of their skills and the requirements of the task or situation at hand. Students who do not have strong problem-solving skills should be taught these skills within the context of existing instructional objectives rather than in isolation (e.g., Baker, Chard, Ketterlin-Geller, Apichatabutra, & Doabler, 2009; Derry & Murphy, 1986). Similarly, students who are deficient in self-regulation or self-monitoring skills may need explicit instruction in these areas (Howell & Nolet, 2000).

Selective attention to task, ability to *recall* information, and *motivation* are three additional student variables that affect learning and that are alterable through instruction. For example, in order for learning to occur, students must selectively attend to important information and ignore irrelevant or unimportant information. Certain instructional techniques (e.g., the use of previewing, prereading questions, and discriminated practice) can help to facilitate selective attention to important aspects of the task (e.g., Good & Brophy, 2007; Kryzanowski & Carnine, 1980). Effective learners are also skilled at recalling important information. Recall of information is important for comprehension tasks, and successful students use strategies (e.g., looking back through text, story webs) to facilitate recall. These strategies can be explicitly taught and embedded within the instructional contexts in which they are useful (e.g., Baker, Gersten, & Scalon, 2002; Pressley et al., 1995; Swanson & De La Paz, 1998). Another important student variable is motivation to learn. Students who persevere (work harder and longer at something despite difficulty or negative feedback) are said to be more motivated than students who tend to give up. Thus, strategies designed to improve sustained engagement in task activities are useful. It is important to note that, although individual differences may exist with respect to the degree to which students have difficulties in each of these areas (i.e., attention to task, recall, and motivation), these task-related skills are *alterable* via various instructional strategies (see Howell & Schumann, 2010). Thus, emphasis should be placed on identifying these deficit areas with the intent to match them with instructional supports designed to improve such difficulties.

Another important student variable is the degree to which a student is proficient in a particular skill, or where the student falls with respect to *skill development* on the learning hierarchy (Haring, Lovitt, Eaton, & Hansen, 1978). Daly, Lentz, and Boyer (1996) describe the learning hierarchy in the following way:

> As the learner is gaining a new skill, he or she will first *acquire* it. The learner then becomes *fluent* in skill use. Next, he or she learns to *generalize* its use to novel contexts. Finally, he or she *adapts* its use to modify the response as necessary according to novel demands. (p. 370)

Different instructional techniques are useful in helping students progress through each stage of the learning hierarchy (Daly et al., 1996; Haring et al., 1978; Howell & Nolet, 2000; Mastropieri & Scruggs, 2009). For example, students who are just acquiring new skills (e.g., beginning reading skills) and who are developing accuracy are in need of modeling, demonstration, prompting, cueing, and corrective feedback. In contrast, students who have mastered a certain level of accuracy with a skill must practice that skill to achieve proficiency and fluency. Strategies for improving fluency include increased opportunities for drill and practice as well as reinforcement for such activities. Instructional strategies have also been developed to promote generalization and adaptation of skills (e.g., Alberto & Troutman, 2009; Alessi, 1987; Stokes & Baer, 1977). When considering a student's level of proficiency from a cognitive psychology perspective, researchers have described this concept as the student's "automaticity" with that skill (e.g., LaBerge & Samuels, 1974). More specifically, "automatic skilled performance develops with extended practice after a level of high accuracy has been reached, and when one is automatic, the skill can be performed with minimum attention and effort" (Samuels & Flor, 1997, p. 109). Evidence indicates that knowledge and skills that are developed to automaticity are retained and that, when students are performing at an automatic level, they are able to devote attention to other tasks. For example, in the area of reading, when students are able to decode at an automatic level, fewer demands are placed on working memory, and they are better able to comprehend what they read (Samuels, LaBerge, & Bremer, 1978). Regardless of the theoretical background of the researcher, much attention in the intervention literature has focused on strategies and instructional techniques that facilitate the development of fluency or the degree to which students are able to perform tasks with some level of automaticity (e.g., Carnine, 1989; Chard, Vaughn, & Tyler, 2002; Fuchs, Fuchs, Hosp, & Jenkins, 2001; Mastropieri, Leinart, & Scruggs, 1999; Mastropieri & Scruggs, 2009).

During the problem-solving process, information collected about a student's prior knowledge (i.e., task-specific knowledge as well as task-related knowledge) can be useful in the development of hypotheses about the reasons why problems are occurring and, subsequently, in selecting appropriate intervention strategies. We have highlighted some important alterable student variables that might be targets of assessment. Processes and procedures for assessing these student variables are available in the literature (e.g., Hawkins, Barnett, Morrison, & Musti-Rao, 2010; Hosp, Hosp, & Howell, 2007; Howell & Nolet, 2000; Howell & Schumann, 2010; Shapiro, 1996, 2004; Witt et al., 2000), and we encourage school psychologists to consult these resources and to become proficient in using a data-driven problem-solving approach to assess student variables and their alignment with curricular variables and instructional strategies (see Chapter 8 for more information).

The Curriculum (What to Teach)

In addition to considering *who* is being taught, teachers need to consider *what* to teach. The *curriculum* is a set of learning outcomes and expectations—the "what" of teaching (Howell & Nolet, 2000; Howell & Schumann, 2010). When thinking about curriculum, Howell and Nolet (2000) argue that it is important to distinguish between the *intended* curriculum (the formally recommended, sanctioned, or adopted curriculum), the *taught* curriculum (the one that is based on what teachers do and use—the actual curriculum), and the *learned* curriculum (what students actually learn). Problems occur when the intended curriculum does not match the learned curriculum. This is evident when discrepancies exist between actual and expected levels of student progress. If students are not making adequate progress in a specific domain, then it is important to ask whether the curriculum is aligned with student needs and instruction.

In a well-designed curriculum, we know when a student is not making adequate progress because student progress in meeting instructional objectives is monitored. A strong curriculum is organized with instructional goals and objectives. According to Howell and Nolet (2000), instructional objectives include the following specifications: (1) content (i.e., what the student is expected to learn), (2) behavior (i.e., what the student does that indicates he or she has learned), (3) criterion (i.e., the expected level of performance), and (4) conditions (i.e., the context or situation in which the student will work). When objectives are established, it is easy to measure student progress and compare it with the criterion to determine whether a problem exists (i.e., a discrepancy between student progress and the criterion).

Part of curriculum development includes organizing and sequencing the content of what is to be taught in a given area. One way to organize content is to think in terms of the "big ideas" in a particular domain of functioning. Big ideas are empirically validated foundational skills and strategies that are prerequisite to later skill development and success in particular content areas or domains (Kame'enui & Carnine, 2001). As we noted earlier in this chapter, for example, certain foundational reading skills (e.g., phonological awareness, the alphabetic principle) are valid indicator skills predictive of later success. Thus, these skills should be part of the "big ideas" found in a reading curriculum (Coyne et al., 2006). Similarly, at the secondary level, "big ideas" have been used to organize a variety of curricula (e.g., earth sciences, history), and this approach has helped to integrate content (see Grossen et al., 2002). To accelerate learning and to proactively address the needs of students, curricula can be organized or engineered around "big ideas" and can incorporate six important principles of accommodation for diverse learners (see Kame'enui & Carnine, 2001; Stein, Carnine, & Dixon, 1998):

- Identifying "big ideas" and organizing curricula around them.
- Teaching explicit problem-solving strategies within the curriculum.
- Preteaching background knowledge.
- Scaffolding instruction (i.e., providing instructional support via coaching, feedback, cooperative learning activities, etc.).
- Integrating new and old skills and concepts.
- Including adequate review that is distributed over time, cumulative, and varied to promote generalization and transfer.

If the curriculum is carefully organized so that it moves along a *sequential hierarchical structure* (i.e., organized so that later concepts and skills build on earlier concepts and skills in a sequential fashion), then assessment of the match between student skills and placement in the curriculum can be very useful (Howell & Nolet, 2000). Further, *what is being taught* (e.g., factual information, conceptual information, rule relationships, strategic knowledge) also dictates to some extent *how* instruction should occur (see Howell & Nolet, 2000; Howell & Schumann, 2010). The structure or format of a lesson should vary as a function of the type of information that is taught (e.g., factual, concept, rule relationships, strategic information). For example, learning of factual information involves memorization and is best achieved via explicit instruction, repeated practice, and error correction. Learning of facts can be hindered when students have difficulties with selective attention and recall. Thus, teachers need to consider how to control the amount of new information to be learned and how to facilitate attention to the task. One procedure for facilitating this process is "folding-in" or "drill-sandwich" procedures, wherein tasks are organized such that students are slowly introduced to unknown material that is embedded with known material (see Shapiro, 1996, 2004). Another important consideration in teaching factual information is facilitating discrimination between new and old facts, and this can be accomplished through the organization of materials such that contrast between new and old facts is at first very large.

Conceptual knowledge (i.e., knowing that certain objects, events, actions, or situations share common attributes) requires abstraction and understanding of rules for defining all relevant features of a member of a category. For example, learning to distinguish the category of "dogs" is best accomplished through presentation of examples and nonexamples that illustrate the full range of attributes that are involved in the concept of "dogs." Discrimination is also important in concept learning. Thus, instructional concepts that are easily confused should be taught separately (see Howell & Nolet, 2000; Howell & Schumann, 2010). Practice in accurately identifying the concept should occur prior to training in discrimination with other concepts. The teaching of rule relationships and strategic information also requires different instructional strategies. As should be evident from our brief description, the curriculum is just one part of the teaching equation, but like student variables and instructional techniques, it plays a significant role in the facilitation or hindrance of academic success (Howell & Nolet, 2000; Kame'enui & Carnine, 2001; Stein et al., 1998).

Further, it is important to note that we have just described one way in which teachers can think about organizing and sequencing the content of what is to be taught, and other empirically grounded descriptions of similar approaches exist in the literature. For example, according to Mastropieri and Scruggs (2009), to promote effective differentiated instruction of students with special needs in inclusive settings, a teacher should consider using the PASS variables:

1. Prioritize instruction.
2. Adapt instruction, materials, or the environment.
3. Systematically teach with the "SCREAM" (i.e., structure, clarity, redundancy, enthusiasm, appropriate rate, and maximized engagement through questioning and feedback) variables.
4. Systematically evaluate the outcomes of your instruction.

School psychologists, who consult with teachers regarding methods for facilitating the inclusion of students with disabilities so that they are able to access the curriculum, should be familiar with the variables discussed in this section and how they relate to effective teaching.

Effective Instructional Approaches (How and When to Teach)

With student issues, we are concerned with "who" is being taught; with curriculum issues, we are concerned with "what" should be taught; and with instruction, we are concerned with "how" and "when" it should be taught. "It is the responsibility of a skilled teacher to make an informed, reasoned decision about which instructional approach is appropriate for a particular student at a particular time" (Howell & Nolet, 2000, p. 71). Some general findings in the effective teaching literature indicate that students who fall behind in the curriculum benefit from instruction that teaches missing prior knowledge in a direct fashion. Further, "students with the least skills, who are making the least progress, need the most instructional support" (Howell & Nolet, 2000, p. 71). Research on effective teaching focuses on defining the qualities associated with maximum instructional support. Teachers can manipulate their use of time, assignments, and actions to match the curriculum and learning needs of the student (Howell & Nolet, 2000; Howell & Schumann, 2010; Mastropieri & Scruggs, 2009). Learning is facilitated via explanation, demonstration, guided practice, timely correction, and task-specific feedback. Teacher actions (e.g., planning for instruction, delivery of information, asking questions, responding to efforts, conducting activities, and evaluating for instruction) should be aligned with objectives in the curriculum. In addition, and as noted in the preceding sections, teachers can align instructional strategies with student needs, with the type of information they teach (i.e., factual, conceptual, rule relationships, strategic information), and with the learning hierarchy (i.e., acquisition, fluency, generalization, adaptation).

Prevention and Intervention Literature on Effective Teaching

An extensive literature exists on empirically supported prevention and intervention practices, and countless resources and books are devoted to this topic. Further, guidelines for selecting EBIs are available within the school psychology literature (e.g., Kratochwill, 2007; Kratochwill & Shernoff, 2004; Kratochwill & Stoiber, 2000a, 2000b, 2002). This wealth of information is both good and bad for school psychologists interested in facilitating the application of prevention and intervention services in school settings. The good news is that, when working with parents and teachers, we do not need to start from scratch in developing specific intervention strategies or selecting techniques that have empirical support. The bad news is that, even when we select interventions from a list of those determined to have empirical support, the list is still quite long, and we have neither the time nor the resources to take a trial-and-error approach to implementing empirically supported practices. Thus, the data-driven problem-solving model is essential to guiding the intervention selection process by linking assessment, intervention, and evaluation services. We also believe that the problem-solving process can be enhanced by knowledge of the literature on how children learn and develop over time as well as by a thorough understanding of how different factors (i.e., student, curricula, and instruction) must be aligned to facilitate learning. As Tilly (2002) notes, effective problem solving involves careful analysis of information on the problem and its context to generate hypotheses and solutions with the least amount of inference. In other words, our knowledge base can help guide our decision-making process so that we can shrink the universe of options to a manageable form. For example, assessment of alterable student and curricular variables can help to narrow the focus of intervention strategies likely to improve learning (see Howell & Nolet, 2000; Howell & Schumann, 2010). Still, it is important that intervention strategies are monitored to determine their effectiveness, feasibility, and acceptability.

In this section, we highlight some prevention and intervention strategies that have been found to have empirical support in addressing important variables related to learning. In a problem-solving approach embedded within an RTI framework, the theoretical or philosophical basis for the intervention is less important than the efficacy of the intervention. Thus, strategies should be selected based on their intended outcome and relevance to the problem situation rather than on their theoretical basis. As you read this section, you will notice that a variety of different intervention strategies are available to address important targeted outcomes. Further, intervention strategies do not necessarily fall neatly within one specific intended outcome category. In other words, one intervention may address multiple problems. For example, an intervention such as peer tutoring may help improve student engagement in task activities by creating increased opportunities to respond and also may improve skill development by providing instructional supports and corrective feedback on a more frequent basis. Our discussion of intervention strategies is brief and intended to provide readers with a *sample* of the range of strategies that might be used to address important learning outcomes. Further, our review is by no means comprehensive. Entire volumes (e.g., Rathvon, 2008; Mastropieri & Scruggs, 2009; Good & Brophy, 2007; Shapiro, 2011; Shinn & Walker, 2010; Stoner, Shinn, & Walker, 1991; Walker et al., 1995) have been devoted to discussion of prevention and intervention strategies and effective teaching methods.

Strategies Designed to Improve Academic Engagement, Motivation, Self-Regulation, and Problem Solving

In 1963, Carroll proposed that learning was a function of time engaged in learning relative to time needed to learn. Since that time, an extensive line of research has shown that there is a direct relationship between the amount of time students are engaged in a task (i.e., paying attention, working on tasks, participating in discussion) and academic performance (Gettinger & Ball, 2008; Seo, Brownell, Bishop, & Dingle, 2008). Differences exist in task engagement rates across classrooms and across students within classrooms. Further, students from lower socioeconomic levels and those with learning problems have been found to have lower rates of task engagement than their peers. In other words, in order for students to learn, they must have both opportunities to do so and access to instruction. Thus, prevention and intervention strategies designed to increase engagement in the learning environment by addressing issues that may hinder such access (e.g., selective attention to task, motivation, self-regulation, and problem-solving skills) can be viewed as a first step in ensuring that students have the opportunity to benefit from the learning environment. Improving attention to task and task engagement involves consideration of the student's skills (selective attention, motivation, self-regulation, problem solving) as well as curriculum and instructional variables. Next, we highlight a few strategies that address this issue (for information, see Gettinger & Ball, 2008; Good & Brophy, 2007; Mastropieri & Scruggs, 2009).

Structuring of the Classroom Environment

One way to facilitate task engagement is to create learning environments that encourage active participation and discourage disruptive and off-task behavior. Research indicates that when teachers are proactive and devote more time to structuring the learning environment at the beginning of the year, students are more engaged in tasks throughout the remainder of the year. Similarly, when teachers spend less time structuring their classrooms to promote academic success, students are less likely to be engaged in tasks and more likely to be disruptive. When students are more disruptive, teachers end up allocating more time to intervening with misbehavior than to instruction, and student task engagement rates drop. Further, it is more difficult for teachers to regain instructional control after losing it than it is for them to maintain it by establishing it proactively and early in the year. Thus, structuring the classroom environment to promote engagement and academic success should be viewed as a prevention strategy that involves several interrelated components best achieved at the beginning of the year. Detailed descriptions of these components are available in the literature (e.g., Gettinger & Ball, 2008; DuPaul, Stoner, & O'Reilly, 2008; Mastropieri & Scruggs, 2009; Paine, Radicchi, Rosellini, Deutchman, & Darch, 1983; Rathvon, 2008).

Contingency Management Interventions

Early on, investigations indicated that providing incentives and contingent feedback resulted in improvements in attention to task (e.g., Ferritor, Buckholt, Hamblin, & Smith, 1972; Hall, Lund, & Jackson, 1968). Hall and colleagues (1968), for example, found that contingent praise was an effective means of increasing study behavior. Ferritor and colleagues (1972) examined the effects of contingent reinforcement on attending behavior and on work completion. Results indicated that contingent reinforcement for completing work affected levels of attention to task, but contingent reinforcement of attending behavior did not consistently affect work completion. Thus, when using contingency-based interventions, it is sometimes necessary to target more specific outcomes of task engagement, such as work productivity (e.g., number of items completed within a time frame) or accuracy (e.g., percent correct). Reinforcement contingencies can be applied to individual students or to groups of students (for a review, see Bear, 2008; Skinner, Skinner, & Sterling-Turner, 2002).

In addition to reinforcement contingencies, researchers have examined the use of contingent punishment (e.g., teacher reprimands or removal of privileges) with individuals and with groups of students. When used properly, punishment procedures have been found to be effective in increasing task engagement (e.g., Abramowitz, O'Leary, & Rosen, 1987; Acker & O'Leary, 1987) and academic productivity (e.g., Abramowitz, O'Leary, & Futtersak, 1988). We have not focused on contingent punishment in this section, however, because of certain complications that may arise with its use (Abramowitz et al., 1988; Bear, 2008; Hall et al., 1968; Kerr & Nelson, 2006).

Increasing Student Engagement through Teaching Strategies

Research indicates that certain teaching strategies are associated with higher levels of student engagement than others (see Gettinger & Ball, 2008). For example, when teachers utilize interactive teaching strategies (e.g., discussion, review, reading aloud), students are more likely to be engaged in task activities. Instruction that occurs at a faster pace is also associated with higher levels of engagement. In addition, evidence suggests that increasing opportunities for students to actively respond results in increased active task engagement. This can be accomplished via peer tutoring and cooperative learning activities and also through high levels of teacher questioning.

Self-Monitoring

As Gettinger and Ball (2008) noted, even when teachers consistently employ strategies designed to maximize student engagement, some students will spend less time than needed on a task as a result of other factors (e.g., low motivation, poor self-monitoring, ineffective problem-solving or self-regulation skills). Students can be taught to self-monitor their attention to task and thus can improve task engagement. According to Shapiro and Cole (1994), self-monitoring involves observing one's own behavior and recording it. It is one component of a set of strategies referred to as self-management.

Other components of self-management are self-evaluation (i.e., comparing information collected about one's own behavior with a criterion) and self-reinforcement (i.e., administering consequences for meeting the criterion). These procedures, together or sometimes in isolation of each other, have been found to improve a variety of target behaviors (e.g., academic accuracy, attention to task) across various target populations (e.g., students with multiple handicaps and developmental delays, preschoolers, students with learning difficulties, students with behavior problems; see Hoff & Sawka-Miller, 2010).

Self-Instruction and Strategy Instruction

Teaching students to use self-instructional strategies as a way to verbally mediate tasks and task situations can facilitate the development of self-control skills (e.g., Meichenbaum & Goodman, 1971). In addition, self-instructional training has been employed to teach social (e.g., Maag, 1990) and academic (e.g., Johnson, Whitman, & Johnson, 1980) skills. Some studies investigating the efficacy of self-instruction have focused on teaching strategies relevant to solving academic problems in the areas of math (e.g., Cullinan, Lloyd, & Epstein, 1981), reading (e.g., Miller, Giovenco, & Rentiers, 1987), and written expression (Baker et al., 2009; Graham, Harris, MacArthur, & Schwartz, 1991). Teaching students strategies for approaching various academic tasks is useful when the type of information being taught involves rule relationships (e.g., "*i* before *e* except after *c*" or when *ie* is sounded as /ay/ as in *neighbor* and *weigh*") or strategic knowledge (e.g., steps in solving arithmetic problems). Thus, this approach to instruction is useful when students have difficulties with problem solving as well as when the type of information being taught involves rules or strategies. In addition to strategy training that is embedded within the context of specific academic tasks, some researchers (e.g., Baker et al., 2002, 2009; Deshler & Schumaker, 1986; Pressley, 1996) have examined the utility of training students in more general learning strategies (e.g., how to study, strategies for memorization, note-taking strategies) rather than those specific to learning a particular academic skill (e.g., long division). For example, strategy instruction can be used to teach students study skills and improve engagement in studying across a variety of academic domains (Harvey, 2002; Lentz, 1992).

Strategies Designed to Improve Skill Development, Fluency, and Retention of Information

Although engagement in instructional activities and tasks is essential to learning, it is not necessarily sufficient (Gettinger & Ball, 2008). In order for learning to occur, there also needs to be alignment of instruction with student skill proficiency on the learning hierarchy and with the nature of the curriculum being taught. As we have noted in earlier sections of this chapter, certain strategies for organizing curricular materials and instruction are recommended in the effective teaching literature. We begin this section with a brief review of this work. Next, we describe a few empirically supported intervention strategies for addressing skill development in important academic domains.

Organization of Material and Instruction to Promote Learning

Teachers can arrange instructional materials (e.g., identify "big ideas" and organize material around them) and employ instructional strategies (e.g., provide feedback and review) to facilitate learning. Some aspects of instruction are dictated by the type of information being taught (factual, conceptual, rule relations, strategies). Similarly, some aspects of instruction should vary to fit the student's skill level with respect to the learning hierarchy. According to Daly and colleagues (1996), instruction during acquisition of a skill should focus on the development of accuracy via demonstration, modeling, cueing, and prompting. Once accuracy is achieved, fluency building can be accomplished through increased opportunities to respond and drill and practice, with reinforcement for high rates of responding in context. When students are accurate and fluent in a particular skill within the learning context in which it was taught, instruction can move toward the development of generalization. This can be accomplished by modeling the skill across contexts, drilling across contexts, and reinforcing skill use across contexts. According to Carnine (1989) and Engelman (1997), some of the most important general considerations during instructional planning that are still applicable today include:

- Introducing information in a cumulative fashion to avoid memory overload.
- Preteaching easier concepts first to reduce errors in training.
- Providing supervised practice in learning to discriminate concepts when topics are introduced that are similar and likely to be confused.
- Spacing discriminated practice trials to reduce interference effects (i.e., introduce one concept and, once it is learned, introduce the other concept with discriminated practice).
- Relating new concepts or skills to learned information to make it more meaningful.
- Providing a delayed review of difficult items.
- Requiring quicker response times to promote fluency and automaticity.
- Teaching to mastery or criterion.

Strategies for Improving Academic Performance

It is important to note that the same effective instructional design principles described previously are applicable across the academic domains (e.g., reading, writing, mathematics, social studies, and science). For each instructional domain, it is important to establish the "big ideas" that need to be taught. For example, in reading, it is important to provide explicit instruction in early foundational skills such as phonemic awareness. In mathematics, *number sense*, or "a child's fluidity and flexibility with numbers, the sense of what numbers mean, and an ability to perform mental mathematics and to look at the world and make comparisons" (Gersten & Chard, 1999, pp. 19–20), seems to be an important foundational skill (see also Gersten, Jordan, & Flojo, 2005). Foundational skills such as phonemic awareness in reading and number sense in mathematics are important because they relate to later success in these important domains. For example, research has indicated an "intricate relationship between conceptual understanding and consistent use of efficient strategies for computation and problem solving" (Gersten & Chard, 1999, p. 26). When students lack proficiency in these important foundational skills, teaching should emphasize explicit instruction such that students acquire and become fluent in them. Numerous intervention strategies have been designed to address particular academic skill areas, and it is not possible to review each of these strategies within this chapter. Instead, we have focused on describing factors important to learning (i.e., student variables, curricular variables, instructional variables) so that readers can consider how these relate to the vast intervention literature. Thus, we encourage readers to consult the literature on intervention strategies designed to address various academic problems (e.g., reading fluency or comprehension) and to see whether they are able to identify the underlying features of the strategy that fit with our discussion of effective teaching. For example, one strategy for improving reading fluency is the use of repeated readings, wherein students are asked to read and reread short passages that contain generally recognizable words several times until a certain criterion is reached (see Chard et al., 2002; Mastropieri et al., 1999). This strategy is useful when students have achieved a certain level of accuracy with regard to reading and when the goal of instruction is to improve fluency. In contrast, reading interventions such as self-questioning or story mapping are designed to improve comprehension (i.e., recall of information or understanding of text), and they involve explicit instruction in strategies and/or rules that are useful to facilitating comprehension (Swanson & De La Paz, 1998; Vaughn & Edmonds, 2006). Examining intervention strategies with an eye toward how they incorporate principles of effective instruction and/or how they fit with the problem context and student learning needs is helpful in narrowing the universe of intervention options during the problem-solving process.

Data-Driven Problem Solving across Levels of Prevention

In Chapter 7, we described the critical features of the data-driven problem-solving model as "outcome focused, data-driven, integrally linked to intervention, and context specific." These critical features are so interwoven that it would be inappropriate to discuss prevention and intervention practices independent of a problem-solving process that includes context-specific assessment and outcome-focused measurement and evaluation. Thus, we instead focus on how prevention and intervention are integrally linked to each phase of the problem-solving process across each level of prevention (i.e., primary, secondary, and tertiary).

As illustrated in the triangle (Figure 7.2), within a multi-tiered, RTI framework, at the level of *primary prevention*, problem-solving efforts (i.e., assessment, analysis, intervention, and evaluation) are focused on *all* students in the school. Primary prevention and intervention efforts are sometimes referred to as *universal supports* because they are applicable to all students. At this level of intervention, it is still important to consider the interaction of population, curriculum, and instructional variables. In other words, the selection of universal supports should involve consideration of *who* will receive these interventions (i.e., the students at the school), *what* will be the structure and content of these services (i.e., curriculum issues), and *how* and *when* instruction and interventions will be implemented (i.e., teaching and intervention delivery and monitoring issues). Further, just as problem solving is data driven when working with individual students, decisions at this level of the problem-solving process should be guided by data (see Van-DerHeyden, 2010).

At the primary prevention level, all students at the school are the targets of universal supports or interventions. Thus, information about the student population is useful in determining intervention needs. In addition, information from the literature on child development and risk and resiliency can be useful in determining domains to target for intervention. Once important domains of functioning are selected as a focus for primary prevention, it is important to gather information about the current school context and general performance of students in the domains of interest. For example, if a school decides to focus on establishing strong prevention and universal supports in the areas of reading and behavior, then it is important to assess how students are currently functioning in these domains. In addition, with regard to questions about curriculum or "what" to teach, it is important to assess whether the intended curriculum (i.e., the curriculum adopted for all students) is designed to address the "big ideas" within various instructional domains and to accelerate learning and meet the diverse needs of students (Kame'enui & Carnine, 2001). This is true when planning the curriculum for young students and for secondary students (Grossen et al., 2002). Further, the same curriculum considerations are needed when planning for basic academic areas (e.g., reading, writing, mathematics) and content areas (e.g., science, social studies) as when planning for behavioral and social skills areas (see Howell & Kelley, 2002; Howell & Nolet, 2000).

Once information is collected about current student performance, curriculum, and instructional practices in the target domain (e.g., reading), this information can be analyzed to determine how students fit within the triangle of need for support and how well instructional practices and curricula are aligned with student needs. For example, information on student performance on foundational reading skills assessments such as the DIBELS (Kaminski et al., 2008) can be used to determine which students are (1) not experiencing problems (i.e., achieving at benchmark or expected levels), (2) at risk for problems (i.e., achieving below expected levels and in need of strategic interventions), and (3) currently experiencing significant problems (i.e., achieving well below expected levels and in need of intensive supports). At this point in the problem-solving process, the information collected helps to determine discrepancies between actual and expected performance as well as gaps in curriculum or instruction. Collecting this information helps to answer the question, What is the problem?

The next step in the problem-solving process is to analyze the information to determine why the problem is occurring and what can be done to improve the situation. At the primary prevention level, the focus is on what can be done to address student needs at a universal or schoolwide level. Interventions at this level consider the curriculum as well as instructional practices and staff development needs. Once universal targets for intervention are selected, it is important to set goals and to plan for monitoring the implementation of interventions as well as for formative assessment of student outcomes. An excellent illustration of the application of these steps of the problem-solving process on a schoolwide or primary prevention level is described by Simmons et al. (2000).

The same problem-solving steps occur at the secondary and tertiary levels of prevention, but the focus of data collection and intervention is on groups of students in need of strategic intervention (i.e., secondary prevention) or individual students in need of intensive supports (i.e., tertiary intervention). Across levels of problem solving, the process of questioning remains the same, but the intensity of prevention and intervention efforts and the frequency of monitoring of student outcomes may increase. Howell and Nolet (2000) argued that students with the fewest skills are often in need of the most support. This is also true of our monitoring efforts. When students are at increased risk for learning and/or behavior problems (i.e., at the top portions of the triangle), it is important to monitor their responsiveness to interventions on a more frequent basis (e.g., Deno, Espin, & Fuchs, 2002).

Conclusions

We believe that school psychologists who have strong foundational knowledge in learning and development, risk and resiliency research, the effective teaching literature, and an RTI framework for data-driven problem solving are in a strong position to facilitate the provision of prevention and intervention services in school settings. As with any learning process, beginning school psychologists should start by acquiring basic foundational knowledge and competencies in the data-driven problem-solving process. They should master the "big ideas" within the empirical literature and build fluency with the problem-solving process prior to attempting to expand their knowledge of the vast prevention and intervention literature. In this chapter, we have attempted to highlight some of the "big ideas" relevant to prevention and intervention issues in school psychology. We encourage school psychologists in training and in practice to continue to expand and refine their knowledge of intervention options once they have established proficiency and fluency in the most robust of these strategies.

DISCUSSION QUESTIONS AND ACTIVITIES

1. Consult the literature on risk and resiliency issues. Imagine that you were asked to design a preschool classroom that promoted the development of academic competence and reduced the exacerbation of risk factors. What would this classroom look like?

2. Visit an elementary classroom and observe instruction for at least one class period. Write a summary of the observation and note as many characteristics of the learning environment as you can in terms of student, curriculum, and instructional variables.

3. Search the empirical literature on a specific intervention topic in this chapter (e.g., reading fluency, comprehension, reading acquisition, strategy instruction, number sense in mathematics, group contingencies). Review the articles and write a brief (i.e., 3–5 pages) summary of the intervention strategy. Include a description of the strategy (e.g., its purpose, target group or skill deficit, procedures, and special considerations) and a summary of the relevant research, with a list of references.

4. Visit a local school or library and obtain a copy of an elementary school reading curriculum. The learning hierarchy would suggest that the curriculum should be sequenced such that concepts and skills build upon earlier concepts and skills in a sequential fashion. Examine the curricular materials and identify aspects of the curriculum that seem to target acquisition of skills and fluency building.

5. Imagine that you are asked to consult with a teacher about a child who is experiencing behavior problems in the classroom. The teacher emphasizes that Joey, who is in her fourth-grade classroom, has difficulty in reading and comprehending stories. She has referred Joey because during reading exercises he is often off task and disruptive in the classroom. What problem-solving strategies would you utilize to effectively assist the teacher and Joey? What questions would you want to ask and what additional information would you gather?

CHAPTER 10

The School Psychologist's Role in Prevention and Intervention
Part 2. Mental Health and Social–Emotional Behavior

In Chapter 9 we focused our attention on the role of school psychologists in prevention of and intervention with *academic* problems. We now turn our attention to the school psychologist's role in addressing students' *mental health* and *social–emotional* needs, specifically in prevention of and intervention with mental health and social–emotional problems. We begin with a brief update on recent advancements in the field. Following this, we provide an overview of the mental health and social–emotional challenges facing today's students. Next, we discuss the application of a data-driven problem-solving approach to the prevention of and intervention with mental health and social–emotional needs of students. In doing so, we highlight the importance of a public health prevention framework, consideration of evidence-based treatments, linking of systems of care, and adherence to a data-oriented problem-solving approach to management activities. We end the chapter with a description of the problem-solving process across levels of prevention, with an emphasis on mental health issues.

Noted Advancements in the Field

As we noted in the previous edition of this text, the social and mental health challenges that faced our children and youth were growing in number, diversity, severity, complexity, and scope as we entered the 21st century. At that time, demands on schools to meet the mental health and social–emotional needs of students were also growing, yet the provision of prevention and intervention services for youth with mental health issues was noted as underutilized (Strein et al., 2003) and fragmented (Greenberg et al., 2003; Hoagwood & Johnson, 2003). More specifically, data at the turn of the century indicated that only a small percentage (i.e., approximately 20%) of children in need of specialty mental health services receive them and that, when they do, the overwhelming majority (i.e., 70–80%) receive these services within school contexts (Hoagwood & Johnson, 2003). With increased recognition that schools were often serving in the role of de facto mental health providers, researchers and policy shapers developed frameworks for the provision of services within an EBP model and policies to address the mental health needs of students in school settings (e.g., Forness, 2003a; Hoagwood & Johnson, 2003; Hunter, 2003; Power, 2000, 2003).

Now, just a few years later as we enter the second decade of this century, although we are seeing positive gains in the range of tertiary level evidence-based psychological interventions (EBI) for clinical dysfunction (e.g., anxiety, depression, and substance abuse), it is unfortunate that, with respect to the provision of mental health services, "we do not reach the vast majority of youth in need with *any* treatment" (Kazdin, 2008a, p. 202). We have seen progress in the exploration of strategies for improving the provision of EBI to children and youth who are already experiencing psychological distress or clinical dysfunction (i.e., intensive or tertiary services), yet even with improvements in providing therapists with training in the implementation of EBI, the traditional model of delivery of mental health services (i.e., one therapist providing services to one child or family or even to traditional groups of children or families) is not sufficient to decrease the prevalence and burden of psychological disorder and dysfunction on a much-needed larger scale (Kazdin, 2008a). As a result, scholars are now arguing for alternative service-delivery approaches that would increase the scope of EBI service provision (Kazdin, 2008a).

In addition to advancements in the identification of EBI and in the provision of tertiary care for mental health disorders, we have seen dramatic growth in the field of school-based prevention, which emphasizes the provision of universal and secondary prevention of social–emotional and behavioral problems (e.g., Collaborative for Academic, Social, and Emotional Learning, 2003; Durlak, Weissberg, Dymnicki, Taylor, & Schellinger, 2011; Greenberg, 2010; Merrell & Gueldner, 2010). In particular, the term *social and emotional learning* (SEL) has been used to describe a variety of skill-based universal prevention programs that emphasize skill development in a variety of domains (e.g., self-awareness, social awareness, responsible decision making, self-management, and relationship management) to build competence in relationships, self-control, healthy values, and resistance to engagement in deviant or dangerous behaviors (Greenberg, 2010). Since the first edition of this text, the literature on SEL programs and prevention of social–emotional and behavioral difficulties has expanded greatly, and the findings are notably promising.

In addition to efforts to improve school-based mental health and social–emotional learning services, mounting research suggests that how and where students spend their time outside of normal school hours has important implications for their development (Durlak & Weissberg, 2007), with estimates indicating that more than 7 million children within the United States are without adult supervision for a portion of their time outside of school, and this unsupervised time places them at risk of learning and behavior problems as well as risky behaviors such as drug abuse (Weissman & Gottfredson, 2001). In recent years, researchers have also explored the effectiveness of after-school programs in addressing these concerns, and recent findings offer empirical support for the conclusion that well-run after-school programs (i.e., those that provide sequential, active, focused, and explicit approaches to skill development) can produce a variety of positive benefits for participating youth (i.e., significant improvement in youth's self-perceptions and bonding to school, increases in positive social behaviors, decreases in problem behaviors and drug use, and improvements in school grades and level of academic achievement; see Durlak & Weissberg, 2007).

Mental Health and Social–Emotional Needs of Students

As many scholars have noted, schools are faced with growing numbers of students with or at risk for learning and/or social–emotional problems (e.g., Greenberg et al., 2003; Kazdin, 2008; OSEP Center on Positive Behavioral Interventions and Supports, 2000). These problems present themselves in varying degrees of severity and complexity. In this section, we provide an overview of the scope of mental health and social–emotional problems among school-age population, as well as the impact of these issues in schools.

Prevalence of Disorders and Range of Problems in School-Age Populations

Kazdin (2004) described the range of student mental health and/or social–emotional concerns as fitting within three major categories: (1) psychiatric disorders, (2) problem and at-risk behaviors, and (3) delinquency.

Psychiatric Disorders

Population-based epidemiological studies have indicated that "16% to 22% of children and adolescents up to the age of 18 have a diagnosable disorder; five to nine percent of youth can be classified as seriously emotionally disturbed" and "approximately 4–8% of children, ages 9–17, had severe psychiatric disorders" (Hoagwood & Johnson, 2003, p. 4). What do these estimates mean exactly? To answer this question, it is important to start with a basic understanding of what is meant by the term "disorder." In addition, it is important to grasp the degree to which these prevalence estimates reflect *actual* rates of disorders and whether they truly represent the range of dysfunction present in children and adolescents (Kazdin, 2004, 2008a).

Various diagnostic systems have been developed that describe criteria for the range of psychological dysfunctions or patterns of behavior associated with impairments in general life functioning, which are referred to as psychiatric or mental disorders. The *Diagnostic and Statistical Manual of Mental Disorders* (DSM-IV-TR; American Psychiatric Association, 2000) and the *International Classification of Diseases* (ICD-10; World Health Organization, 1992) are two prominent diagnostic systems that catalog the range of disorders that individuals might experience in childhood, adolescence, and/or adulthood. The DSM is the most commonly used system, and it includes 10 broad categories of disorders that are first evidenced in infancy, childhood, or adolescence: *mental retardation, learning disorders, motor skills disorder, communication disorders, pervasive developmental disorders, attention-deficit and disruptive behavior disorders, feeding and eating disorders of infancy or early childhood, tic disorders, elimination disorders,* and *other disorders of infancy, childhood, or adolescence.* The DSM also includes a range of broad categories of disorders that are not unique to childhood but that are also relevant because they can arise throughout the life span (e.g., *anxiety, mood, substance-related,* and *eating disorders*). It is important to note that although systems such as the DSM provide specific criteria for diagnosing disorders, criteria differ across different diagnostic systems, and they have been revised and changed considerably in various editions of the same diagnostic system. For example, the DSM-5 is scheduled for release in 2013, and although final decisions have not yet been made, there are a number of proposed changes with the infancy, childhood, and adolescence category, including possible new disorders as well as reclassification and/or renaming of current disorders (see *www.dsm5.org* for more details).

In addition to the taxonomies of disorders available in formal diagnostic systems such as the DSM, some general categories of dysfunction are widely recognized by researchers and practitioners, and these are often used to categorize disorders in treatment studies. Kazdin (2004) describes five general categories: *externalizing disorders, internalizing disorders, substance-related disorders, learning and mental disabilities,* and *severe and pervasive psychopathology.* Externalizing disorders, which are problems directed toward others or the environment (e.g., oppositional behavior, aggression, hyperactivity, and antisocial behavior), are the most common reason for clinical referrals in children and adolescents, followed by internalizing disorders, or problems directed internally (e.g., anxiety, depression).

When looking at prevalence rates of various psychiatric concerns and when considering outcomes of treatment studies, Kazdin (2004) notes several important considerations. First, he argues that general categories of disorders (e.g., internalizing disorders and externalizing disorders) are often more useful than specific diagnostic categories, because some treatment studies do not adhere to strict criteria for inclusion. This way of looking at general categories is also referred to as the *broad-band* approach (Merrell, 2008), which has its roots in multivariate statistical studies for classification of children's behavioral and emotional problems. In addition, Kazdin notes that, regardless of which classification system is used to determine diagnosis, different assessment methods can result in different prevalence rates. Also, prevalence rates for different disorders do not necessarily capture the scope and severity of problems. More specifically, prevalence rates of disorders may underestimate problems, because a number of children may exhibit symptoms that approach but do not fully meet criteria for disorders (i.e., subsyndromal or subthreshold), yet these children still show significant impairment in functioning (Kazdin, 2004, 2008a). Similarly, some children may meet criteria for severity of symptoms but may not meet criteria for duration or age of onset of symptoms. Finally, prevalence estimates may not capture the severity and complexity of problems, because many children and youth who meet criteria for one psychiatric disorder also qualify for a second or comorbid disorder.

Problem and At-Risk Behavior

Research indicates that approximately "30% of 14- to 17-year-olds engage in multiple high risk behaviors that jeopardize their potential for life success" (Greenberg et al., 2003, p. 467). During adolescence, students are more likely to engage in a range of behaviors (e.g., risky sexual behavior, violence, truancy, drinking and driving, substance use) that are likely to place them at risk for psychological, social, and health concerns. Although many children who engage in such activities also meet criteria for a disorder, many more students engage in such behaviors but are able to manage daily functioning and do not meet criteria for a disorder (Kazdin, 2004, 2008a). Regardless of whether these behaviors co-occur with a diagnosable disorder, the risk associated with such acts is often sufficient to warrant intervention.

Delinquency

The third category of problem behavior, delinquency, is "a legal designation that includes behaviors that violate the law" (Kazdin, 2004, p. 546). Within the category of delinquency, some behaviors are deemed illegal for adults and juveniles. These are called *index* offenses and include such acts as robbery, drug use, aggravated assault, and homicide. Other acts, referred to as *status* offenses, are designated as illegal for certain age groups (e.g., juveniles). Some examples of status offenses include running away, underage drinking, and truancy. Prevalence estimates are more difficult with delinquent behavior, because many of these offenses go undetected or unreported. As Kazdin (2004) notes, studies have indicated that a fairly large percentage of adolescents (e.g., 70%) engage in some form of delinquent behavior. Most of these youth engage in status offenses such as underage drinking or substance use and do not continue to engage in such behaviors. A much smaller percentage (e.g., 20% to 30%) are involved in more serious offenses, and only about 5% are responsible for committing greater than 50% of officially documented offenses.

Issues of Complexity and Comorbidity: Need for Early Detection and Intervention

Children and youth who meet criteria for one psychiatric disorder, problem, or at-risk behavior and/or delinquency often meet criteria for an additional disorder or problem category. The co-occurrence of psychiatric disorders among children and youth is termed *comorbidity* and has been well established in the empirical literature (Angold, Costello, & Erkanli, 1999; Kazdin & Whitley, 2006). In community samples, for example, roughly 50% of youth who meet criteria for one psychiatric disorder also meet criteria for a second, and rates are much higher for clinically referred samples (Kazdin, 2004). As problems increase in severity, it seems that a concomitant increase in comorbidity occurs. For example, the overlap between delinquency and psychiatric disorders is reportedly high, with estimates indicating that between 50 and 80% of delinquent youth meet criteria for at least one diagnosable disorder, the most common of which are ADHD, conduct, and substance abuse disorders (Kazdin, 2004). Research also indicates that the prevalence of mental health disorders is higher for students who are receiving special education services (i.e., 70.2%) than for any other group, including students who are served in the mental health system or the drug and alcohol treatment systems (Hoagwood & Johnson, 2003). Thus, it should not be surprising that large numbers of students with mental health concerns and/or deficiencies in their social–emotional competence also have difficulty learning and may disrupt the learning of others (Greenberg et al., 2003). Studies of child treatment have shown that children with comorbid diagnoses have greater impairments at home, at school, and in interpersonal relationships than those with single diagnoses (Ezpeleta, Domenech, & Angold, 2006)

The issue of comorbidity among psychiatric disorders and other problems can be illustrated with an example. ADHD is now recognized as the most *common* neurobehavioral disorder of childhood and among the most chronic health conditions affecting school-age children (American Academy of Pediatrics [AAP], 2001). Estimates of the prevalence of the disorder range from 4 to 12% in nonreferred, school-age community samples (AAP, 2001), with higher estimates in clinically referred children. According to Barkley (2006), children with ADHD account for a significant percentage (i.e., 30–40%) of referrals to mental health practitioners. Among children and adolescents with ADHD, there is a high prevalence of associated disorders, including anxiety, LDs, depression, and disruptive behavior disorders (Brown et al., 2001; Jensen et al., 2001). With regard to the co-occurrence of other psychiatric disorders, estimates indicate that approximately 44% have one, 33% have two, and 10% have three other disorders in addition to ADHD (Root & Resnick, 2003). The most common comorbid diagnosis is oppositional defiant disorder, followed by conduct disorder, anxiety disorder, and depression (Barkley, 2006;

Root & Resnick, 2003). Estimates indicate that approximately 80% of children with ADHD experience academic difficulties and that approximately 50% are eligible for and are receiving special education or related services (Reid, Maag, Vasa, & Wright, 1994; Root & Resnick, 2003). Thus, it is safe to say that school psychologists will be involved with children and adolescents who meet criteria for ADHD, and likely for comorbid disorders or learning difficulties, on a fairly regular basis. This does not mean, however, that *all* students with diagnoses of ADHD will have learning problems or comorbid psychiatric disorders. Instead, this means that, at a group level, children and/or adolescents who meet criteria for ADHD are more likely to experience learning or comorbid disorders than those who do not meet criteria for ADHD.

When psychiatric disorders such as ADHD co-occur with other psychiatric disorders, with problem or at-risk behaviors, with delinquency, and/or with learning and behavior problems, failure to detect such comorbidity may affect response to treatment. For children with ADHD, for example, findings from a large-scale, 14-month comparative study conducted by a national consortium of researchers (MTA Cooperative Group, 1999a, 1999b) suggested that the presence of some comorbid disorders (e.g., anxiety) moderated the effects of medication treatment (Jensen et al., 2001). According to Forness (2003b), "By not attending to emergence of a psychiatric diagnosis and of possible comorbid diagnoses, we may not only be potentially mismanaging treatment resources but also may be missing critical opportunities for determining the most effective course for treatment-resistant disorders" (p. 322). Despite widespread recognition of the common co-occurrence of academic, social–emotional, and mental health concerns within the empirical literature, underidentification and misidentification rates for mental health problems in school settings appear to be fairly common (for a discussion, see Forness, 2003a, 2003b). Forness (2003b) cites primary prevention research that demonstrates how classwide interventions in preschool have been found to result in significant improvements in symptoms and functional behavior of at-risk children (e.g., Serna, Lambros, Nielsen, & Forness, 2002) as well as possibly forestalling the actual development of psychopathology for those at highest risk (e.g., Serna, Nielson, Mattern, Schau, & Forness, 2002). Forness (2003b) argues that we must attend to comorbidity issues and early signs of pathology. In addition, he comments that educators in general and school psychologists in particular are guilty of "back-loading" our efforts and providing only reactive or tertiary care for mental health concerns rather than working from a public health or primary prevention framework wherein services are "front-loaded" to address the earliest signs of problems. We agree with this criticism and believe that the field of school psychology has great potential to make inroads in mental health promotion by moving increasingly toward a prevention and early-intervention mode of service delivery, and preliminary evidence in this area has been promising (Greenberg, 2010).

Addressing Mental Health Issues from a Problem-Solving Stance

Stepping back for a minute from the gravity of the mental health and social–emotional issues we described in the previous section, let's revisit the problem-solving approach to school psychology service delivery that we outlined in Chapter 7. To start, we argued that the traditional refer–test–place model of school psychology practice, wherein the school psychologist's role is that of diagnostician, was inadequate. More specifically, we described how assumptions in the philosophically based system that dominated early practice (i.e., that diagnosis informs treatment) were questionable (e.g., Deno, 2002;

Tilly, 2002) and how school psychologists had been faced with enough practice failures from this approach to begin to consider alternatives. Next, we argued that school psychologists might approach problems from a data-oriented problem-solving approach that focused on using the scientific method to determine what works, in contrast to the traditional model, which was more likely to produce recommendations based on diagnosis. We highlighted the fact that a problem-solving approach is outcome focused, data driven, integrally linked to intervention, and context specific. Further, it follows a specific line of questioning: (1) What is the problem? (2) Why is it occurring? (3) What can we do about it? (4) Did it work? The decision-making process in this model is guided by data with an emphasis on formative assessment (see Chapter 7) to determine the effectiveness of our prevention and intervention efforts. Thus, in a problem-solving approach, "instead of measuring student performance to find disabilities our purpose is to diagnose the conditions under which students' learning is *enabled*" (Tilly, 2002, p. 29). Further, from this perspective, "failure to profit from general education is relatively common and results to some extent from idiosyncratic, inappropriately arranged environmental events" (Lentz & Shapiro, 1985, p. 199). In Chapter 9, we described how a problem-solving model was applicable to addressing academic concerns. In particular, we described how learning problems are best solved through consideration or *diagnosis* of the alignment and interaction of student, curriculum, and instructional variables rather than from consideration of any one of these factors in isolation (Howell & Nolet, 2000).

In the beginning of this chapter, we described the scope of mental health and social–emotional issues facing our youth. In doing so, we used diagnostic terms (e.g., ADHD) and labels (e.g., delinquency) that are based on structural taxonomies. When reading our description of mental health concerns, one might ask, Why should we place an emphasis on structural, diagnostic taxonomies of behavior, when we argued in Chapter 7 that diagnosis does not necessarily inform treatment? This is an excellent question, one that we believe warrants further discussion prior to describing the application of a data-oriented problem-solving approach to addressing mental health and social–emotional problems. So, we ask ourselves, What is the utility of a structural, diagnostic classification system such as the DSM and how can it possibly fit within a functional, data-oriented problem-solving approach to school psychology?

According to Scotti, Morris, McNeil, and Hawskins (1996), "A basic first step in any scientific endeavor is classification" (p. 1179). Theories are often developed through deductive methods that start with observations of typical and atypical behavior, with efforts to sort these observations into categories of similarity and dissimilarity. Taxonomies that result from this process are again observed, and over time theories can be developed about these observations. The application of inductively derived theories and classification schemes must then be deductively applied in order to determine their practical use. This process and its importance in applied sciences are described by Scotti et al. (1996):

> Once we have amassed a number of critical observations about the behavior of many individuals, we summarize them (i.e., construct and theory development) and then apply these generalizations to the specific case. Without such a process, we would need to rediscover the principles of behavior anew for each client who seeks our services. "In effect, syndromal categories … provid[e] fundamental guidance to the *beginning* of a functional analysis" (Hayes & Follette, 1992, p. 352); that is, we begin an analysis at the nomothetic level and proceed deductively from what we know about persons with

similar patterns of behavior (e.g., etiology, response covariation, prognosis, treatment design) to a focus on the target person in question. (p. 1179, emphasis added)

Thus, one way to look at diagnosis and how it might fit within a problem-solving model is to consider these terms as describing constellations of covarying behaviors that can help to inform the "what" of behavior (i.e., delineating specific clusters of covarying behaviors [syndromes] and setting criteria for the duration of their occurrence).

Scotti and colleagues (1996) argued that the DSM structural categories are open to two levels of analysis. First, they can be viewed descriptively, because they point to other symptoms and/or behaviors to investigate and, therefore, can be helpful in defining problems (i.e., discrepancies between expected levels of functioning and developmentally inappropriate levels that meet criteria for a diagnosis). Second, when a syndrome or set of covarying behaviors is present across individuals, it is possible to raise more causal questions of common etiology, mechanism, or function. This is to say that, with continued research on the developmental trajectories of certain syndromes (i.e., clusters of systematically covarying behaviors), we might be able to come to some general conclusions regarding common etiologies, response covariation, associated risk factors, prognosis, and potentially common treatment strategies to address the covarying set of behaviors or symptoms. Currently, however, the utility of the DSM classification system in meeting this second aim is questionable.

Scotti and colleagues (1996) argued that there is much to be done before we can attempt to move in the direction of linking intervention strategies to certain clusters of covarying behaviors but that with continued research this might become possible. For example, at a descriptive or structural level, the behaviors of children with panic disorder resemble the behaviors of children with social phobia, yet at a functional level differences can be noted. Children with panic disorders and those with social phobia often exhibit a cluster of behaviors that is referred to as a "panic attack" (i.e., physiological responses and thoughts of losing control or being embarrassed that are associated with behavioral avoidance that significantly interferes with daily functioning). On a purely structural level, these two disorders appear very similar. Yet, at a functional level, this pattern of behaviors tends to be situation specific for children with social phobia and more closely triggered by internal and physiological cues for children with panic disorders. In other words, a similar pattern of behavior can be triggered by different antecedents for different syndromes, and these functional relations (i.e., between the syndrome and the antecedent cue) can be useful in directing treatment for the different groups. Still, this analysis leaves out other potentially relevant functional relationships that may contribute to or exacerbate patterns of behavior exhibited by individuals (e.g., consequences connected to avoidance of social situations, skill deficits that may have contributed to the initial development of the social avoidance pattern). These finer-grained analyses might be accomplished through functional assessment methods conducted at the level of the individual child. Scotti and colleagues (1996) argue that we consider a melding of structural and more problem-solving or functionally based approaches to treatment by "augmenting the DSM with a system of functional analysis, using the best of both methods by moving from broad and nomothetic classification of the person to fine-grained idiographic analysis of the case, which includes the person and relevant social systems" (Scotti et al., 1996, p. 1187).

We now return to the problem-solving model and its application to prevention and intervention for mental health and social–emotional issues. As we noted in Chapter 7, the purpose of schooling is to alter development (cognitive, affective, social, and physical) from its natural or unschooled course (Deno, 2002). For example, from an academic learning standpoint, we expect that students' reading, writing, and math performances will be altered through the course of schooling. In addition, we recognize that students will learn to read at different rates and that problem solving will be necessary to determine proper alignment of student, instructional, and curriculum variables to facilitate literacy development. Although we often think of schooling in terms of academic development, it is also true that most of us (e.g., educators, parents, students, teachers, and community members) expect schools to address broader issues for students.

Greenberg and colleagues (2003) capture this broader educational agenda:

> In addition to producing students who are culturally literate, intellectually reflective, and committed to lifelong learning, high-quality education should teach young people to interact in socially skilled and respectful ways; to practice positive, safe, and healthy behaviors; to contribute ethically and responsibly to their peer group, family, school, and community; and to possess basic competencies, work habits, and values as a foundation for meaningful employment and engaged citizenship. (Greenberg et al., 2003, pp. 466–467)

In other words, schools are expected to alter student development from its unschooled course across a wide range of domains, including mental health and social–emotional competence. Just as individual differences exist in how students develop literacy skills, the development of social competence is not a uniform process across students. Problems arise when gaps exist between current and expected levels of mental health and social–emotional well-being. As we described earlier, taxonomies of mental health problems, such as the DSM, can help to organize our thinking about what constitutes a significant discrepancy between expected and actual performance in domains of mental health and social–emotional functioning. In other words, they help us determine whether or not a problem exists (i.e., whether the child's functioning is discrepant from developmentally normal levels of functioning), and, from a structural standpoint, they assist us in a description of *what* the problem looks like and can potentially help direct the nature of additional inquiries (Scotti et al., 1996). When we move on to problem analysis, however, and we ask "why" or "what for" questions about problem behaviors, the utility of diagnostic classification systems is reduced, and we need to consider assessment procedures that have been found to be more directly linked to intervention development (e.g., functional assessment, functional analysis). Thus, departure from structural classification systems begins in the second step of the problem-solving process when we ask why the problem is occurring. When we begin to think about intervention strategies (i.e., what can we do about the problem?), we may return to consideration of syndrome and the EBIs that have been found to be effective for groups of students with particular disorders (e.g., the use of psychostimulants for children with ADHD or the use of cognitive-behavioral therapy [CBT] for children with anxiety problems). We do so with caution, however, knowing that we need to carefully consider issues of contextual fit and individual responsiveness to intervention. Thus, during the fourth step in the problem-solving process (i.e., did it work?), it is important to directly evaluate the effectiveness of the intervention.

As we entered the 21st century, school psychologists were and still are faced with growing social–emotional and mental health concerns of students. These problems are often complex and rarely occur in isolation from other problems. In order to properly address these issues, we believe school psychologists need to be:

1. Aware of the nature, scope, complexity, and developmental trajectories of student mental health and social–emotional issues that point to the need for early detection, primary prevention, and intervention.
2. Knowledgeable about EBI for addressing these concerns and also knowledgeable about universal and secondary SEL prevention programs.
3. Prepared to interact with professionals from medicine, clinical psychology, and community care to ensure access to treatment.
4. Experts in the application of a data-oriented problem-solving approach to management of primary, secondary, and tertiary prevention and intervention efforts.

In the remaining sections of this chapter, we describe how the integration of a public health prevention model, emphasis on evidence-based prevention and intervention practices, coordination of systems of care, and adherence to a data-oriented problem-solving approach to school psychology practice provides a promising framework from which to address the mental health and social emotional needs of students.

Adaptation of a Public Health Prevention Framework to Schools

The adaptation of public health models to developing systems of support for students within school settings will clearly play an integral role in the shaping of the future provision of prevention and intervention services for children and youth with or at risk for mental health concerns. Public health notions of primary, secondary, and tertiary prevention, which grew out of public concern over medical threats (e.g., communicable diseases), are currently being used across a variety of disciplines. For example, these approaches were adapted for use in the field of community psychology (e.g., Adams, Hampton, Gullotta, Wiessberg, & Ryan, 1997; Cowen et al., 1996; Edelstein & Michelson, 1986) and also have been applied to educational settings and school psychology (e.g., Greenberg, 2010; Hoagwood & Johnson, 2003; Strein et al., 2003).

Returning to the river parable that we presented in Chapter 7, a public health prevention framework considers not only the needs of students who are already experiencing difficulties (i.e., children in the river) or at risk for experiencing difficulties (i.e., children close to the river) but also those who are not at risk or experiencing difficulties (i.e., children who are safely on dry land). Using a triangle of support (e.g., Figure 7.2), primary prevention services or universal supports are delivered to all students. Secondary prevention services are targeted toward students who are identified as at risk for the development of problems, and more intensive tertiary prevention efforts are directed at children who are already experiencing problems (i.e., children at the top of the triangle).

Arguably, the bulk of school psychology and special education practice has focused on the provision of tertiary services to children who are already experiencing difficulties (Forness, 2003a; Hoagwood & Johnson, 2003; Kazdin, 2008a; Shapiro, 2000). As Shapiro (2000) aptly noted, "The difficulty with a child-by-child focus is that while we are solving little problems, we are missing the big problem" (p. 561). Shapiro argues for a shift in our approach to solving instructional problems from a reactive stance to a proactive and preventive position that considers the instructional needs of *all* students and emphasizes the prevention of academic problems through primary and secondary prevention efforts. The same argument can and has been made regarding the provision of mental health and social–emotional services to students in school settings (e.g., Greenberg, 2010; Hoagwood & Johnson, 2003; Strein et al., 2003; Walker et al., 1996). One potentially positive outcome of this shift in focus is the likelihood that through prevention and early intervention efforts we may reduce the number of students with or at risk for the development of more severe problems. This is indeed a meaningful goal when one considers the enormous amount of time and resources that are spent in reactive management of the most severe problems. For example, students with severe behavior problems account for a relatively small portion of the school population (1–5%), yet they are often the focus of greater than 50% of office/discipline referrals and may take up a significant amount of educator and administrator time (Sugai, Sprague, Horner, & Walker, 2000). Further, with early prevention and intervention efforts in place, it may be possible to alter developmental psychopathology trajectories in such a way that we reduce the incidence of psychopathology in our children and youth (Forness, 2003a, 2003b).

The public health framework also fits nicely with a data-oriented problem-solving approach for several reasons. First, "the framework for constructing levels of risk, causality, and health promotion depends upon data-based decision making" (Strein et al., 2003, p. 25). Second, in addition to being data driven, emphasis is placed on the development of prevention and intervention strategies. The focus of "research" in this approach is to gather information to determine relationships among variables (e.g., biological, physiological, genetic, behavioral, social, economic) "with the explicit aim of ascertaining causality and developing interventions to promote health" (Strein et al., 2003, p. 25). Finally, research is conducted within the natural context to promote generality of findings to target settings and populations, and, consistent with a data-driven problem-solving model, there is a strong reliance on the scientific method rather than expert judgment to determine what works.

Evidence-Based Practice Movement

Evidence-based practice (EBP) is another movement that has gained momentum and that is directly relevant to applying data-oriented problem solving to students' mental health and social–emotional needs. According to the American Psychological Association (APA) Presidential Task Force on Evidence-Based Practice (2006), EBP in psychology is defined as "the integration of the best available research with clinical expertise in the context of patient characteristics, culture, and preferences" (p. 273). Although much of the discussion regarding EBP was initially focused on evidence-based/empirically supported *treatments* (e.g., Chambless et al., 1998) and evaluating the research support for specific interventions, EBP is a more comprehensive term, taking into account not only the research but also the specifics about the client and the treating professional (APA Presidential Task Force on Evidence-Based Practice, 2006).

The concept of EBP is not unique to psychology. In fact, much of the initial literature and discussion on EBP came from the medical field. In particular, David Sackett, who along with his colleagues instituted the Centre for Evidence-Based Medicine (*www.cebm.net*), is often considered to be one of the primary leaders in this area. Other disciplines, including psychology, speech–language–hearing, and education (including special education), have provided definitions and guidelines for EBP in more recent years.

As noted, the initial discussions in psychology related to defining what was first termed "empirically validated treatments" and later changed to "empirically supported treatments" (EST). A group of professionals from Division 12 of APA worked to develop criteria for what constituted an EST. Treatments are divided into "well-established" and "probably efficacious" categories. According to Chambless et al. (1998), a well-established treatment is one that has

> at least two good between group design experiments demonstrating efficacy in one or more of the following ways: A) Superior (statistically significantly so) to pill or psychological placebo or to another treatment; b) Equivalent to an already established treatment in experiments with adequate sample sizes OR a large series of single case design experiments demonstrating efficacy. (p. 4)

A probably efficacious treatment is one that has been shown to be superior to a wait-list control group in at least two experiments; one that meets the primary criteria for a well-established treatment but has not been evaluated by at least two different research groups; or one that has a small series of single-case designs for support (Chambless et al., 1998). This list was later expanded to include "possibly efficacious treatments," where at least one good study supports the intervention, and "experimental treatments," which are untested treatments (Silverman & Hinshaw, 2008).

Within the field of school psychology, the Task Force on Evidence-Based Interventions in School Psychology was in place from 1999 to 2008 (see *www.indiana.edi/~ebi*). The purpose of this task force was to identify evidence-based interventions to address behavioral, emotional, and academic needs of children in school settings (e.g., Kratochwill, 2007; Kratochwill & Shernoff, 2004; Kratochwill & Stoiber, 2000a, 2000b, 2002). The task force in school psychology has aimed to "improve the quality of research training, extend knowledge of evaluation criteria for evidence-based interventions (EBI), and report this information to the profession of school psychology" (Kratochwill & Shernoff, 2004, p. 34). Several coding manuals were developed by the task force but, as noted on its website, as other professional groups became more involved in reviewing interventions to summarize the literature, the task force moved away from this as a specific goal but instead focused on promoting research related to interventions in school psychology. Currently, there are several websites hosted by professional organizations that summarize treatments that have empirical support. For example, the Society of Clinical Psychology (Division 12 of APA) hosts a website (*www.div12.org/PsychologicalTreatments/ treatments.html*) that lists treatments and their evidence for a variety of psychological problems (mainly focused on adults). The Association for Behavioral and Cognitive Therapies and the Society of Clinical Child and Adolescent Psychology (Division 53 of APA) have a website listing EBI for disorders of childhood and adolescence (see *www. abct.org/sccap/?m=sPro&fa=pro_ESToptions*). Another website worth noting is What Works Clearinghouse (*ies.ed.gov/ncee/wwc*), which was established by the U.S. Department of Education's Institute of Education Sciences in 2002 as a trusted source for scientific evidence of what works in education. Journals have also devoted special issues to covering EBI. For example, in 2008 the *Journal of Clinical Child and Adolescent Psychology* published a special issue on EBI with reviews covering nine different problem areas, and in 2005 *School Psychology Quarterly* published a special issue on evidence-based parent and family interventions.

Although a complete synopsis of the literature on EBI or practices is beyond the scope of this chapter, a few of the major issues and findings are worth noting. School psychologists who are new to the field should be aware of some of the criticisms that have been raised, particularly initially when the focus was more exclusively on research evidence without taking into account other factors. For example, within the EBP literature, an important distinction has been made between the concepts of *efficacy* and *effectiveness* whereby *efficacy* refers to standards for evaluating treatments in controlled research studies and *effectiveness* standards require demonstrated utility in the practice context (Kratochwill & Shernoff, 2004). According to the school psychology task force, "an intervention should carry the *evidence-based* designation when information about its contextual application in actual practice is specified and when it has demonstrated efficacy under the conditions of implementation and evaluation in practice" (Kratochwill & Shernoff, 2004, p. 35). In other words, school psychologists should concern themselves with interventions/practices that have met standards for *effectiveness* (as well as *efficacy*). As the concept of EBP as a comprehensive model has grown, these ideas have been take into consideration with greater frequency.

In addition to the distinction between efficacy and effectiveness, a host of other issues are relevant to the integration of EBP into school-based practice. Kratochwill and Shernoff (2004) highlight four of these. The first issue they raise is the difficulty in reviewing and summarizing the literature despite attempts to delineate clear criteria. The literature and the groups who are attempting to summarize the evidence are diverse, and this makes it difficult to organize a unified, consistent approach. Second, organizational and systems issues present in practice may not be considered in controlled research studies. This factor limits the generality of some research findings to school settings. Third, as we noted in Chapter 7, school psychology is a relatively immature profession, and as such practitioners may be more likely to rely on clinical judgment rather than the scientific method or the empirical literature to determine what works. Thus, movement toward the adoption of an EBP model will require a shift in this tradition. We find this shift a positive one, yet we recognize that any shift in tradition is often met with resistance. Finally, bridging the research-to-practice gaps in the implementation of EBI (once they are identified) is likely to require additional training in these practices. Similar training issues are likely to arise for teachers and special educators.

Given the greater emphasis on accountability in education, we believe that the EBP movement will likely continue to gain momentum in practice in school psychology training programs. Thus school psychologists should engage in continued professional development activities to keep abreast of the treatment research as new findings are integrated. In addition, EBI should be implemented with careful adherence to a problem-solving model that incorporates a formative assessment process to determine whether, in fact, the intervention was effective for the individual or group of individuals in the practice context. This approach is not unlike Cronbach's (1975) argument for the use of "short-run empiricism," as discussed in Chapter 7.

In the sections that follow, we highlight some interventions that have been found to have empirical support in addressing the problems associated with the most common mental health and social–emotional needs of students. This is not an exhaustive list of evidence-based interventions. Instead, we have attempted to describe a range of interventions that illustrate the diversity of this literature and capture some of the major issues that arise. First, we discuss parent management training as a well-established treatment for aggression and oppositional behavior. This treatment is also indicated as an EBI for children with ADHD (Kazdin, 2003a, 2004) and incorporates the application of operant principles not unlike those found in another supported intervention for ADHD: classroom contingency management, which we discussed in Chapter 9. Next, we describe CBT and its application and evidence in treating a variety of disorders (i.e., anxiety, depression). We end with a description of the evidence for the use of psychostimulant medication in the treatment of problems associated with ADHD. Forness (2003b) argues that educators have virtually ignored the psychopharmacology literature and that doing so places us "at risk of not choosing the most effective intervention for children in our care" (p. 322). Of course, school psychologists are not in a position to prescribe medication. The point Forness is making is that we need to be careful not to ignore or argue against potentially efficacious treatments such as the use of psychostimulants for children with ADHD. We include this example because it raises important questions regarding the current limitations of our practice and the need to link systems of care. Although additional examples are beyond the scope of this chapter, readers are encouraged to examine the literature, including the websites mentioned earlier, for a wider range of evidence-based interventions. Finally, it is important to recognize that any list of such interventions is essentially a work in progress and will need to be altered to accommodate and integrate more recent findings.

Parent Management Training for the Treatment of Aggression and Oppositional Behavior

Parent management training (PMT) is perhaps the most well-researched treatment for oppositional and aggressive behavior in children and adolescents (Eyberg et al., 2008; Hood & Eyberg, 2003; Kazdin, 1997, 2003a, 2004, 2008b; Maughan, Christiansen, Jenson, Olympia, & Clark, 2005; Sanders, 1999; Sanders, Markie-Dadds, Tully, & Bor, 2000; Webster-Stratton, Reid, & Hammond, 2004; Weisz, Hawley, & Doss, 2004). Within the literature, one can find a number of empirically based PMT programs. Some of these programs are more generally targeted toward children with externalizing or disruptive behaviors (e.g., McMahon & Forehand, 2003; McNeil & Hembree-Kigin, 2010; Kazdin, 2008b; Webster-Stratton et al., 2004), whereas others focus on children with specific diagnoses, such as ADHD (e.g., Barkley, 1997; Barkley, Edwards, & Robin, 1999). Although specific procedures may vary across programs, the majority of PMT approaches emphasize teaching parents to use contingency management techniques to effectively manage their child's behaviors. Underlying this approach is a fundamental assumption that oppositional and aggressive behaviors are established and maintained by maladaptive parent–child interactions. Much of this emphasis is grounded in the work of Patterson and colleagues (e.g., Patterson, 1982; Patterson, Reid, & Dishion, 1992). PMT instructs parents in behavior management strategies (based on principles of operant conditioning) and teaches parents to be more positive, predictable, and consistent with their children. The goal is to shift interaction patterns so that prosocial, positive, and compliant behaviors are reinforced. Most PMT interventions follow a similar format wherein parents are taught techniques to increase positive behaviors (e.g., positive attention) before moving on to discipline strategies (e.g., time-out). This format is based on a two-part model originally developed by Hanf (1969) and subsequently adapted by others (e.g., Barkley, 1997; McMahon & Forehand, 2003; McNeil & Hembree-Kigin, 2010). The process generally involves having parents meet with a therapist, who trains them in a variety of specific parenting behaviors (e.g., establishing rules, administering positive reinforcement for appropriate behavior). Program duration varies and may be dependent on the severity of presenting problems. For example, for young children with milder oppositional problems, PMT may last approximately 4 to 8 weeks, but for more complicated problems (e.g., clinically referred conduct disorders) it might last as long as 12 to 25 weeks (Kazdin, 2003a).

As noted, there is significant support for parent training as an intervention to reduce disruptive behaviors. However, not all children treated do improve following parent training. Although increasingly researchers are evaluating the components of parent training programs as well as mediators and moderators of effectiveness (e.g., Kaminksi, Valle, Filene, & Boyle, 2006; Reyno & McGrath, 2006), it is important for practitioners who are implementing parent training programs to engage in the problem-solving model so that they are taking data and evaluating whether the intervention is having the intended effect on the child and his or her parents.

Although PMT began as more of a tertiary intervention, in recent years it is increasingly being implemented as a primary prevention technique. For example, the Triple P Positive Parenting approach (Sanders, 1999, 2008), which has significant empirical support, incorporates different levels of prevention/intervention. The first level is a universal prevention program geared toward all parents. At this level, information regarding parenting is shared via a variety of methods, including the media. Level 2 is geared toward parents who are interested in learning more or who have some concerns about their child and is typically delivered in the context of routine health care visits. Level 3 is focused on parents with specific concerns who need more detailed guidance. Levels 4 and 5 focus on children who are currently exhibiting problem behaviors, with greater supports provided at Level 5 for families who are experiencing additional stressors (e.g., parental mental health problems). In addition to these five levels, there are two more specialized intervention modes: Stepping Stones (geared toward families of preschool children with disabilities) and Pathways (geared toward parents who are at risk of child maltreatment).

CBT for the Treatment of Internalizing Problems

CBT is currently recognized as an EBI and treatment of choice for internalizing problems such as child and adolescent anxiety and depression (e.g., Barrett, Farrell, Ollendick, & Dadds, 2006; Compton et al., 2004; David-Ferdon & Kaslow, 2008; Silverman, Pina, & Viswesvaran, 2008). This approach focuses on cognitive distortions or maladaptive cognitions and their role in problems of anxiety (Kendall, Panichelli-Mindel, Sugarman, & Callahan, 1997) and depression (Lewinsohn & Clarke, 1999). In addition, there is a concomitant focus on modification of patterns of behavior and the development of more adaptive skills (Compton et al., 2004; Kazdin, 2003a, 2004). It is worth noting that although CBT is effective in treating anxiety and depression, several recent large-scale randomized controlled trials have provided evidence that combining CBT with medication may be the most effective treatment for many youth (Walkup et al., 2008; TADS Team 2004, 2007).

CBT and Anxiety

In the treatment of anxiety, CBT employs a variety of techniques, including psychoeducation, relaxation, problem solving, reinforcement, modeling, and exposure-based interventions to promote the use of cognitions and behaviors resulting in habituation or extinction of inappropriate fears (Compton et al., 2004; Kazdin, 2003a, 2004; Kendall & Suveg, 2006). The exposure-based component of the intervention rests on the notion that "anxiety is a set of classically conditioned responses that can be unlearned or counterconditioned through associative pairing with anxiety-incompatible stimuli and responses" (Compton et al., 2004, p. 941). With systematic desensitization, for example, stimuli that are anxiety arousing are paired gradually and systematically with competing stimuli that produce relaxation (e.g., food, praise, cues for muscle relaxation). This can be accomplished through imagery or *in vivo* exposure. Treatment also involves modeling and direct reinforcement of new skills and behaviors designed to mediate anxiety. For example, children are taught to recognize the physiological symptoms (e.g., muscle tension) and the internal dialogue (e.g., negative "what if" statements) associated with anxiety. Therapy focuses on the development of coping skills, including strategies for recognizing and reconceptualizing anxiety-provoking situations as well as problem-solving alternatives for coping with the situation. Emphasis is placed on generating alternative explanations to correct maladaptive self-talk. In addition, children are taught to generate alternative actions or plans for how to cope with anxiety-provoking situations. Finally, children are taught to evaluate their alternative coping plans through self-evaluation and self-reinforcement procedures. CBT for anxiety problems typically involves 12 to 20 individually administered sessions. The first six to 10 sessions are devoted to learning new coping skills, and the second 6–10 sessions focus on application of these skills to varying levels of anxiety-producing situations.

A substantive research base supports the utility of CBT for the treatment of child anxiety (Compton et al., 2004; Kazdin, 2003a, 2004; Kendall & Suveg, 2006; Walkup et al., 2008). This treatment has been evaluated in both single-case and randomized control trials with children and adolescents. Multimethod and multi-informant outcome data indicate improvements in anxiety, as well as other areas (e.g., depression, aggression, social problems, hyperactivity). Further effects of treatment have been replicated by independent investigators, and effects have been maintained for periods of up to 7 years. Although not all children are diagnosis free following treatment with CBT, studies have often found that about 60 to 70% of children are diagnosis free immediately following treatment. In addition, treatment gains may be maintained for up to 7 years (Kendall & Suveg, 2006; Silverman et al., 2008)

One of the best know (and well-researched) cognitive-behavioral interventions for anxiety disorders is the Coping Cat program, developed by Kendall and colleagues (Kendall & Hedtke, 2006a, 2006b). In a recent NIMH funded study involving almost 500 children ages 7 to 17, the efficacy of the Coping Cat program was compared to Sertraline (as well as a combination of the two and a placebo group). Although the combination treatment was the most effective, the CBT Coping Cat program and Sertraline by itself also produced positive effects compared with the placebo condition (Walkup et al., 2008).

CBT and Depression

In the treatment of depression, CBT focuses on reinstating behavioral patterns associated with pleasant experiences and confrontation of maladaptive cognitions such as helplessness or hopelessness (Compton et al., 2004; Kazdin, 2004). CBT for depression is based on an assumption that "symptom change is most likely to occur through interventions that modify patterns of behavior through skills acquisition and patterns of cognition, with changes in depressed mood following in turn" (Compton et al., 2004, p. 952). Some aspects of CBT are standard (i.e., psychoeducation about depression and its causes, goal setting, general problem-solving skills), whereas others are tailored to the specific skill deficits and needs of the individual (e.g., addressing negative self-attributes, poor self-assertion skills, failure to attribute positive outcomes to internal, stable, or global causes). In addition, current CBT packages integrate parent and family sessions with individual CBT (Compton et al., 2004).

Research also supports the use of CBT in the treatment of depression (Compton et al., 2004; David-Ferdon & Kaslow, 2008; Kazdin, 2004). These studies adhere to the same methodological rigor as CBT studies focused on anxiety disorders, but there are fewer studies that focus on youth with depression. In the largest outcome studies on the use of CBT for depression to date involving more than 400 youth ages 12 to 17, the TADS Team, a group of researchers from a number of different sites, evaluated the efficacy of CBT and of fluoxetine (Prozac), as well as the combination of the two, in comparison to each other and a placebo control condition (TADS Team, 2004, 2007, 2009). Results immediately posttreatment found that the combined treatment was most effective but that Prozac alone was also more effective than a placebo treatment (TADS Team, 2004). When looking at results 36 weeks out (with the placebo condition discontinued), response rates were similar across the three treatment conditions. Interestingly, although CBT initially was not superior to the placebo treatment, CBT "caught up" with fluoxetine by 18 to 24 weeks and with the combined treatment by 30 to 36 weeks (TADS Team, 2007). These results were maintained at a 1-year evaluation point (TADS Team, 2009), and only 6 to 33% of all youth demonstrated a worsening of symptoms after treatment was discontinued.

Psychostimulants for the Treatment of ADHD Symptoms

Psychostimulants are a well-established treatment for the symptoms of ADHD (Kazdin, 2003a, 2004). When compared with nontreatment controls, psychostimulant medication has proven effective in approximately 70 to 80% of children with ADHD (e.g., Barkley, 2006; Greenhill et al., 2001; Spencer et al., 1996). Further, in cases in which multiple psychostimulants are employed (i.e., a second medication is tried when a child does not respond to the first medication), response to medication has been shown to reach as high as 90% (AAP, 2001).

The largest study to date on the use of stimulant medication was an NIMH-funded study conducted by a national consortium of researchers with more than 500 children. Intensive medication management was compared with intensive behavioral treatment, a combination of the two, and community care. Following the 14-month treatment period, medication management (alone and in combination with the behavioral intervention) was most effective in reducing core ADHD symptoms, and the combined treatment had better outcomes for other symptoms, including internalizing symptoms, academic achievement, social skills, and parent–child relations (MTA Cooperative Group, 1999b). However, over time, the more positive effects for the medication and combined groups decreased so that by 2 years posttreatment children in all four groups showed improvements over time, with no differences among groups (Jensen et al., 2007). The most recent report from the MTA group follows up on children in the study 6 to 8 years after the beginning of treatment (Molina et al., 2009). Children in the MTA study did show improvements over time; however, in comparison to a group of children without ADHD, children with ADHD had worse functioning, providing "evidence that the differential effects of the ADHD treatments, evident when the interventions were delivered, attenuated when the intensity of treatment was relaxed (Molina et al., 2009, p. 494). The authors go on to note that initial symptom presentation "including severity of ADHD symptoms, conduct problems, intellect, and social advantage, and strength of ADHD symptom response to any treatment, are better predictors of later adolescent functioning than the type of treatment received" (p. 494).

Currently, literature documenting the short-term effectiveness of psychostimulant medication on symptoms of ADHD represents the largest body of treatment literature for any childhood psychiatric disorder (Spencer, Biederman, & Wilens, 2000).

Psychostimulants are also associated with positive gains in academic, behavioral, social, emotional, and physical functioning (for reviews, see Bennett, Brown, Craver, & Anderson, 1999; Connor, 2006; DuPaul & Stoner, 2003). To date, however, long-term benefits on academic achievement have not been documented (e.g., Greenhill, Halperin, & Abikoff, 1999), yet some scholars have suggested that this may be partly because some academic outcome measures (e.g., standardized achievement tests) may not be specific enough to capture differences in academic performance (DuPaul & Stoner, 2003).

The issue of side effects of stimulant medication has also been studied extensively. Research has indicated that psychostimulants can have adverse side effects that may be short or long term and that the severity of adverse effects tends to increase linearly with dosage increases (Brown & Sammons, 2002). Approximately 4 to 10% of children experience adverse effects to stimulant medication with more common side effects, including headaches, insomnia, and decreased appetite. Such adverse side effects are typically transient and dissipate after medication is discontinued (AAP, 2001; Barkley, McMurray, Edelbrock, & Robbins, 1990; Brown & Sammons, 2002; Connor, 2006). A smaller percentage of children (i.e., < 1%) may be affected by tics as a result of psychostimulant use, particularly if the child has Tourette syndrome, another tic disorder, or a family history of such symptoms. More recently, concerns have been raised regarding cardiovascular side effects and the potential for sudden death, particularly in children taking Adderall (Connor, 2006; Pliszka, 2007).

Although a recent study indicated there was a greater risk of increased death in children taking stimulant medications (Gould et al., 2009), the Food and Drug Administration (2009) noted multiple limitations of this study and called for more research and review. Increased psychosis in individuals with a preexisting condition or risk for such a condition may also be a rare but serious side effect (Connor, 2006; Pliszka, 2007). Concerns with growth suppression have been discussed for many years. A recent review of the literature on this topic (Faraone, Biederman, Morley, & Spencer, 2008) indicated that stimulant medications do seem to reduce expected height and weight, although whether this leads to a meaningful difference in adulthood is not clear. Although serious side effects of stimulant medications are rare, as with all medications it is important that children taking simulants be monitored over time to evaluate both positive and adverse outcomes.

Concluding Comments Regarding EBP

In the preceding sections, we described three EBIs for the treatment of mental health or social–emotional concerns of children and youth. Our examples (i.e., PMT, CBT, and psychopharmacology) are intended to illustrate some of the commonly used strategies that have been found to be efficacious as well as effective for a variety of commonly occurring problems. They also illustrate the need to coordinate services across systems of care, a topic that we discuss in more detail in the next section. Other interventions have been identified in the literature (e.g., multisystemic therapy, classroom contingency management, problem-solving skills training) for the treatment of various problem domains, and the list is constantly evolving with additional research. Thus, school psychologists should keep abreast of the literature and frequently update their knowledge and skills. For information on the current state of our knowledge of EBIs and other issues relevant to mental health and social–emotional issues of children, readers should consult the recent literature.

Linking Supports across Service Delivery Systems and Providers

Limitations associated with traditional approaches to training psychologists to work in specific settings and to restrict their work to addressing the needs of individuals who are experiencing difficulties have led scholars to argue for changes in the manner in which we deliver services (e.g., Power, Shapiro, & DuPaul, 2003) and train psychologists (Power, 2000; Power et al., 1995). Beyond important issues of the adoption of public health frameworks for prevention and the need to consider EBI is the need to consider how we can link health, educational, community, and family systems to better meet the diverse needs of children and adolescents (e.g., Power et al., 2003). To build capacity for linking services across these systems, it is important that service providers (including school psychologists) build competencies in particular domains that will promote integration of services. For example, in an attempt to facilitate the linking of systems to address the prevention and management of chronic health conditions, Lehigh University and the Children's Hospital of Philadelphia have embarked on a joint endeavor to train doctoral-level pediatric school psychologists (see Power et al., 2003, for a description). Competency domains in training include (1) interventions for chronic illnesses (e.g., knowledge and application of assessment and intervention methods), (2) prevention programming (e.g., knowledge of risk and protective factors related to chronic health problems and ability to apply core prevention programming components), (3) program evaluation (e.g., use of single-case and quasi-experimental research methods in program evaluation, use of participatory action research), and (4) intersystem collaboration (e.g., expertise in addressing health problems across settings, knowledge of methods for promoting interdisciplinary collaboration). Training is accomplished via coursework, practicum experiences, and research training that mirror the notions behind linking systems by providing integrated training experiences (e.g., practicum experiences occur across school and health care settings). This movement toward explicit training in competencies relevant to linking systems of care is promising. It is likely that school psychologists will continue to work with other service providers (e.g., physicians, community agency personnel, clinical psychologists) and that efforts to facilitate coordination of services will enhance the delivery of mental health prevention and intervention services to children and youth. This work is still in its infancy, yet we believe it will play an integral role for school psychologists of the future.

Data-Driven Problem Solving across Levels of Prevention

In Chapter 9, we discussed the application of a problem-solving model to various levels of prevention in addressing academic problems. The same process applies to the application of this model to address levels of prevention of mental health and social–emotional health. The work of Sugai, Horner, and colleagues provides an excellent example of prevention and intervention efforts aimed at addressing violence prevention through a positive behavioral support (PBS) process (e.g., Sugai, 2003; Sugai & Horner, 2002a, 2002b; Sugai et al., 2000). PBS is a process through which schools begin to improve services for all students by creating systems wherein intervention and management decisions are data driven and guided by what has been demonstrated in the empirical literature to be effective.

As we noted earlier in this chapter, it is perhaps an understatement that student learning and social–behavioral needs are increasing. Longitudinal research points to the chronic nature of such problems and the critical need for early intervention if we are to offset negative long-term outcomes. The poor prognosis for students who experience early academic or behavior problems has been well documented. Irrespective of whether or not students receive special education or related services from schools, both academic and learning difficulties are associated with increased risk of negative outcomes, with a high cost to society (e.g., school dropout, substance abuse, unemployment, and incarceration). Moreover, when efforts toward intervention are provided in a crisis or reactive manner, the chronic nature of learning and behavior problems becomes more pronounced and is potentially more resistant to change (Forness, 2003a, 2003b).

With regard to social–behavioral difficulties, although students with severe behavioral problems account for a relatively small percentage of the student population, their needs tend to be chronic as well as time and resource intensive (Sugai et al., 2000). Further, research reviews suggest that the rise in adoption of "zero-tolerance" discipline policies, which rely heavily on suspension and expulsion practices, are not working and may, in fact, be exacerbating these problems (see Skiba & Peterson, 2000). Thus, there is a need to shift our efforts from reactive and punitive methods to the development of more proactive, preventive, and educationally focused methods. PBS approaches are responsive to these issues. More specifically, PBS employs a public health prevention framework in providing a continuum of supports and prevention for (1) students who currently are not experiencing learning and/or social–behavioral difficulties (*primary prevention*); (2) students determined to be at risk for the development of learning and/or social–behavioral difficulties (*secondary prevention*); and (3) students who currently are experiencing significant learning and/or social–behavioral difficulties (*tertiary prevention*).

Primary prevention efforts, or universal supports, are provided to all students through schoolwide reform that involves the consistent use of research-based effective teaching and behavior management practices, ongoing monitoring of these practices and student outcomes, staff training and professional development, and systems-level decision making. The goal of primary prevention is to create school and classroom environments that promote student learning and ultimately decrease the number of students at risk for learning and/or social–behavioral problems. The selection of universal supports should involve consideration of *who* will receive these interventions (i.e., the school population and risk and protective factors in the local community), *what* will be the structure and content of these services (i.e., EBI for prevention of mental health and social emotional problems), and *how* and *when* instruction and interventions will be implemented. Further, just as problem solving is data driven when we are working with academic concerns, decisions at this level of the problem-solving process should be guided by data.

Within PBS, secondary prevention and tertiary prevention efforts often involve the employment of a data-driven problem-solving process that includes the use of functional behavioral assessment (FBA) procedures. As we discussed in earlier chapters (i.e., Chapters 7 and 8), FBA has been defined as a structured problem-solving process through which a broad range of information is gathered through various methods (e.g., teacher interviews, rating scales, direct observations) to develop hypotheses regarding the "functional" or "causal" relationship between specific events (e.g., teacher attention) and the occurrence of problem behaviors (e.g., disruptive behavior).

The same problem-solving steps occur at all levels of prevention, but the focus of data collection and intervention is on varying numbers of students at each level (i.e., school, small group, individual). Like the application of this process to academic problems, problem solving to address students' mental health and social–emotional needs follows the same line of questioning at each level, yet the intensity of prevention and intervention efforts and the frequency of monitoring of student outcomes may increase with the intensity of student needs. When students are at increased risk for mental health or social–emotional problems (i.e., at the top portions of the triangle), it is important to monitor their responsiveness to interventions on a more frequent basis and to coordinate services across systems of care (Power et al., 2003).

Conclusions

In this chapter, we have highlighted some of the important issues relevant to prevention of and intervention with mental health and social–emotional concerns in school settings. We believe school psychologists are in a unique position to make a significant contribution to prevention and intervention efforts. In order to do so, we believe there needs to be a shift in intervention focus from one that is predominately tertiary in nature to one that addresses primary and secondary prevention from a public health framework. Further, it is essential that practicing and preservice school psychologists are knowledgeable about (1) developmental trajectories relevant to various social–emotional and mental health problems, comorbidity issues, and risk and resiliency factors associated with such concerns; (2) EBIs for the treatment of such problems; and (3) strategies to link systems of care to support such endeavors. Finally, we consider a data-driven problem-solving model approach to be essential in comprehensively addressing the growing mental health and social–emotional needs of students in school.

DISCUSSION QUESTIONS AND ACTIVITIES

1. Interview a teacher and ask him or her to describe some of the current mental health and social–emotional challenges that are affecting children and youth in school settings. Consider how the problems described fit within the categories discussed in the beginning of the chapter (i.e., psychiatric disorders, risky behaviors, delinquency).

2. What is comorbidity, and why is it an important consideration when working with children with or at risk for mental health and social–emotional concerns?

3. Should school professionals be concerned with psychiatric diagnoses and diagnostic classification systems such as the DSM? Why or why not? Support your answer. If your answer is yes, how can diagnostic classification systems fit within a data-oriented problem-solving approach to school psychology?

4. What is an evidence-based intervention? Describe the distinction that is made between *efficacy* and *effectiveness* in the outcome literature. Why is this distinction important to school psychologists?

5. Interview a practicing school psychologist about the role that he or she plays in addressing students' mental health and social–emotional issues. Ask about his or her involvement in primary, secondary, and tertiary levels of care. Does the role involve linking to other systems of care? If so, how does this occur? What interventions does he or she employ? Does he or she use a data-driven problem-solving model in his or her approach to addressing these issues?

CHAPTER 11

The School Psychologist's Role in Collaboration, Consultation, and Facilitation of Systems Change

In earlier chapters of this volume, we mapped our vision for the future of school psychology practice with a focus on the roles that we believe school psychologists should pursue. Thus far, we have provided an overview of a data-oriented problem-solving approach to defining problems, assessing problems, and linking these activities to the provision of evidence-based prevention and intervention services. We now consider the manner in which school-based psychologists interface with school personnel, families, and community members via *consultation* and *collaboration*. Further, and as we noted in Chapter 7, in order for any shifts in practices to be adopted and sustained, the question of how new practices will fit within existing organizational structures and systems must be addressed. Thus, we also consider the *context* in which these practices occur and the *systems* issues important to their use.

In this chapter, we start by briefly describing the role of consultation and collaboration as it relates to school psychology as a problem-solving endeavor. Although space does not permit a thorough review of the literature on this topic, we recognize the importance of effective consultation and collaboration in problem solving. Following our brief discussion of consultation and collaboration, we provide an overview of the systems-change literature and its relevance to schools and to school psychology. We describe how the current school context and the challenges facing educators highlight the need for effective consultation, collaboration, and systemic reform efforts. Next, we discuss systems-change theory and its application to school systems. Emphasis is placed on viewing school organizations as systems and addressing levels of performance and performance needs within these systems. Drawing from lessons learned from previous attempts at systems change, as well as from best practices in the literature on this topic, we describe important stages of successful systems-level change in schools. We end this chapter with a discussion of the school psychologist's role in these endeavors.

Consultation and Collaboration

School psychologists do not apply their skills as problem solvers in isolation or within a vacuum. In order for school psychologists to be successful problem solvers, they must be able to effectively collaborate and consult with parents, teachers, other service providers, and other individuals who work directly with students. Further, the use of a collaborative consultative problem-solving process is an integral part of the RTI model of service delivery, as a consultative problem-solving process is applied at the level of the larger system (e.g., school or district), the smaller system (e.g., grade level, classroom or group), as well as the individual (child). In this section, we provide a brief description of consultation and its importance to the provision of school psychology as a problem-solving endeavor.

Many models of consultation have been described within the literature, and among these some of the major models include mental health consultation, behavioral consultation (direct, indirect, and conjoint formats), and organizational development consultation (for more information, see Dougherty, 2009; Kratochwill, 2008). Despite various differences noted across models of consultation, all emphasize the consultant's expertise in problem solving within a triadic relationship that, in school-based applications, includes the consultant (e.g., school psychologist or other professional with problem-solving expertise), consultee (e.g., teacher and/or parent), and client (Kratochwill, 2008). Collaboration is "a structured, recursive process in which two or more people work together toward a common goal" (Sheridan, Magee, Belvins, & Swanger-Gagne, 2010). Thus, a collaborative consultative problem-solving process can be defined as involving two or more individuals working together to apply the problem-solving process (as described in chapter 7) to improve outcomes for students. When collaborative consultation occurs within an RTI framework, then the targeted outcome occurs at an individual, small-group, or large-group level, depending on whether the focus is primary, secondary, or tertiary prevention.

Consultation is often viewed as an *indirect* service, wherein the consultant works with the consultee (e.g., teacher or parent), and the consultee then provides services directly to the child. Thus, the consultant's service to the child is indirect. Beyond simple triadic consultative relationships involving the consultant–consultee–child, the problem-solving consultation process can also be applied to groups of teachers, administrators, or teams of individuals (Kratochwill, 2008). One touted advantage of the indirect nature of consultation is that the consultant's expertise has the potential to improve services to more students, assuming that the consultee is able to generalize the use of a problem-solving process to improve outcomes for other students (for discussion of potential problems with the indirect nature of consultation and for a description of a direct consultation alterative approach, see Watson & Sterling-Turner, 2008). Of course, and as with any indirect service, it is important to clearly define problems, articulate the goals and intended outcomes of the consultation process, and carefully monitor such outcomes to ensure that the process is carried out with integrity and that intended student outcomes are achieved. In addition, because consultation is a process that involves a relationship between the consultant and consultee, interpersonal interaction and communication skills are thought to play a role in contributing to the effectiveness of the consultation process (Kratochwill, 2008; Sheridan & Kratochwill, 2008). Much has been written about consultation and collaboration that is beyond the scope of this introductory text. Readers are encouraged to explore the literature on this important topic, with particular emphasis on its application in school settings (Dougherty, 2000; Kratochwill, 2008; Sheridan & Kratochwill, 2008).

The School Context: Challenges Facing Schools

Schools are faced with an array of interrelated challenges as they try to address the academic, social–emotional, and mental health needs of students. In this section, we highlight some of the most salient contextual issues facing schools today, including (1) technological advances and changing dynamics of the workforce; (2) increased heterogeneity of the student population and increased number, severity, and complexity of student needs; (3) the push for EBP and increased accountability despite diminishing resources; and, (4) current global economic challenges. Consideration of the interplay of these challenges helps to illuminate the need for coordinated and systemic reform efforts.

Technological Advances and Changing Dynamics of the Workforce

Greenberg and colleagues (2003) noted several societal changes that affect life circumstances of today's children and youth, including "increased economic and social pressures on families; weakening of community institutions that nurture children's social, emotional, and moral development; and easier access by children to media that encourage health-damaging behavior" (p. 467). These external, economic, and sociopolitical factors can alter the development of students who enter our school systems and play a role in shaping the heterogeneity of student needs. Just as the climate in schools is constantly changing as a function of an increasingly diverse student body, competencies required to enter the workforce have become a moving target in response to changing global dynamics and exploding informational and technological advances. Clearly, schools are struggling as they attempt to prepare an increasingly diverse student population for constantly changing demands in the workplace.

Changes in the Student Demographics and Student Needs

Schools in the 21st century are faced with rising numbers, increasing diversity, and greater severity and complexity of student needs. In comparison to schools that were formed in the 1900s, today's schools serve significantly larger student bodies. Higher enrollments and class sizes can affect the general culture within a school setting and thus have an impact on how services are provided (Greenberg et al., 2003). In addition, student populations are increasingly heterogeneous (Greenberg et al., 2003; Greenberg, 2010; OSEP Center on Positive Behavioral Interventions and Supports, 2000). This is true with respect to social and economic disparities, ethnicity, race, range of abilities, and motivation (Greenberg et al., 2003). Not only are schools challenged with meeting the needs of an expanding and increasingly diverse student population, but, as we noted in earlier chapters, they are also faced with growing numbers of students with or at risk for learning and/or social–emotional problems (OSEP Center on Positive Behavioral Interventions and Supports, 2000). In sum, the rapidly changing nature of student characteristics creates new contextual demands on schools. As a result of these changes, educational systems must adapt and change if they are to be effective in meeting the needs of a complex and diverse student population.

Increased Demands for EBP and Accountability Despite Diminishing Resources

As Fullan (2000) aptly notes, "Forces that were previously outside are now in teachers' faces every day" (p. 3). In an era of EBP and accountability, schools are increasingly expected to do more to address the needs of students (academic, social–emotional, and mental health) despite diminishing resources (Greenberg, 2010; Greenberg et al., 2003; Kazdin, 2008a; OSEP Center on Positive Behavioral Interventions and Supports, 2000). In order to address the increasing numbers, diversity, and severity of student needs, schools must create systems of support that, on the one hand, work proactively to anticipate and prevent problems before they occur and, on the other hand, provide a responsive continuum of secondary and tertiary supports for students with or at risk of developing more severe problems. The level of intensity of problem-solving and intervention efforts required to ameliorate concerns must vary as a function of the durability, complexity, and severity of the presenting problem. Thus, increasingly more resources are necessary to match the growing issues in school settings. Given the finite nature of resources available for such efforts, schools must be proactive in anticipating needs and flexible in making adjustments to new challenges and changing demands as they present themselves. The RTI framework provides one example of a model that has mechanisms for being responsive to varying problems and changing demands in the school setting.

Current Global Economic Challenges

Economic downturns have been felt at a global level in recent years, and in keeping with such times of economic unrest, the challenges that present themselves trickle down to the social systems, including schools, as well as the individuals served by them (i.e., students). In addition to a general sense of diminishing resources, there is potential for the pressures associated with economic stress to affect students' well-being in myriad ways. For example, the loss of parental employment, loss of health care insurance, home foreclosure, and other such stressors can affect families broadly. Further, one only has to open a newspaper to see the various affects that budget cuts can have on schools, such as increased class sizes, fewer aides and specialized supports for students, less money for supplies, and so on. School psychologists may be called in to assist in supporting school staff, students, and their families as they cope with diminishing resources, increased demands, and the uncertainties associated with such times.

Change as a Unifying Feature of the Challenges Facing School Systems

When one considers the top challenges facing school systems today (i.e., technological advances and changing dynamics of the workforce, increased heterogeneity of the student population and growing student needs, push for EBP and increased accountability) and current economic issues, it is noteworthy that one unifying feature of these challenges is "change." Just as the pressures facing managers (e.g., global competition, increasingly demanding customers, and technological advances) are in a constant state of change—"relentless, multifaceted, unforgiving, blindingly rapid change" (Rummler & Brache, 1995, p. 1)—the pressures and challenges facing school systems are a moving target. Schools, like businesses, are evolving systems. Thus, they are affected by and reciprocally influence the contexts in which they exist. When contextual factors are changing at a rapid pace, pressures on the system to adapt are great. This situation exists because organizations respond to their external environments in an attempt to seek equilibrium. In the business world, "A processing system (organization) will either adapt to its environment, especially its receiving system (market), or cease to exist" (Rummler & Brache, 1995, p. 12). In a similar vein, "Organizational change and strategic planning should be natural, necessary, and ongoing components of any healthy, evolving school" (Knoff, 2008, p. 905).

It is important to note that "adaptation is a process, not an event" (Rummler & Brache, 1995, p. 13). Systems that are healthy continually "demonstrate the capacity to analyze problems and to solve them in a manner that facilitates the attainment of their goals" (Curtis, Castillo, & Cohen, 2008, p. 889). Thus, the concept of *lasting change* is an oxymoron. Problems occur when the focus of change is on an *innovation* (e.g., EBP, piecemeal solution) rather than on the *healthy evolution of the system* (e.g., Grimes & Tilly, 1996). This distinction is paramount to the development of school systems that are responsive to the changing contextual demands that we described earlier. School psychologists who are involved in systemic reform efforts will need to keep abreast of the demands and challenges that affect school systems. They also need to have knowledge and skills in a problem-solving approach to systems change.

Problem Solving, Systems Change, and School Psychology

As the river parable described in Chapter 7 illustrates, we must consider primary and secondary prevention if we are to address the continuum of students' needs adequately. In the past, school psychology practice has almost exclusively focused on tertiary care (e.g., Forness & Kavale, 2001; Reschly, 2000; Shapiro, 2000; Ysseldyke, 2000), and current practices consistent with RTI emphasize the need to consider prevention of problems at primary, secondary, as well as tertiary levels (e.g., Reschley, 2008; Tilly, 2008). Thus, it should not be surprising that systems-level change has not been a focus of service provision within our profession until more recent years.

Despite the limited focus on systems change within our field, some scholars in school psychology have long been proponents of systems change as an integral part of practice (e.g., Curtis, Castillo, & Cohen, 2008; Knoff, 2002, 2008). They have argued that school psychologists are well suited to a systems-change role, as they are likely to "understand human behavior within the ecology of the school as part of a larger system" (Curtis, Castillo, & Cohen, 2008, p. 888). When discussing the competencies necessary for school psychologists to engage effectively in this process, the following descriptions have been offered:

> In order to effectively facilitate system-level change, school psychologists need to call upon three areas of expertise: an understanding of human behavior from a social systems perspective, an ability to use collaborative planning and problem-solving procedures, and a familiarity with principles for organizational change. (Curtis, Castillo, & Cohen, 2008 p. 888)

To coordinate and facilitate a school-based organizational change and strategic planning process, school psychologists must have expertise in four primary areas: (a) the evidence-based components, activities, and interactions underlying effective school and educational practices; (b) the data-based problem-solving and decision-making processes, including the planning and development cycles, of schools and districts from an organizational perspective; (c) how to guide or support strategic planning processes such that effective, functional school improvement plans are written and executed; and (d) the consultation skills to facilitate proactive organizational change, effective group processes, student-focused academic and behavioral skills and mastery, functional assessment, and strategic and intensive interventions. (Knoff, 2008, p. 905)

Drawing from these two descriptions, one can identify several key competencies for school psychologists interested in the systems-change process. These competencies include knowledge of systems theory and the principles of organizational change, a basic understanding of schools as systems (e.g., their social ecology, structural aspects, and component parts), and skills in collaborative planning and problem solving. We believe that school psychologists of the future will play an increasingly integral role in the systems-change process and, therefore, should build competencies in these areas. Further, preparation and practice in systems-level influence and change are included in the most recent *Standards for Graduate Preparation of School Psychologists* (NASP, 2010c) and *Model for Comprehensive and Integrated School Psychological Services* (NASP, 2010a). In addition, emphasis on knowledge and skills in understanding and changing systems appears in NASP's *School Psychology: A Blueprint for Training and Practice III* (Ysseldyke et al., 2006). In the sections that follow, we discuss the systems-change literature and its application to school settings.

Systems-Change Theory

One important prerequisite for serving in the role of a systems-change agent is a basic understanding of systems and systems theory. According to Curtis, Castillo, and Cohen (2008), general systems theory provides the theoretical foundation for systems-level intervention and organizational development. Early applications of general systems theory focused primarily on military and industrial settings, and extensions were made to behavioral sciences in the 1950s and to schools in the early 1960s (Curtis et al., 2008).

A *system* can be defined as "an orderly combination of parts that interact to produce a desired outcome or product" (Curtis, Castillo, & Cohen, 2008, p. 888). For example, at a very small level, a human system might be defined as "the orderly combination of two or more individuals whose interaction is intended to produce a desired outcome" (Curtis, Castillo, & Cohen 2008, p. 889). Further, and in contrast to mechanical systems, which are inorganic and more static or fixed, schools are organic or "living" systems. One manner in which living systems differ from inert systems is the way in which these systems are influenced by and in turn influence the environment and other systems. This *reciprocal influence* is captured in the manner in which some scholars have described child development. Bandura (1978) and Bijou (1993), for example, have suggested that from a systems or ecological perspective the child is influenced by and in turn influences the environment or system of which he or she is a part.

All living systems also are considered "open systems" wherein each part is interconnected with and reciprocally influences all other parts of the system as well as the system as a whole (Curtis, Castillo, & Cohen, 2008). For example, school building systems are part of larger systems (e.g., a school district) and contain inner systems or "subsystems" (e.g., classrooms, intervention assistance teams, school improvement teams). When change occurs in one aspect of the system (e.g., change in personnel, change in student needs), the system is affected. In a similar fashion, changes in the surrounding contexts or larger systems affect the system as well as its subsystems. For example, policy changes (e.g., mandated testing for *all* students) or catastrophic events (e.g., a student suicide) can affect the system at all levels (e.g., policy, staff, administrator, and student levels).

The broad nature of the interlocking contingencies that govern living systems is captured within the following often-cited statement attributed to the pioneering environmentalist John Muir: "When we try to pick out anything by itself, we find it hitched to everything else in the universe." Learning how various aspects of the system are interconnected and how they work together is one challenge that presents itself in systemic reform efforts. According to Curtis, Castillo, and Cohen (2008), *organizational development* is "the planned and sustained effort to bring about system-level improvement through self-assessment and problem-solving methods" (p. 892). For this process to be effective it must be planned and systematic.

As we noted in the preceding section, the early application of systems theory to real-world settings focused primarily on industrial and military settings. Thus, the literature on improving performance within business settings is quite extensive. This section draws from this literature to describe the important distinction between viewing an organization from a vertical and functional standpoint and viewing it from a horizontal or systems perspective (Rummler & Brache, 1995).

Rummler and Brache (1995) argued that most business managers view their organizations from a fundamentally flawed perspective. More specifically, the typical view of an organization is *vertical* and *functional*, in which separate units within the organization (e.g., research and development, manufacturing, marketing and sales) are depicted as operating independently from one another and vertically via reporting relationships to other entities such as managers (see Figure 11.1). Within this vertical and functional view of an organization, the structures built around units are referred to by Rummler and Brache (1995) as "silos (tall, thick, windowless structures)" (p. 6). A similar picture could be drawn of a school organization, wherein grade-level units are depicted as separate entities that report vertically to the principal (see Figure 11.2). In high school settings, the units might be organized according to content areas (e.g., science, mathematics, social studies, language arts, music) or grade-level instructional teams. Regardless of how the units are organized, this vertical and functional approach to viewing organizations is limiting because it fails to depict how work flows. Further, it does not illustrate what happens, for whom, or how. When managers and/or school leaders have this view of an organization, they tend to manage each unit separately (e.g., meeting separately with grade-level teams, or area units). This approach can result in a perpetuation of the vertical and functional view and can create competition across units. Conflict can arise when decisions are made that have implications across units. In school settings, for example, decisions such as scheduling or additional resource allocation can result in conflict. When units function independent of each other, it is difficult to address these broader, schoolwide issues in a comprehensive manner. For example, a principal who is given additional funding and personnel to address reading at an elementary school must decide how best to utilize those resources. If the units within the school are viewed vertically and functionally independent from one another, then each grade-level unit might make a separate case for the use of these resources with little integration of information

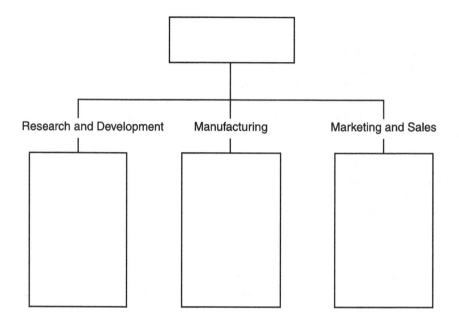

FIGURE 11.1. Traditional (vertical) view of an organization. From Rummler and Brache (1995). Copyright 1995 by John Wiley & Sons, Inc. Reprinted by permission.

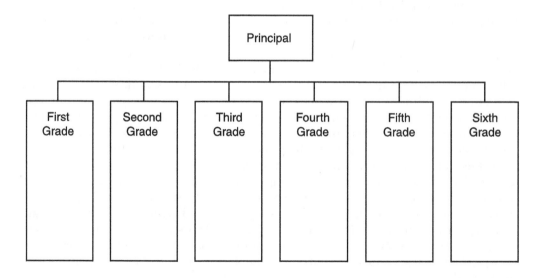

FIGURE 11.2. Vertical view of a school organization.

across grades. The result is that the principal must make some hard decisions, and some grade-level units will no doubt be unhappy with the outcome.

An alternative to viewing organizations vertically and functionally is to view them *horizontally* and from a *systems perspective* (Rummler & Brache, 1995). Figure 11.3 is an example of a systems or horizontal view of a business organization. This view helps to illustrate the flow of work and includes a description of what the organization does and for whom. Further, it allows one to see how the work is done by illustrating the connections between components of the system. Viewing systems in this manner allows one to examine where potential problems might arise in the flow. It also allows managers to adapt to change proactively by anticipating its impact on the flow of work within the system. Systems charts can be drawn to illustrate the flow of work for organizational systems as well as for the subsystems that operate within organizations. As we described in an earlier section, healthy organizations adapt to changing demands. "If an organization survives, it has adapted," yet "its health is a function of *how well* it has adapted" (Rummler & Brache, 1995, p. 12). From a systems perspective, managers can contribute to the health of an organization by using the systems framework to anticipate and adapt to change in a proactive manner.

Beyond this level of analysis, systems approaches to solving organizational performance problems also examine the connections between an organization's internal and

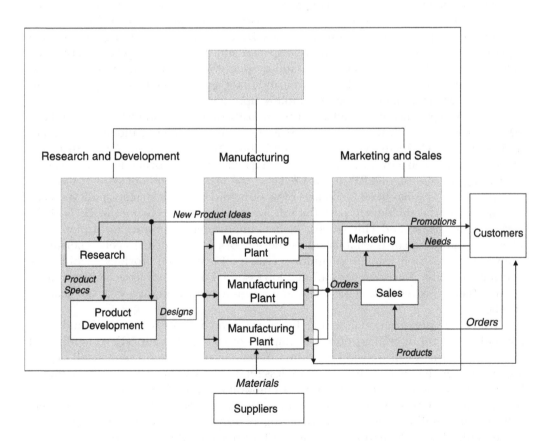

FIGURE 11.3. Systems (horizontal) view of an organization. From Rummler and Brache (1995). Copyright 1995 by John Wiley & Sons, Inc. Reprinted by permission.

external ecosystems and how these connections can be understood by examining how three *levels of performance* (i.e., organizational, process, and job/performer) interact with three *performance needs* (i.e., goals, design, and management). According to Rummler and Brache (1995), "The overall performance of an organization (how well it meets the expectations of its customers) is the result of goals, structures, and management actions at all Three Levels of Performance" (p. 17). A discussion of these interactions is beyond the scope of this chapter, but readers interested in systems-change issues are encouraged to explore this literature further (see Rummler & Brache, 1995).

Lessons Learned from Past Systemic Reform Efforts

Some of what we know of the systems-change process is a result of lessons learned from past attempts at implementing and sustaining innovations in school settings (e.g., Fullan, 2000; Fullan, Bertani, & Quinn, 2004; Gersten, Chard, & Baker, 2000). In an effort to address gaps between research and practice in school settings, attempts have been made to import "research-based" models into school settings (e.g., Fuchs et al., 1996). Unfortunately, and despite initially positive results, follow-up data indicated that projects often fail to sustain innovations when external supports were removed (Fuchs et al., 1996; McDougal et al., 2000). For example, one study conducted by Fuchs and colleagues (1996) trained schools to employ mainstream assistance teams (MATs) to support students experiencing learning problems. Despite providing training and ongoing support to 120 general educators and 30 special educators, school psychologists, and guidance counselors over several years and despite evidence that the MATs were successful in improving outcomes for children and that they could be run independently by school staff, MATs were not sustained at follow-up.

Failures to produce sustained adoption of EBPs, such as the study by Fuchs and colleagues, point to a critical need to understand systems and organizational issues (Curtis & Stollar, 2002; Fuchs et al., 1996; Knoff, 2002; McDougal et al., 2000). In recent years, there has been a shift in the focus of some educational reform efforts from simply advocating for the use of EBPs toward *building the capacity* for school systems to adopt such practices. This has been facilitated by working directly with systems, policymakers, and important stakeholders to pave the way for lasting change (Grimes & Tilly, 1996). According to Grimes and Tilly (1996), "School improvement becomes institutionalized when: (a) improvement is established as the school's direction; (b) agency personnel contribute to new policies that will guide services; (c) leadership provides ongoing support for innovative practices; (d) staff develop essential skills, knowledge, and attitudes; and (e) agency procedures, goals, roles, and assignments are aligned with the change" (p. 466).

Within the organizational change literature, two concepts have been found to be particularly useful in guiding efforts to implement change namely: (1) recognition of the distinction between individuals within an organization who are interested or willing to consider change and those who are less ready or resistant and (2) understanding how individuals' levels of concern toward an innovation can affect their commitment to the procedures necessary to implement that innovation (see Curtis, Castillo, & Cohen, 2008, for further discussion of the work of Rogers, 1995; Hall & Hord, 2006). Continued research like this on the nature of change and factors that influence readiness for adoption of new practices should help to facilitate efforts to promote the adoption of effective intervention and instructional strategies in school settings.

Phases of the Systems-Change Process

Adelman and Taylor (1997) analyzed the psychological and organizational literature to delineate a working framework for *scaling up* reform efforts in school settings. In a scale-up model, the framework that guides the systems-change process includes four overlapping phases: (1) *creating readiness* by enhancing the climate or culture for change; (2) *initial implementation*, whereby well-designed guidance and support structures are utilized to carry out replication in stages; (3) *institutionalization*, wherein there is a focus on ensuring that an infrastructure exists to sustain and enhance productive changes over time; and (4) *ongoing evolution*, which involves the development of mechanisms to improve quality and to provide continuing support in the face of new challenges and changing contexts.

We work from this framework and integrate additional concepts from the literature as we describe the phases of systems change in school settings. Before we start this discussion, however, we acknowledge an additional step that may be necessary prior to embarking on any systems-change initiative. According to Carnine (1999), important changes in professional practice are usually triggered by some *catalyst*. For example, potential catalysts for change in school systems include increasing global economic competitiveness, growing diversity in student demographics, and the fact that educational performance determines economic well-being for individuals and society. Carnine argues that it may be necessary to *campaign* for systemic reform efforts in education prior to initiating these changes. He defines a campaign as "any course of systematic aggressive action toward a specific purpose [that is] concrete, comprehensible, and to some degree urgent" (Carnine, 1999, p. 3).

A campaign involves six important steps. First, the campaign should *target visible problems* that are important and of broad interest to stakeholders. For example, issues such as literacy, school violence, and math or science performance are known to the general public and affect schools and the community broadly. Thus, it is more likely that stakeholders will support systems-level initiatives that target these issues. The second step in a campaign is *establishing a coalition of groups* (e.g., private and public sector groups, advocacy groups) dedicated to the issue. Third, this coalition should be headed by a prominent credible leader to help ensure that a critical mass is built. *Staffing the campaign* is the fourth step in the process. The staff is responsible for lobbying, for translating research findings into practical summaries, and for disseminating information to relevant groups (e.g., researchers, policymakers, practitioners, community members). The fifth step is to *assemble the right information*. Information should be organized on the basis of its importance, trustworthiness, practicality, and accessibility. The sixth and final step in the campaign process is to *launch the campaign*. Like the problem-solving process we described in Chapter 7, this final step is outcome or solution focused.

Where Carnine (1999) leaves off in the final step in a campaign initiative (i.e., launching the campaign) is where the phases in systems-change process begin in the scale-up model described by Adelman and Taylor (1997). A scale-up project includes "a necessary organizational base and skilled personnel for disseminating a prototype, negotiating decisions about replication, and dispensing the expertise to facilitate scale up" (Taylor, Nelson, & Adelman, 1999, p. 306). Thus, the process will typically be facilitated by a core team (i.e., two to four individuals), with additional members added when necessary to assist with new curricula, advanced technology, restructuring of education support programs, and other processes. Further, the scale-up process will likely require the addition of temporary infrastructure mechanisms to facilitate changes. The first phase of the process begins by laying the groundwork for change: creating an "official and psychological climate for change" (Taylor et al., 1999, p. 306). We believe that school psychologists should be involved in core teams focused on systems change. Following our discussion of the phases of change in a scale-up model of reform, we highlight the potential role that school psychologists might play in this process.

Phase 1: Creating Readiness

As a first step in initiating the systems-change process, it is important to create a culture or context of readiness. According to Elias, Zins, Graczyk, and Weissberg (2003), "Genuine collaboration is a form of collective ownership and it takes time to develop.... Thus, when an initiative begins it may signal not the beginning of change, but, at best, the beginning of readiness for change" (p. 312). Taylor and colleagues (1999) describe the tasks associated with creating readiness as follows: (1) disseminating the desired prototype and pursuing activities to build interest and consensus for change, (2) negotiating a policy framework and agreements for engagement, and (3) modifying institutional infrastructure. These tasks should be undertaken in a manner that reflects an understanding of the nature of the organization and its stakeholders. Stakeholders should play an integral role throughout the process. In particular, they should be involved in the decision-making process and in the redesign of mechanisms of the systems infrastructure. Further, in developing a sense of community and commitment, it is important that efforts be made to clarify potential benefits of the change efforts, with an emphasis on their personal relevance to stakeholders. Taylor and colleagues (1999) describe the steps in this process as well as the potential barriers or pitfalls.

When creating readiness for change, the first consideration is the development of *vision* and *leadership*. It is important to have a vision of what the new approach would look like as well as an understanding of how to facilitate necessary changes to move in that direction. Major objectives in this part of the process include the careful delineation of desired outcomes of the intended change, anticipated costs, and potential incentives and establishing which aspects of the prototype are nonnegotiable to change and which aspects can be adapted. A variety of assessment tools can be useful in this process (e.g., Smith & Freeman, 2002). For example, diagnostic evaluation methods that attempt to identify the needs of the system through multiple sources (e.g., surveys, questionnaires, interviews and observations, and input evaluations) can be useful in identifying potential goals (e.g., Curtis, Castillo, & Cohen, 2008). Input evaluations that focus on the assessment of skills and available resources for addressing needs identified in diagnostic evaluations are also helpful in this regard. Knoff (2008) describes additional activities (e.g., external environmental scan and analysis, internal organizational scan and analysis, stakeholder perceptions and expectations analysis, and a community education process) that are useful in this stage of the process.

An important part of this process is involving a critical mass of stakeholders (e.g., policymakers, staff, and parents) in the development of a vision. In fact, "*all* stakeholders should be meaningfully involved in every aspect of system-level change efforts, beginning with initial discussions regarding *potential* change and continuing through implementation" (Curtis, Castillo, & Cohen, 2008, p. 893). Some stakeholders function as "gatekeepers" in the system. They hold decision-making power and authority within the system, so their participation and sanction of the change are essential. It also is important to involve other stakeholders and, in particular, members of the system who will be affected by the change (e.g., teachers, parents). One strategy for gaining support from practitioners is to demonstrate innovations (Curtis, Castillo, & Cohen, 2008) and encourage staff to experiment with new practices that may eventually become policies (Grimes & Tilly, 1996).

Leadership and policy commitment are important because they help to ensure the availability of appropriate resources to support the change initiative (e.g., time, space, funding, and administrative support), and they also provide safeguards for risk taking (Taylor et al., 1999). Administrators and policy statements should identify reform efforts as a high priority. Taylor and colleagues (1999) recommend the negotiation of formal agreements among the various stakeholders at each jurisdictional level. They suggest that this process be accomplished through three essential steps. First, to establish a basis for consensus, the scale-up team should provide in-depth information by building on introductory presentations. The goal should be to ensure informed and voluntary consent for participation. Second, a policy framework and set of rules for engagement should be negotiated. This should include a realistic budget. Third, representatives of all major stakeholders should ratify the agreements and policies in an informed and voluntary manner. The aspects of the systems-change process (e.g., principles, components, standards) that fall into the category of *nonnegotiable* considerations should be stated up front (e.g., need for the establishment of temporary infrastructures to facilitate change).

Another essential consideration in a scale-up model is *infrastructure redesign* to ensure ownership, support, and participation. Five fundamental components to redesigning infrastructure are (1) governance, (2) planning and implementation of specific organizational and program objectives, (3) coordination and integration, (4) daily leadership, and (5) communication and information management (Taylor et al., 1999). Each of these endeavors involves a time commitment. In fact, time is one of the most common barriers to the change process.

Problems may occur if enough time is not set aside to create readiness and lay the groundwork needed for substantive change (Taylor et al., 1999). For example, considerable time and resources are needed to develop policy agreements, yet these are essential to sustained change. In addition, consensus and capacity building among key stakeholders is also time consuming, yet critical, as is establishing time for planning. Thus, restructuring of time is one of the most difficult problems associated with any scale-up method.

Phase 2: Initial Implementation

The next phase in the scaling-up process is initial implementation of the prototype (Taylor et al., 1999). Temporary mechanisms are added in the redesign of the organizational infrastructure to provide guidance and support as the prototype is adapted and phased into the system. The first of these mechanisms is the addition of a site-based steering team that works with the scale-up team (from Phase 1) to guide program development and to provide support for implementation and replication. This team works directly with the school's administration, specific planning groups, and other stakeholders and is responsible for determining the sequence for change as well as the strategies to facilitate implementation. The second mechanism involves having a change agent from the scale-up team work together with stakeholders on a change team. Curtis, Castillo, and Cohen (2008) identify this person as the on-site facilitator, whose purpose is to monitor implementation and refocus the group when necessary. Finally, mentors and coaches are trained to model and to subsequently teach elements of the prototype.

During this initial implementation phase, emphasis is placed on capacity building, which is accomplished through intensive coaching or mentorship, as well as follow-up consultation and technical assistance. Another critical feature of the implementation phase is the use of formative evaluation procedures to provide ongoing feedback for program development. Formative assessment information is collected on the implementation of the prototype (i.e., implementation integrity, acceptability) as well as on changes in processes (e.g., planning processes, governance structures, policies, and resources) and initial outcomes (e.g., student outcomes). Summative assessments are less useful here, because sufficient implementation time is required to fully implement and adapt the prototype to fit within the existing context.

Some common problems during initial implementation result from a failure to create readiness in Phase 1. If there is a failure to establish consensus and commitment from stakeholders directly involved in the implementation process, for example, the result may be implementation of form rather than substance of the change. Top-down or administratively mandated policies that are established without active and meaningful involvement of staff members can lead to resistance to change, lack of understanding, and fault-finding behaviors on the part of staff members (Grimes & Tilly, 1996). Thus, a failure to establish readiness in Phase 1 can have serious deleterious effects on initial implementation. Other potential difficulties in this phase might be those associated with the establishment of temporary infrastructures. If these mechanisms are not sufficiently in place, it may be difficult to facilitate productive working relationships and to anticipate and address problems promptly.

Phase 3: Institutionalization

The integration of an innovation into an organization is called *institutionalization* (Sigurdsson & Austin, 2006). According to Taylor and colleagues (1999), "Institutionalizing a prototype entails ensuring that the organization assumes long-term ownership and that there is a blueprint for countering forces that can erode the changes" (p. 317). Thus, in addition to maintaining implementation over time, emphasis is placed on creating mechanisms to address the evolution or enhancement of the system in the face of changing contextual demands. In order for this to occur, it is important that the organization assumes ownership and program advocacy (e.g., taking over the temporary steering group's functions, addressing ongoing policy and long-range planning concerns, and maintaining financial support). Institutionalization, however, is not ensured through ownership alone. "Over time, mechanisms for planning, implementation, and coordination are maintained by ensuring the activity is an official part of the infrastructure, has appropriate leadership, and is effectively supported" (Taylor et al., 1999, p. 318). Accomplishing these goals requires a critical mass of team members so that there is a broad base of involvement and the workload is manageable. Adequate resources (e.g., time, technical support, recognition and incentives for participation, continued professional development) are needed to support the institutionalization process. When approaches are newly institutionalized, it is also important to provide mechanisms for ongoing capacity building, particularly with regard to addressing staff turnover.

Phase 4: Ongoing Evolution

"Ongoing evolution of organizations and programs is the product of efforts to account for accomplishments, deal with changing times and conditions, incorporate new knowledge, and create a sense of renewal as the excitement of newness wears off and the demands of change sap energy" (Taylor et al., 1999, p. 319). The key to fostering this process is the use of formative and summative evaluation—that is, data. These data are used to document accomplishments and to provide information to guide decision making. Beyond data on the efficacy of outcomes for students, formative data to facilitate program development and organizational change must be gathered (Earl & Fullan, 2002). For schools to sustain this process without support, it is essential that mechanisms be in place for collecting, analyzing, and interpreting evaluation data (Stecker, Fuchs, & Fuchs, 2005). Thus, the scale-up team should help to establish an evaluation team and should build capacity for this team to conduct evaluations. Although this aspect of the systems-change process may appear straightforward, this evaluation process may be financially costly, and it has the potential to have a "negative psychological impact on those evaluated, and the ways it can inappropriately reshape new approaches" (Taylor et al., 1999, p. 321). In particular, overemphasis on *accountability* tends to result in negative reactions, regardless of the type of organization or its focus. With this potentially problematic issue in mind, it is important to emphasize the use of formative evaluation methods to guide problem-solving efforts.

The Role of the School Psychologist

As we have described in this chapter, the work of school psychologists does not occur in a vacuum or in isolation. School psychologists play a role in school systems. Thus, their work influences and is influenced by the people with whom they consult as well as the systems in which they work. In Chapter 1, we introduced our vision for school psychology practice in the 21st century. The roles we described included data-oriented problem solving, assessment, prevention and intervention, systems-level change, and being involved as a consumer and producer of research. These roles are interrelated, and the context in which they occur is a living, open, constantly evolving school system.

As we described in this chapter, school systems also exist as part of larger systems (e.g., districts, communities) and contain smaller subsystems (e.g., classrooms). These systems are complex and integrally interconnected. They provide the context for our work. School psychologists who are data-oriented problem solvers cannot and should not attempt to disconnect the problems they solve from the contexts in which they occur. We believe that school psychologists who possess knowledge and skills in systems change are in a position to play a role in problem-solving efforts designed to facilitate the development of healthy, evolving school systems. In this chapter, we provided a brief introduction to some of the important concepts that are relevant to systems-change theory and its application to school settings. In addition, we described some of the phases of the systems-change process.

Practicing school psychologists and those who are new to the profession should seek opportunities to develop their knowledge and skills in consultation and systems change, as we believe that competencies in this area can only enhance our effectiveness in other roles. We also believe that some of the skills and competencies that are already well developed in school psychologists (e.g., consultation, collaborative problem solving, assessment, research, and intervention skills) make school psychologists ideal participants in the systems-change process. In fact, we might argue that one potentially promising shift in our professional roles is from that of diagnosticians who primarily work in a tertiary care role to data-oriented problem solvers who address prevention and intervention across all systems of care (i.e., primary, secondary, and tertiary) and work to facilitate the development of healthy, evolving school systems. We are convinced that knowledge of systems and possession of systems-level change skills are becoming increasingly important for the effective practice of school psychology.

DISCUSSION QUESTIONS AND ACTIVITIES

1. What are some of the major challenges facing schools today?

2. What is a system? What kind of systems are schools? Describe the subsystems that make up the school system as well as the larger systems of which this system is a part.

3. Interview a principal and ask for a description of the organization of the school. Does the description given provide a vertical or horizontal view of the school organization?

4. The school principal you are working for would like to implement a research-based program to promote social competence. She attended a conference and learned of a packaged program that helped a school in another district. She wants you to take the lead on the project. Given your awareness of the systems-change literature, how would you go about this process? Who would you involve in the process? Where would you start? What questions would you have?

5. Find an article in the school-based literature that describes attempts made to produce lasting change or adoption of a process or EBI in a school setting. Was the approach successful or unsuccessful? Critique the article and identify components that were consistent with a systems-change approach to facilitating lasting change. What would you recommend to improve the process?

CHAPTER 12

The School Psychologist's Role in Research and Evaluation

A s indicated in Chapter 5, most school psychology practitioners do not spend a significant amount of time engaged in research activities. Although research may not be a key role for the majority of practitioners, it is nevertheless important for all school psychologists to have a basic understanding of research methods. Even school psychologists who do not formally conduct research must be good consumers of research in order to stay up to date on effective practices and to answer questions from parents and teachers regarding best practices in educational and psychological issues. For school psychologists to respond knowledgeably to such questions, they must read and be able to critically evaluate research-based articles, including methodology and research design. All school psychologists, in addition to being consumers of research, should utilize some aspects of research design methodology to engage in data-based decision making in their everyday practice. It is essential that data-based decision making occur to ensure that students are actually benefiting from the services they receive. Of course, some school psychologists will also conduct formal research studies. For those who wish to engage in research, the schools are a prime place to conduct research studies, including applied research and program evaluation. Although program evaluation has traditionally received little emphasis in school psychology training programs, we believe that well-trained school psychologists have the potential to play an important role in evaluating the impact of educational and mental health programs in schools and related settings. In this era of increasing accountability, it is essential for those in educational systems to be able to conduct evaluations of their programs to provide evidence for their continued use to various stakeholders, such as school board members, administrators, and community members. School psychologists who have basic training in program evaluation can provide an important service in this regard. In this chapter, we provide an overview of the different aspects of research and evaluation in the schools. We encourage all school psychologists to use these skills to help improve outcomes for the students, families, and teachers they serve.

School Psychologists as Consumers of Research

School psychologists must be able to understand and critically evaluate journal articles so that they can stay abreast of changes in the fields of education and psychology and share this information with parents and teachers as appropriate. School psychologists should be familiar with the four primary school psychology journals: *School Psychology Review* (the official NASP journal), *School Psychology Quarterly* (the official journal of Division 16 of APA), *Psychology in the Schools*, and *Journal of School Psychology*. Other journals related to school psychology include *School Psychology International*, *Journal of Applied School Psychology*, and *Journal of Evidence-Based Practices for Schools*. In addition to these journals, numerous others are available on topics of interest to school psychologists. These include journals focused on assessment (e.g., *Journal of Psychoeducational Assessment*), consultation (e.g., *Journal of Educational and Psychological Consultation*), early intervention (e.g., *Journal of Early Intervention*), and single-subject design studies (e.g., *Journal of Applied Behavior Analysis*) and journals devoted to a multitude of applied topics related to mental health issues in children and adolescents (e.g., *Journal of Clinical Child and Adolescent Psychology*, *Journal of the American Academy of Child and Adolescent Psychiatry*). Obviously, it is impossible for school psychologists to subscribe to all journals that may be relevant to the field. However, we encourage school psychologists to subscribe to at least a couple of journals. School psychologists who are members of NASP will automatically receive *School Psychology Review*, and those who are members of Division 16 of APA will automatically receive *School Psychology Quarterly*.

Of course, subscribing to a journal is only the first step in keeping up to date with developments in the field. Plenty of journals sit on bookshelves and desks without ever being opened. Sometimes this is due to a lack of time to read; often, though, it is due to being intimidated by research-based articles. We admit that these articles are not always the most scintillating pieces of literature and that evaluating the merits of a research article can be difficult, especially if it has been a long time since one has taken a research methods or statistics course. However, this skill is important because not all published articles are of high quality. Although all of the journals mentioned here are peer reviewed (i.e., the research is evaluated by members of the journal's editorial board, who offer opinions regarding the quality of each manuscript), this does not mean that the research that appears in these journals is without flaw. In fact, no research is perfect. Later in this section, we provide some guidelines to assist in evaluating research articles, but first we turn to the general types of journal articles school psychologists are likely to read.

Types of Journal Articles

Journals generally contain three types of articles: original research studies, meta-analyses, and narrative reviews. Each of these is discussed next.

Original Research Studies

Original research studies provide data in an attempt to answer specific research questions. There are numerous types of research studies that vary in their complexity and the stringency of their research methods and designs.

Some less complex original research studies involve survey research in which data are analyzed mainly via descriptive statistics (e.g., frequencies, means, and standard deviations). Such studies typically attempt to describe a general population. For example, many of the studies on the roles and functions of school psychologists that were cited in Chapter 5 were survey studies in which the researchers mailed survey questionnaires to school psychologists. These surveys contained questions regarding basic demographic information about school psychologists as well as questions regarding how much of their time is spent engaged in various professional activities (e.g., assessment, consultation, intervention). Survey research can provide useful information regarding trends and practices in the field of school psychology, but it is less useful in guiding practice, because the purpose of such research is to describe what is currently being done or to evaluate perceptions of what should be done rather than to evaluate what assessment methods or intervention procedures might be the most valid for a certain population.

Correlational studies, which look at the relationships between different variables, are another common type of research. Much of the research on assessment instruments is correlational in nature. For example, when creating a new measure of anxiety, the developers would correlate the new measure with existing measures of anxiety: The higher the correlation between these measures, the stronger the relationship, and the more confident we can be that the new measure is assessing the same construct as the existing measures. Correlational studies can also be used to obtain information related to possible contributing factors to problems. For example, many studies examine how parent factors (e.g., parenting style, psychopathology, stress) relate to child behavior problems. When high correlations are found between parent factors and child behavior problems, we can say that these two constructs are related (e.g., the more behavior problems the child exhibits, the more stress parents report). However, as everyone who has taken a basic statistics course should remember, we *cannot* infer *causation* from correlational data. For example, even given a high correlation between parent stress and child behavior problems, we cannot conclude that high levels of child behavior problems *cause* parents to experience greater stress. It may be that this is the case. However, it also may be that parental stress leads to child behavior problems or that a third variable contributes to both stress and behavior problems. For example, a difficult child temperament may be related to the expression of both behavior problems in children and increased stress in parents.

Only from a true experimental study can one draw conclusions regarding causation. However, true experimental studies are often difficult to conduct on many of the topics of interest in school psychology. For example, because of legal and ethical constraints, researchers cannot assign some children to receive certain services and others to receive no services. What is sometimes possible, however, is to assign some children to receive "services as usual" and others to receive a different instructional method that shows promise in targeting a particular area. However, if students who are taking part in an intervention study are receiving special education services, it is important to ensure that all interventions would be in compliance with the child's IEP.

Experimental studies can be either group design studies or single-subject design studies. Because of the prominence of single-subject design methodology in the practice of school psychology, these designs are covered later in a separate section of this chapter. Group design experimental studies involve random selection of participants (in which potential participants within the population of interest have an equal chance of being selected to participate) and random assignment of the participants to the different experimental groups (in which participants have an equal chance of being assigned to any of the groups in the study). These designs can be either between-group studies (in which different groups of participants are compared) and/or within-group studies (in which participants are compared with themselves, as in pretest and posttest design studies). In addition to true experimental designs, there are quasi-experimental designs in which the researchers cannot truly randomize participants (e.g., a researcher plans to examine the effects of different bilingual education programs but children are placed in the different programs based on the schools they attend).

Within the field of psychology, intervention or treatment studies are some of the most common types of studies that involve an experimental design. For example, if a researcher were conducting a study designed to evaluate the effectiveness of an intervention for anxiety, children with anxiety would be selected from the general population (ideally this selection is random, but rarely is this truly the case) and randomly assigned to either an active treatment group (e.g., CBT) or a control group in which children do not receive a treatment thought to affect anxiety (e.g., an attention-only group). Children in the study would be assessed at pre- and posttreatment. If children in the active-treatment group improved and those in the control group did not, the researcher could tentatively conclude that the treatment led to the improvements. However, various threats to the design of studies (outlined in more detail later in this section) may hinder conclusions and need to be considered when evaluating data.

Meta-Analyses

In addition to original research studies, meta-analyses, which are quantitative reviews of the literature, have gained in popularity over the years, and a well-done meta-analysis can be extremely valuable in integrating a variety of previous findings. When conducting a meta-analysis, the researcher examines original research studies on a certain topic. Results from individual studies are quantified using a common metric so that results from these individual studies can be combined and compared (Kazdin, 2000). For example, if one were conducting a meta-analysis on the effectiveness of medications versus CBT for anxiety, studies using each of these treatment modalities would be collected and coded so that all studies using medications could be compared with all studies using CBT. It should be noted that this is a simplistic explanation of meta-analyses, because there are many issues to consider when conducting this type of research. For example, how studies are selected for inclusion is an issue; typically, studies are excluded if their methodology is deemed to be inadequate. In addition, different researchers may define constructs differently (e.g., CBT may be defined as including different components in different studies), and results obtained via different assessment measures are combined. Different methods for quantifying outcomes of studies can also influence the outcomes of the meta-analysis and the conclusions reached (Kazdin, 2000). Even given these issues and the difficulties inherent in combining multiple studies in a common, quantifiable manner, the meta-analysis is the best method we currently have for summarizing information across studies in a meaningful way.

The use of effect sizes is the most common way of quantifying and comparing outcomes across studies in meta-analytic reviews. An effect size reflects the magnitude of a finding. Although there are different methods of calculating effect sizes, the most common method involves subtracting one mean from another mean (e.g., the CBT group mean from the medication group mean) and dividing by the pooled standard deviation. The result is a number expressed in standard deviation units that has a mean of 0 and a standard deviation of 1 (Kazdin, 2000). Higher effect sizes indicate a greater difference between groups. Cohen (1988) offered guidelines for interpreting these mean difference effect sizes. He suggested that effect sizes of 0.80 and greater are large; those from 0.50 to 0.80 are medium, and those from 0.20 to 0.50 are small.

Narrative Reviews

Although meta-analyses offer a way to quantify findings from different studies, narrative reviews of the literature are also commonly conducted. In such a review, the researcher gathers original research articles on a certain topic area and summarizes the results in a qualitative fashion without attempting to create a common metric to combine results across studies. Narrative reviews are not as useful as meta-analyses because they provide no way to easily summarize and compare results across studies. In narrative reviews, it is more likely that studies of varying quality will be included and less likely that the authors will have specific criteria for the inclusion and exclusion of studies.

Evaluating Research

As noted earlier, good consumers of research must be able to critically evaluate the research they read. In the following sections, we address some of the specific issues that should be considered (i.e., validity and clinical significance) when evaluating research articles as well as general steps one can take when reading research to help evaluate the quality and contribution of the research.

Internal Validity

Internal validity refers to the extent to which the results of a study can be attributed to differences in the independent variable in the study (e.g., the type of treatment) rather than to factors unrelated to the study. For example, if following an intervention intended to decrease depression children's depression decreases, then the stronger the internal validity of the study is, the more confident we can be that it was the intervention that led to the decrease in depression rather than some other factor (e.g., simple passage of time). In their classic text, Cook and Campbell (1979) outlined a number of threats to internal validity. Some of the more common threats are listed here, with brief definitions and examples related to an intervention study for children with depression. These threats are also summarized in Table 12.1.

TABLE 12.1. Threats to Validity

Threats to Internal Validity

- History: an event unrelated to the study occurs during the study
- Maturation: events that occur with the normal passage of time
- Testing: repeated testing at different times intervals during the study
- Instrumentation: changes in methods or measures used
- Statistical regression: tendency of extreme scores to regress to the statistical mean on repeated testing
- Selection: participants in one group differ from those in another group
- Mortality attrition: participants withdraw from the research study
- Selection interactions: methods of selecting participants or assigning participants to conditions interact with other threats

Threats to External Validity

- Sample characteristics: lack of similarity of participants to general population of interest
- Setting characteristics: lack of similarity of research setting to settings of interest
- Context characteristics: lack of similarity of participant behavior in research setting to behavior in natural setting

- *History*—an event unrelated to the study occurs and influences the results of the study (e.g., a popular student commits suicide right before the postassessment period, and all children report increased symptoms of depression; obviously, this influences scores in the opposite direction than we would want to see).

- *Maturation*—events that occur with the normal passage of time (e.g., children report improvement on measures of depression simply as a result of the passage of time).

- *Testing*—repeated testing may influence results (e.g., children complete depression inventories every week, become bored with them, and begin answering all questions the same way).

- *Instrumentation*—changes in methods or measures used (e.g., children are rating how "down" they feel on a weekly basis; however, over time some children begin to interpret this term differently than they did originally).

- *Statistical regression*—the tendency of scores to get closer to the statistical mean on repeated testing (e.g., one would expect that a child who scored very high on a measure of depressive symptoms would not score as high at a second testing simply because scores tend to regress to the mean).

- *Selection*—participants in one group may differ on some variables from participants in another group (e.g., children in the intervention group are primarily from high-socioeconomic-status [SES] backgrounds, whereas those in the control group are primarily from low-SES backgrounds).

- *Mortality*—participants may withdraw from the research study (e.g., more children in the intervention group drop out than in the control group, leaving only the children most motivated to change in the intervention group).

- *Selection interactions*—methods of selecting participants or assigning participants to conditions may interact with any of the previously listed threats (e.g., children in the control group are all from the same classroom and children in the intervention group are from a different classroom; a child in the control classroom passed away during the intervention, possibly contributing to increased emotional distress in this group).

Given these threats to internal validity, what can be done to increase internal validity of research, and what should consumers of research look for when attempting to evaluate the internal validity of a study? In studies using different groups of participants, random assignment to groups is important. Random assignment helps to equalize the effects of these potential threats across the groups. Of course, this does not always occur. Participants in one group may drop out at a higher rate than those in another group, even though random assignment was used. Historical events may also differentially affect the groups. An additional difficulty in applied studies, as noted, is that true random assignment is often difficult, and sometimes impossible, to achieve. For example, when conducting research in the schools, often classrooms rather than students are randomly assigned to conditions. This situation leaves open the possibility that differences between classrooms, rather than the intervention, are contributing to the results. When random assignment is not possible (or even in cases in which it is), participants in the different groups may be "matched" on certain characteristics to ensure that the groups are equivalent (e.g., students in the intervention and control groups may be matched based on gender, SES, and grade point average).

External Validity

Even if a study has strong internal validity, the results may not be useful if they do not generalize beyond the experimental setting of the research study. External validity refers to the extent to which results from one study will generalize to other populations, settings, and so forth. Evaluating the external validity of a study is important because it helps consumers of research know to what extent the findings of the study may apply to the settings in which they work. Various factors have been noted to affect the external validity of research studies (Cook & Campbell, 1979; Kazdin, 2003b; Scotti, Morris, & Cohen, 2003), and these are summarized in Table 12.1. One group of factors to consider are the characteristics of the sample used in the study. The more similar the participants in the research are to the individuals in the general population one wishes to know about, the more likely the results will generalize. For example, if a researcher were interested in crisis intervention practices of school psychologists in the United States, it would be best to obtain a sample of school psychologists from all areas of the United States rather than a sample of school psychologists from the specific state in which the researcher works. Alternatively, if one were interested in crisis intervention practices of school psychologists in rural areas, only school psychologists who work in rural school districts should be selected for participation.

The extent to which results will generalize also has to do with how the study was conducted. For example, if a study on the treatment of depression in children was conducted in a clinical setting with trained graduate student therapists following specific manuals, the results may not generalize to a school setting in which the school psychologist would be implementing the intervention without specific manuals and reliability checks.

How participants react to being in a research study can also limit the ability to generalize findings. For example, if a study on child compliance is conducted in a clinical setting, it is likely that children will be more compliant than if they are in their home settings. Findings from this study may indicate that children are compliant with the majority of parental commands. However, because of the difference between the laboratory (clinic) setting and the home setting, this number is not likely to be reflective of the true rate of compliance in children across different settings. Thus, the results would not generalize to other settings and would be specific to parent–child interactions in a clinic setting.

In order to attempt to produce results that will generalize, researchers should strive to randomly select participants from the population to which they are interested in generalizing and ensure that the methods of the study are similar to settings to which they wish to generalize. However, this is easier said than done—it is difficult to truly select participants randomly. For example, in selecting potential participants to be in the study on crisis intervention practices, a researcher might obtain a list of 500 school psychologists across the United States, randomly selected from NASP's and APA Division 16's membership lists (this being the simplest way to obtain a random sample of school psychologists across the country). Although this sample of potential participants may be a random sample of NASP and APA members, it is not truly a random sample of school psychologists because only NASP or APA members could be selected. It may be that there is something different about school psychologists who are NASP or APA members compared with those who are not (e.g., NASP and APA members may be more likely to seek continuing education opportunities and, therefore, be more knowledgeable about crisis intervention). Thus, the results may generalize only to school psychologists who are members of NASP or APA. In addition, obtaining a random sample of individuals to whom the researcher will mail the survey does not guarantee that a random sample of surveys will be returned. Perhaps those school psychologists who are more involved in crisis intervention will be more likely to respond to the survey. Thus, although the target sample was randomly selected, those who responded are different from those who did not respond. Typically, there is no way to evaluate how those in the obtained sample may have answered differently from those who did not respond. However, in some situations it may be possible to compare those who responded with those who did not respond on certain characteristics (e.g., years of experience as school psychologists). Because true random selection can be difficult to achieve, when evaluating research studies one should attend to the extent to which random selection was attempted to help better understand the population to which the results will most clearly generalize.

Construct Validity

The construct validity of a study has to do with the intervention (or experimental manipulation) in the study and its definition. If threats to internal validity have been ruled out, one can assume that the experimental intervention was responsible for the effect. Questions of construct validity relate to the extent to which factors considered not to be part of the intervention interfere with the interpretation of the intervention (Finger & Rand, 2003; Kazdin, 2003b). For example, did children who received a CBT for depression improve more than those in a wait-list control group because of the cognitive-behavioral intervention specifically (as we might assume) or because they were receiving extra attention from a supportive adult? Threats to construct validity include experimenter contact with participants, demand characteristics, and experimenter expectancies. As in the preceding example, experimenter contact with participants may threaten the construct validity of a study if the experimenter has more contact with one group than with the other group. Demand characteristics can influence study outcomes when participants in research studies respond differently than they would naturally simply because they are in a research study. Participants may attempt to respond in a manner consistent with what they think the researcher wants or expects. For example, parents whose children are in a treatment study for depression may report that their children's symptoms are better because they know that the goal of treatment is to decrease symptoms of depression. Expectancies of the researcher can also limit the construct validity of a study. For example, a researcher may expect the children in the treatment group to improve and those in the control group not to improve. Because of this expectancy, the researcher may unknowingly and subtly treat the children in the two groups differently (e.g., being more positive with the children in the treatment group), and this difference may influence the outcomes of the study (Kazdin, 2003b; Scotti et al., 2003).

To help reduce threats to construct validity as well as internal validity, the gold standard when conducting intervention studies is to use double-blind placebo-control designs. In such studies, participants are randomly assigned to either a treatment group or a no-treatment placebo group, but neither the researchers nor the participants know who is in which group. This type of design is frequently used when evaluating the efficacy of medications. For example, if a new medicine for social phobia is being evaluated via a double-blind placebo-control study, half of the children in the study would be assigned to take the new medication and half to receive a placebo pill (a sugar pill), but neither the researcher nor the participants would know who was receiving the placebo pill and who was receiving the "real" medication. (Obviously, someone knows, via coded links, who has received what medication; however, this person is not involved in running the study or interacting with the participants.) By using this design, the researcher can control for expectancy effects on the part of the participants and the researcher. Participants in both the placebo group and the medication group may expect that they will improve, but expectancy will not differentially affect the groups. In addition, the researcher will not treat those on medication differently from those taking a placebo because medication status is also unknown to the researcher.

Although double-blind placebo-control studies are relatively easy to implement when evaluating the efficacy of medications, such studies are much harder to implement when evaluating psychological or educational interventions. As of yet, no one has developed an adequate psychological placebo. Some researchers use an attention-control group as a placebo treatment. In this situation, a study therapist meets with the participants but does not engage in the active therapy being evaluated (e.g., CBT). Instead, he or she engages in nontherapeutic activities (e.g., play activities, academic tutoring if the treatment focus is not on academics). However, given that the relationship between therapist and client seems to be an important factor in predicting who will improve in therapy, it is questionable as to whether this method truly represents a placebo treatment. In addition, it is very difficult to double-blind psychological or educational intervention studies. Although participants may not be aware of whether they are receiving the active treatment, researchers most likely will be aware because the difference between an active treatment and a placebo treatment can be observed (whereas a placebo pill can be made to look just like the real medication).

Statistical Conclusion Validity

This type of validity relates to errors in the use of measurement and statistical analysis techniques. Threats to statistical conclusion validity include unreliability of measures, low statistical power, subject heterogeneity, and increasing the study error rate by making multiple statistical comparisons (and, therefore, likely getting a result that is statistically significant simply because of chance; Finger & Rand, 2003; Kazdin, 2003b). The use of appropriate assessment methods and statistical procedures can help reduce threats to statistical conclusion validity.

Clinical Significance versus Statistical Significance

In addition to evaluating the validity of a study, consumers of research should evaluate the clinical significance of the findings. Kazdin (2000) defines clinical significance as "the practical value or importance of the effect of an intervention, that is, whether it makes a real difference in everyday life" (p. 117). This issue of clinical significance and how it differs from statistical significance is one that has been receiving an increasing amount of attention in recent years. Statistical significance refers to conclusions reached about significance based on statistical hypothesis testing. This is the classic "p value" with which one becomes familiar in introductory statistics courses. A p value refers to the probability that the finding was obtained by chance. In order to be considered statistically significant, p values have traditionally needed to be less than .05 (i.e., $p < .05$). This statement asserts that there is only a 5% probability that the obtained result was due to chance. However, statistical significance testing does have drawbacks. One drawback is that it is heavily influenced by sample size. If a study has a large sample size, statistical significance is relatively easy to achieve. Conversely, if a study has a small sample size (and, therefore, low power—the ability to detect a meaningful effect when the effect is present), statistical significance is difficult to achieve. In addition, statistical significance tells the reader nothing about whether the obtained result is meaningful in the real world. For example, if a researcher utilizes statistical significance testing to compare CBT with an attention-control "treatment" for children with anxiety and if those in the CBT group have a significantly greater reduction in anxiety symptoms at the posttest than children in the control group, we only know that, as a group, children in the CBT group improved more than children in the control group. We do not know whether children in the CBT group showed a meaningful decline in symptoms. It is possible that children in both groups were still experiencing high levels of anxiety at posttreatment.

Effect sizes (as discussed in the Meta-analyses section of this chapter) have been used frequently as measures of clinical significance. However, although effect sizes are not influenced by sample size and do provide information about the magnitude of change, they still have limitations when evaluating the meaningfulness of a certain outcome. This issue is particularly relevant in treatment studies in which the question is whether a certain treatment is effective. In order to truly evaluate the effectiveness of a treatment, some measure of whether participants are functioning at a normative level is generally needed, given that the goal in treatment is typically to return symptoms to a "normal" level. In addition to examining the effect size from pre- to postintervention for a given change, researchers can also determine whether scores at posttreatment fall in the normal range (as defined by normative information for that measure) and determine whether diagnostic criteria for the disorder for which the child was receiving treatment are still met (Kazdin, 2000). Jacobson and Truax (1991) proposed the idea of utilizing a *reliable change index* (RCI) in combination with statistically derived cutoff scores to help evaluate the clinical significance of results. The RCI involves determining whether reliable change took place from pre- to posttest and takes into account the standard error of measurement of the instrument used to assess change. A cutoff score denoting whether an individual is in the functional or dysfunctional range (obtained via various formulas presented by Jacobson and Truax) is used in combination with the RCI to determine whether an individual has achieved meaningful change.

Although methods of assessing clinical significance are increasingly being applied in studies (particularly therapy outcome studies), Kazdin (1999) argues that we should not assume that a person must be in the normal range on an outcome measure to conclude that change is clinically significant. He argues that, in some cases, change can be clinically significant when an individual shows some changes even though symptoms are not normalized (e.g., a child with severe separation anxiety, which led to school refusal, can now attend school even though he or she still has significant anxiety) or when the person is better able to deal with his or her symptoms even though no change has occurred (this would be especially true in the case of chronic problems such as tic disorders).

The topic of clinical significance and how to evaluate it is likely to continue to evoke much discussion. Consumers of research should be aware of this issue and, when reading research articles, attend to whether the authors have reported measures of clinical significance. This will help in the evaluation of whether the article provides meaningful information that can be applied to everyday practice.

What to Look for When Reading Research Articles

In the preceding sections, we have mentioned some aspects of research that the consumer should attend to when evaluating research studies. We now provide more details on how to evaluate the entirety of a research study. Pyrczak (2008) provides detailed information on evaluating research articles, and we have drawn extensively from his discussions. Consumers of research should begin their critical evaluation of an article with the introduction and review of literature. The literature review should include recent research on the topic area (although often older research of a seminal nature is also important to include), and the research should be discussed in an evaluative fashion so that both strengths and weaknesses or studies cited are clear. When discussing the previous literature, the authors should distinguish between theory-based or opinion literature and empirical literature. Literature reviews should be neither too broad nor too narrow but should provide sufficient background information to understand the importance of the study currently being conducted. The literature review should make it clear how the present study builds on previous studies and should lead directly to the research questions or objectives for the current study. After reading the literature review, the reader should understand how the current study will help advance knowledge and understanding of the particular topic area.

The method section follows the literature review. This section typically includes three subsections that provide detailed information on the participants involved in the study, the measures used, and the procedures followed. A close examination of the method section is important in assessing both the internal and the external validity of a study. Participants should be adequately described, and the general population these participants were selected to reflect should be specified. Information on the number of participants and the demographic characteristics of participants should be included. Readers should evaluate whether the sample size is appropriate given the expectations of the study and the methods used to evaluate the results. In general, the more comparisons being made, the larger the sample size that is needed. For example, if a researcher is evaluating the outcome of a treatment program for depression and wants to look at outcomes for males versus females and children from two-parent homes versus one-parent homes, a larger sample size would be needed than if the researcher just wanted to examine overall outcomes. Measures used should be described and their psychometric properties mentioned. If the measures used were not psychometrically sound, the results may be questionable (e.g., findings may have been due simply to the unreliability of the measures used rather than the intervention). The procedures section should provide adequate details so that the reader is able to understand how the sample was chosen, how many eligible individuals participated, and what the dropout rate was. The uses of both random selection of participants and random assignment of participants should be clear from the method section.

Within the results section, the reader must attempt to determine whether appropriate methods of analysis were used and appropriate conclusions reached based on the results of these procedures. The analyses should be tied to the research questions proposed by the study authors, and it should be clear how each research question was addressed. Researchers should also include general descriptive statistics that describe the sample prior to presenting their main data analyses. For example, means and standard deviations for all measures used should be presented. If there are different groups in the study, this information should be presented for each group and compared in some manner. If the groups are not equivalent on these variables prior to the implementation of an intervention, the researchers should attempt to account for this in their data analysis. Statistical procedures used should be clearly described and limitations noted. In addition to evaluating the statistical significance of the results, the researchers should also discuss the practical or clinical significance of the findings and make clear when results may not be clinically significant even if they are statistically significant.

The discussion is the last section in an empirical research-based journal article. In the discussion, the authors summarize the findings and tie them back to the literature previously reviewed. Readers should attend to whether the discussion accurately reflects what is presented in the results. Researchers will sometimes overstate findings or play up significant findings while downplaying nonsignificant findings. In addition, the limitations of the study, including issues related to whether the results are likely to generalize, should be noted in the discussion. Conclusions that are based on data should be clearly differentiated from authors' hypotheses regarding what the results may mean. Because discussion sections do not always fully and accurately depict the actual results of a study, consumers of research should avoid skipping the results section and reading just the discussion section, although we realize it may be tempting to do this (especially in an analysis-heavy article).

The more one reads journal articles, the more familiar one will become with the different components of articles, and the easier it will become to evaluate research studies. We encourage school psychologists to take their journals off their shelves and read at least one article of interest each month.

Conducting Applied Research in the Schools

Thus far in this chapter, we have focused on the school psychologist as a consumer of research. As important as it is to be a savvy consumer, we also believe there are great opportunities for school psychologists to become involved in conducting research. School psychologists have access to large populations of children, and children with a variety of difficulties are referred to them. This situation provides school psychologists with great opportunities to conduct research related to children. These opportunities may include intervention studies (e.g., do repeated readings with no corrective feedback increase children's reading fluency?), studies on assessment methods (e.g., is a new measure of depression psychometrically sound?), and studies that attempt to more fully describe a population (e.g., how do the social skills of children with depression differ from the social skills of children with anxiety?).

Although most school psychologists receive some training in research methods in graduate school, those in specialist-level programs and PsyD doctoral programs typically are not exposed to research as a primary focus of their training. If school psychologists wish to become involved in conducting research but are unsure how to proceed, it may be beneficial to contact faculty members in school psychology training programs to collaborate on projects.

If a school psychologist wishes to conduct research in the schools, he or she must take several steps before beginning the research. All research conducted in schools must be approved by the school district. Districts have different procedures for approving research, but most have an individual or a committee that reviews proposals to conduct research in the schools. In addition to obtaining district-level approval, it is also important to obtain building approval through the school principal. If a school practitioner is conducting research in collaboration with a graduate student or faculty member at a university, approval from the university's Institutional Review Board for the Protection of Human Participants (IRB) will also need to be obtained. In addition to following required district procedures for conducting research, the school psychologist must adhere to ethical guidelines for conducting research. Ethically, participants must take part in the research voluntarily and must be allowed to cease participation at any time without consequence. For example, a student's grade cannot be dependent on the student participating in a research study. Informed consent must be provided by a child's parent or guardian prior to the child's participation in the study. For parents to provide *informed* consent they must be fully informed of the procedures involved in the research as well as the risks and benefits to them and their children of participating in the research. Child assent should also be obtained directly from the child prior to study participation. Above all, school psychologists should ensure that the welfare of the children they serve takes priority over their research agendas. For more information on research involving human participants, the website of the Office for Human Research Protections (*www.hhs.gov/ ohrp*) offers a variety of information. In addition, the IRBs at all universities should have their own websites containing information specific to that institution.

When developing a research study, school psychologists should review the literature in the area in which they are interested and develop specific, testable research questions they wish to answer (Keith, 2008). Broad questions should be clarified and broken into smaller, targeted questions. For example, the question "How can the social skills of children with ADHD be improved?" is a large and vague question with no specific testable research questions. Specific questions related to this global question might be:

1. Does a classwide social problem-solving skills intervention lead to increases in prosocial behavior in children with ADHD?
2. Does a pullout group program for children with ADHD that focuses on social problem-solving skills increase prosocial behavior in children with ADHD?
3. Does individual social problem-solving instruction result in an increase in prosocial behaviors in children with ADHD?

A research project might focus on just one of these questions or might attempt to answer all of them and to make comparisons between the three methods of intervention. In addition to developing research questions, the researcher needs to define what is being measured and how the measurement will occur. For example, the researcher interested in social skills programs for children with ADHD would need to decide how to measure prosocial behaviors (e.g., observations of the students, teacher report, student self-report) and what specifically is defined as prosocial behavior. Obviously, in this case, the intervention program(s) would also need to be identified.

Single-Subject Research

Although the previous example is likely to lend itself to a group design study, as noted earlier in this chapter, single-subject design research is particularly applicable in the school setting. There are a variety of single-subject designs (as discussed later in this section), but all such designs have some commonalities. Freeman (2003) outlines four characteristics of single-subject designs. Single-subject designs involve *using participants as their own controls*, with the performance of participants being compared across several conditions, which at a minimum include a baseline and an intervention phase. In addition, single-subject designs involve the *repeated measurement* of the participants in the different conditions. Often observations are conducted in single-subject research, but this is not a necessary aspect of such research. Dependent variables can also be measured via other means that lend themselves to repeated use (e.g., words read correctly on a curriculum-based measure). Single-subject designs also involve *replication*. Instead of simply conducting a pre- and postassessment, there is some replication of the intervention condition. This strategy allows the researcher to be more confident that it is the intervention that is leading to any observed changes. Within single-subject designs, only *one variable is manipulated at a time*. This practice allows the researcher to make stronger conclusions regarding the effects of an intervention. For example, in an intervention to increase reading fluency, participants might initially be offered a tangible reinforcer for a certain rate of fluency. This would be the only change made, so that the researcher can determine whether this intervention leads to changes in fluency. Because single-subject designs, unlike typical group designs, use participants as their own controls and do not require large sample sizes, they are well suited to research in the schools. School psychologists can obtain data on interventions they are implementing across just a couple of students and be able to draw strong conclusions. In addition, one of the appealing aspects of single-subject designs is the ease with which one can determine whether the intervention was effective. By simply graphing the pattern of responses under the different experimental conditions, one can *see* whether the intervention had an effect. There are no concerns with complicated statistical analyses, as there can be with group designs. School psychologists can use single-subject designs to do research without having to access large populations of certain children, which may be difficult given the low prevalence rates of many disorders. For example, it would be unusual for a school psychologist to have more than a handful of children with school refusal at any one time. Thus, utilizing a group design study to evaluate an intervention for school refusal would be difficult. However, using single-subject methodology, the school psychologist can research effective interventions for these children. The basic single-subject research designs are outlined subsequently. These designs are discussed in much more detail in a variety of sources (e.g., Cooper, Heron, & Heward, 2007; Freeman, 2003; Kazdin, 2001, 2003b).

As noted previously, almost all single-subject designs begin with a baseline phase (typically referred to as A). Prior to beginning the intervention phase, it is important to ensure that the baseline data are stable. Baseline data should continue to be collected until such stability is achieved. Stability is typically reflected by a relatively flat line (indicating little change in the occurrence of the behavior) when data are graphed. The simplest single-subject design is a baseline phase followed by a treatment phase (an *AB design*). However, this design lacks internal validity, because it does not allow the researcher to see whether the intervention or another factor accounted for the change. Therefore, this design is not typically used in research published in the more prestigious journals, but variations on this design that have stronger internal validity are commonly utilized. In an *ABAB design*, baseline data are collected and the intervention implemented; then a return to baseline occurs and, after achieving a stable baseline a second time, the intervention is reimplemented. To conclude that the intervention is effective, the behavior should improve during the first treatment phase, reverse to close to initial baseline levels in the second baseline phase, and improve following the implementation of the second treatment phase. Figure 12.1 provides a hypothetical example of an ABAB design in which an intervention was implemented to decrease a young child's aggressive acts (e.g., hitting, kicking, biting). As can be seen in this graph, aggressive acts decreased in the B (intervention) phases compared with the A (baseline) phases. On the basis of a graph such as this, a researcher could conclude that the intervention had the desired effect. Variations to the ABAB design are numerous and include adding additional treatment components to study the effects of more than one intervention (e.g., ABACABAC, with B and C being different interventions).

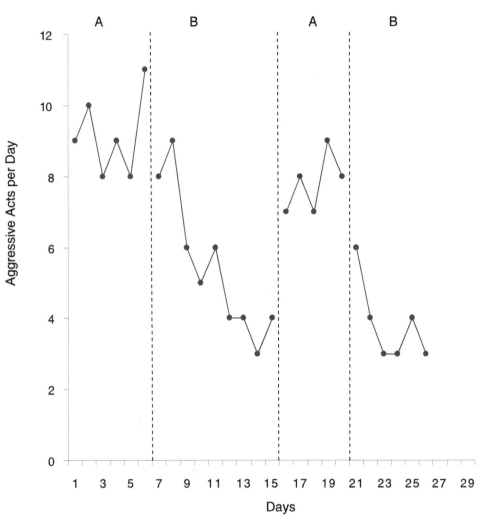

FIGURE 12.1. ABAB design example.

Multiple-baseline designs are also commonly used in single-subject research. In this type of design, instead of withdrawing a treatment, the treatment is implemented across multiple behaviors, settings, or individuals at different points in time. If the treatment has an effect, the behavior should remain stable until the treatment is implemented for that behavior, setting, or individual. Figure 12.2 presents a hypothetical example of a multiple-baseline design across individuals. In this example, second-grade students struggling with reading were initially provided with no intervention (baseline phase). A reading intervention was then implemented for one child, and this child's reading performance improved whereas the reading performance of the other two children remained stable at baseline levels. The intervention was then implemented for the second child, whereas the baseline condition remained in effect for the third child. Again, once the intervention was implemented, this child's reading performance improved. Finally, the intervention was implemented for the third child and, as with the other two children, reading performance improved from baseline levels. Because for each child

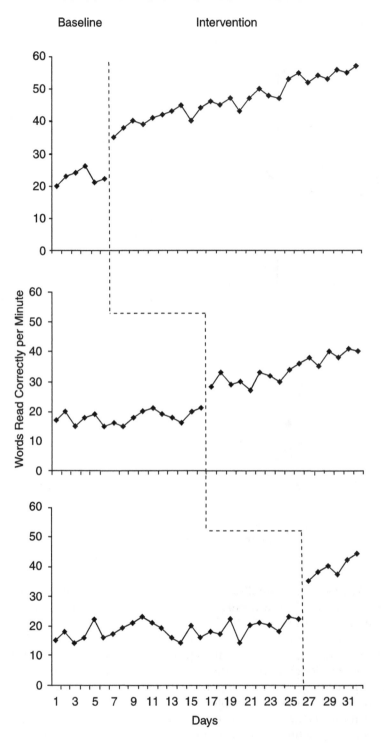

FIGURE 12.2. Multiple-baseline design example.

reading performance improved only after the intervention was implemented, we can conclude that it was likely the intervention that led to this change.

If a researcher wishes to compare the effectiveness of two or more treatments, an *alternating-treatment design* may be appropriate. In such a design, two or more treatments (both intended to address the same target behavior) are presented in a random fashion (so that B does not always follow A) across observation periods. This procedure allows the researcher to determine whether one intervention produces more of an effect than another intervention. Although baseline phases are not required in alternating-treatment designs, they are frequently included prior to the presentation of the alternating treatments. Another variation on the alternating-treatment design is to include a final phase in which only the "best" treatment from the alternating-treatment phase is included.

Changing-criterion designs are used to evaluate the effectiveness of an intervention through making the criterion for success (and the associated reinforcement for this success) increasingly more stringent. In this design, the individual must reach a certain criterion to earn a reinforcer during the treatment phase. Once this initial criterion is met on a consistent basis, it is altered to require an increased level of performance. Once the second criterion level is met, the criterion is increased again, and so on. If the behavior changes only after the criterion is adjusted, the researcher can conclude that it was likely the intervention that resulted in the behavior change. For example, a child who is completing no math problems may initially have to complete five math problems to earn a reinforcer. Once he is consistently completing five math problems, the criterion may be changed to 10, and then 15, and so on until the child is regularly completing an entire math sheet of 25 problems.

Once a researcher has collected the data in a single-subject design, the data must be evaluated. Unlike with group-design methods, there are no statistical significance testing methods appropriate for single-subject data. Data from these studies are typically graphed, and a visual analysis of these graphs is used to interpret the data and determine whether a meaningful change in behavior occurred and whether this change can be attributed to the intervention (Cooper et al., 2007; Kazdin, 2001). This visual inspection typically involves assessing the overall pattern of change in the data via examination of variability in the data, changes in the level or mean rate of responding, and trends (or directional paths) in the data. In some cases, it is quite easy to see that there was an effect. For example, if data are stable within each condition and no data points overlap between the baseline and treatment conditions, the researcher can conclude that the intervention had an effect. This is the case in the multiple-baseline example provided in Figure 12.2; for each child, there is no overlap between data points in the baseline and intervention phases. However, often there will be significant variability within phases and overlap in data points between phases (as there is in the ABAB design example shown in Figure 12.1). The more variability there is in the data within a certain condition, the greater is the need for additional data to help spot a pattern of responding. Without a stable pattern of responding within each phase, drawing conclusions becomes more difficult, especially if there is a large overlap between data points in the different phases. The level of responding during each phase can also be examined to determine whether there is a difference in the behavior across conditions. For example, when switching from baseline to treatment, there may initially be a very dramatic change in level of the behavior. In an ABAB design, the same dramatic shift may also occur when returning to the baseline phase. The mean rate of behaviors in each condition is one method used to evaluate the level of responding. However, this method has drawbacks, particularly when there is significant variability in the data within conditions and a mean level line would not accurately reflect what was happening in each condition. When examining the trend in data, an evaluation of the overall pattern of responses is conducted. This may be accomplished via examination of a trend line for each phase. For example, in the ABAB design in Figure 12.1, although there is some variability in responses in each of the phases, in general there is little change in the trend of the data in the baseline phases but a clear decreasing trend in the data following implementation of the intervention. In this example, there is both a change in the level of behavior and a change in the trend of the behavior between the baseline and treatment conditions. As is discussed in more detail in the final section of this chapter, single-subject designs can be utilized not only when conducting formal research but also when evaluating the effects of interventions for individual students. As such, all school psychologists should be familiar with the basic single-subject designs and how to evaluate change when using these designs.

Program Evaluation

An additional type of applied research in which school psychologists may become involved is program evaluation. Program evaluation involves evaluation of social intervention programs (Rossi, Lipsey, & Freeman, 2004). At the heart of program evaluation is the idea of accountability at the systems level. Given that accountability has been an increasingly emphasized concept in education in general and school psychology specifically, this type of research is an important activity (Godber, 2008). A variety of ongoing programs are implemented in schools (e.g., academic intervention programs, drug abuse prevention programs, bully prevention education), and evaluation of these programs is imperative to ensure that the outcomes are at the desired level. Unfortunately, it seems that programs have often been implemented with little research to support them, and then little research is conducted to evaluate these programs once they are in place. In some cases, programs may become exceedingly popular without any data to indicate that they are making the impact they are intended to make. One notable expert in special education and school psychology research has stated that "educators are notorious for embracing programs that look good but do no actual good" (Walker, 2001, p. 2). An example of this phenomenon of popular programs that are thin in supporting evidence is the Drug Abuse Resistance Education (DARE) program, a well-intentioned program geared toward preventing substance abuse. Although DARE programs have been implemented in numerous schools across the country, outcome data on these programs have not been impressive. However, schools, families, and communities look favorably on this program and have expressed great distress in areas where this program has been replaced with different drug abuse prevention programs, including those that have more supportive evidence behind them (e.g., Lynam et al., 1999).

Program evaluation is a broad and complex area. There are different types of evaluations as well as numerous evaluation activities. One distinction that is often made is between formative and summative evaluations. Formative evaluation is ongoing and intended to provide feedback on how a program is working so that changes can be made, if needed. Summative evaluation is conducted after the program has been in place for some time or at the end of a program to determine how effective the program has been (Fitzpatrick, Sanders, & Worthen, 2004; Godber, 2008). Often an evaluation incorporates both formative and summative activities. A distinction between internal and external evaluations is also often made. Internal evaluations are those completed by staff members from the agency running the program (e.g., a school psychologist employed by the school district evaluates the effectiveness of the school's drug education program). External evaluations are those completed by a group or individual outside of the agency (e.g., a group of researchers from the state department of health evaluates the school's drug education program). There are advantages and disadvantages to both internal and external evaluations. External evaluators are likely to be more objective about the program they are evaluating, whereas internal evaluators are more likely to be familiar with the program and the context in which it operates (Fitzpatrick et al., 2004).

The activities within any type of evaluation are numerous. Many experts in program evaluation promote the idea of working from a logic model to clarify and link information regarding the proposed evaluation activity. A logic model links together (1) needs/problems with (2) goals/objectives for addressing the problem, (3) program activities related to these goals and objectives, and (4) outcome measures that will allow the evaluators to determine whether progress has been made (Chinman, Imm, & Wandersman, 2004; Godber, 2008). Each of these four aspects of the program evaluation process are discussed in more detail next.

Targets/Needs Assessment

The main question to be addressed at this phase is whether there is a problem. Assuming that a problem is present (e.g., children are being bullied at school), the evaluator must clearly define the problem. This definition includes who is affected by the problem (e.g., children in middle school and high school) as well as the severity of the problem (e.g., about one-quarter of middle and high school children are victims of bullying). The identification of the problem can be achieved through a review of previous literature (including government reports) and by obtaining information directly from those involved in the organization. For example, in defining the bullying problem, we might look at previous research (which suggests that many middle school and high school students are bullied) and also obtain information directly from those in the schools in which we are considering implementing a program. We might conduct interviews with teachers, school staff, and students and review disciplinary records. In defining the problem, we should also ensure that the identified problem is an important issue for those involved. For example, if students indicate that bullying is a problem but rank alcohol use and school crime as greater problems, it may be better to address one of the more salient issues instead of bullying. It is also important to assess the demand for a program. For example, we may wish to implement a bully prevention program that includes both a schoolwide component and a parent education component about recognizing the signs of bullying and/or bully victimization and how parents can respond. However, it may be that parents (even those who perceive bullying as a problem) are not interested in actively participating in such an education program.

Identifying Goals and Objectives

Once the need has been identified, more specific goals and objectives are developed. For example, if a bully prevention/intervention program is to be implemented, goals might include decreasing the amount of bullying in the hallways between classes and increasing response times when students report a problem with bullying. Objectives would then be developed that relate to the goals (e.g., when a bullying episode is reported to a school administrator, counselor, or teacher, the incident will be responded to within one school day). The objectives are important because these will help guide the evaluation process.

Program Activities

The activities are the specific prevention/intervention services that are being delivered to meet the stated goals and objectives. For example, program activities might include providing classwide information on bullying, conducting pull-out groups with victims of bullying, and providing trainings to school staff on what to look for related to bullying problems.

Assessing Process and Outcomes

At this stage of the evaluation process, the program has been implemented and data are collected to help determine whether the program is being implemented as intended and whether the program outcomes are positive. Questions related to the process of implementation might include the following: Is the program reaching those in need? Are program participants receiving the level of services intended? Are the needed resources available and are these being used appropriately (Rossi et al., 2004)? Returning to the bullying program example, let's assume that, based on our needs assessment, we have chosen to implement a schoolwide intervention, with components that address student and staff outcomes and objectives as well as small-group interventions for selected individuals. It is likely that this program is reaching those in need because of the broad nature of the program. To evaluate whether participants are receiving the level of services intended, we could evaluate how much time was being spent in intervention activities, whether students/staff were attending trainings as intended, whether lesson topics are being appropriately covered, and so on. In terms of evaluating whether needed resources are available and being used appropriately, we could interview teachers who are implementing the intervention and ask about coverage of certain issues as well as their perceptions of whether they have the resources necessary to conduct the intervention (e.g., Are they receiving needed training in the intervention? Do they receive release time for preparing the intervention materials?).

When assessing program outcomes (also referred to as impact assessment; Rossi et al., 2004), evaluators should determine whether the specified objectives are being met. In addition, it is often important to evaluate the efficiency of the program (the costs related to the benefits; Rossi et al., 2004). These activities can be quite complicated because there are numerous ways in which a program can be evaluated. The key idea behind assessing the outcomes of a program is determining whether the program produced the desired effect (e.g., a decrease in bullying) and whether this effect was greater than what would have occurred without the program or what would have occurred with an alternative program (Rossi et al., 2004). Outcome measures (e.g., school discipline records, rating scales, observations) as well as the group that will provide outcome data (e.g., students, parents, teachers) must be identified. It should also be recognized that the program may have an impact on more people than just the program participants. The families of participants as well as staff members at the school where the program is implemented may be affected. In addition, the immediate impact of the program may differ from its long-term impact (Greene, 2003). Thus, the evaluator must decide who will be the focus of the impact assessment as well as the time intervals that will be used to evaluate the impact. In addition, the evaluator must ensure that the design of the evaluation study allows the evaluator to draw conclusions regarding the effects of the evaluation (i.e., that there is internal validity). Rossi et al. (2004) discuss a variety of specific designs and techniques for evaluating program impact/outcomes.

The efficiency of a program may be evaluated through cost-effectiveness or cost–benefit analyses (Greene, 2003; Rossi et al., 2004). In cost-effectiveness analysis, the cost of a program is evaluated relative to the results of the program. This allows comparison across programs (e.g., one bullying program, which cost $10 per student to implement, reduced bullying rates by 50%; another program costing $50 per student reduced bullying rates by 75%; thus, the cheaper program is more cost-effective). In cost–benefit analyses, the cost of the program is compared with the monetary value of the result. In this method, the outcome is expressed purely in monetary terms (e.g., difference in dollars expended on the anti-bullying program vs. dollars saved from reduced negative consequences associated with bullying). The actual calculations of the efficiency of a program can, obviously, get quite complicated, especially when attempting to assign a monetary value to outcomes that are not easily quantifiable.

As should be evident from this brief discussion, program evaluation is an important yet complex activity. Rossi et al. (2004) stressed this point when they stated, "Program evaluation is not a cut-and-dried activity like putting up a prefabricated house or checking a document with a word processor's spelling program" (p. 18). Programs often have many more components, individuals involved, and desired outcomes than experimental research studies. In addition, programs tend to be ongoing rather than time limited, as traditional research studies are. Because program evaluations are complex, they are rarely carried out by a single person. School psychologists who wish to become involved in program evaluations should seek information on what is already being done in their districts and attempt to collaborate with individuals currently involved in such activities. In addition, school psychologists could collaborate with university faculty in developing and evaluating programs designed to address school-based issues.

Data-Based Decision Making

Although not all school psychologists will be engaged in formal research activities, all school psychologists should be engaged in data-based decision making. Particularly with RTI procedures being implemented with increasing frequency, it is imperative that school psychologists understand how to make data-based decisions. As discussed in detail in Chapter 7, the data-driven problem-solving model requires school psychologists to examine discrepancies between how a child is currently performing (what is) and how the child should be performing (what should be). Under this model, discrepancies are domain specific (e.g., a child may have a discrepancy in social skills but not in reading skills) and context dependent (e.g., the problem may be present during independent seat work but not small-group activities), and the assessment of the discrepancy is specific to the situation (e.g., using CBM probes to assess reading fluency). Interventions are then developed that target the discrepancy within the context in which the problem is occurring. Interventions should target the specific reason why the problem is occurring, as outlined in the overview of problem analysis in Chapter 7 (e.g., Is the work too difficult for the student? Does the student "get" something out of not doing the work?). Once the intervention is in place, it should be monitored via continuous collection of objective data (e.g., CBM probes, behavioral observations) to determine whether the intervention is having the intended effect and is, in fact, decreasing the discrepancy between "what is" and "what should be" for the student. At each of the steps in the problem-solving model, the school psychologist is required to use data to inform his or her decision-making process.

Data-based decision making as used within the problem-solving model closely parallels research activities but also has some differences. Research activities are geared toward drawing conclusions that may generalize to other settings, individuals, and so forth. Research activities typically begin with specific research questions and hypotheses. Participants who meet certain criteria are then recruited to answer these questions. Data-based decision making is more focused on the individual student or client. The "question" to be answered is whether an intervention is having the intended effect for a specific individual in a specific situation. For example, Ella, a child with reading difficulties, is referred to the school psychologist for an evaluation. The evaluation is conducted, and recommendations are made for improving Ella's reading performance (e.g., conducting reading drills with overcorrection procedures). The question of interest in this case is, "Do reading drills increase Ella's reading fluency?" In data-based decision making, the focus is on addressing the problem (i.e., discrepancy), and the question is whether or not the discrepancy was reduced by the intervention. When the presenting problem involves an individual child, the methods of evaluation are much the same as they are in single-subject research designs: We want to be able to draw an informed conclusion regarding whether the intervention is having the desired impact on the student.

To obtain a baseline level of Ella's reading fluency prior to implementing the reading drills, the school psychologist could administer CBM probes. Following the baseline phase, the reading intervention is implemented, and the school psychologist continues to evaluate Ella's reading fluency through regular CBM probes. Assuming Ella's reading performance improves, the school psychologist may be satisfied and conclude that this intervention is having the desired effect. If Ella's reading fluency does not improve, the school psychologist would likely conclude that the intervention is not having the desired effect and would implement another intervention. If Ella's performance is evaluated in this manner, the basic AB design described earlier is followed. However, as noted, with this design the school psychologist would be unable to attribute improved performance to the intervention specifically, because there might be something else influencing the outcomes. For example, in this case, perhaps it was noted that Ella's vision seemed to be poor, that she recently started wearing glasses, and that it was actually her improved vision that led to her improvement in reading. To be confident that it was truly the intervention that led to the improvement, the school psychologist would need to implement one of the other single-subject designs (e.g., an ABAB design) discussed earlier.

In addition to making data-based decisions regarding the effectiveness of specific interventions for children, school psychologists should also assist in making data-based decisions regarding students' educational programs. As discussed in Chapter 6, all students who are receiving special education services must have IEPs that outline specific goals they are to achieve. However, all too often there is little done to evaluate whether children are meeting their IEP goals. If it is unclear whether goals are being met, it is also unclear whether the special education program is having a positive impact on the child. Thus, it is imperative that IEP goals be evaluated. For this to occur, IEP goals must be stated in measurable terms, and the child's performance on these goals must be evaluated on an ongoing basis. IEPs need to be reviewed only once a year. However, progress toward goals should be monitored much more frequently to determine whether the child is making adequate progress. Baseline levels of performance, as well as expected levels of performance, must be clear, and a system to measure change over time must be in place. If the child is not progressing, modifications may need to be made to that child's educational plan.

In addition to using data-based decision making to evaluate the outcomes for individual students, school psychologists who are involved in secondary or primary prevention efforts with groups of students (as discussed in Chapter 7) should also engage in data-based decision making. This data-based decision making may encompass both evaluation of the prevention program as a whole (which would parallel program evaluation methods discussed earlier in this chapter) as well as evaluation of individual student progress. As noted in Chapter 7, not all children respond in the same manner to prevention efforts. Thus, for some children more intensive services may need to be implemented, whereas for others the services provided through a prevention program may be adequate to prevent learning or behavioral problems. Without monitoring of student progress, it becomes impossible to know which students involved in a primary prevention program may benefit from secondary or tertiary prevention and intervention efforts. In addition, if data are collected in a proactive manner (i.e., data are obtained on all students) on important domains of functioning (e.g., reading), then this information can help inform decisions regarding in which areas schools should focus their prevention efforts and which students should be the targets of secondary- and tertiary-level prevention and intervention.

Implementing interventions without evaluating their effectiveness is poor practice and is much less likely to lead to positive change for students than interventions that are evaluated in an ongoing fashion and are modified as needed. As noted in Chapter 7, there is significant concern that traditional special education services are not effective in reducing the performance gap between children with and children without disabilities. If this is the case, clearly we are doing many students a disservice by not providing them with the skills they need to succeed within our school systems. We believe that by following the data-based problem-solving model in their daily practices, school psychologists can make a difference and can help students close that gap between where they are performing and where they should be performing. We strongly encourage all school psychologists to engage in this data-based decision-making process so that children are receiving the services most likely to meet their needs.

DISCUSSION QUESTIONS AND ACTIVITIES

1. Obtain a copy of a recent issue of one of the four main school psychology journals. Examine the articles published in this issue and identify whether each is an original research article, a meta-analysis, or a narrative review. What differences do you see in the structure of these different articles?

2. Using a group design experimental study from one of the main school psychology journals (or another journal focused on children), identify the possible threats to internal validity in the study. Also note whether the authors mention these in the discussion section of the article.

3. Locate a group-based intervention study focused on children (the *Journal of Clinical Child and Adolescent Psychology* is one good source of intervention studies). Do the authors evaluate the clinical significance of their results? If so, what method(s) do they use? Do you agree with their conclusions regarding the meaningfulness of their findings?

4. Locate a single-subject design study (*Journal of Applied Behavior Analysis* is one good source of such studies). What type of design do the researchers use? How do they evaluate the meaningfulness of the effects of their intervention?

5. Ask around in your school district about the types of programs that are run and the types of evaluation activities that occur. Are all programs evaluated? Do you see areas for improvement in the way programs are evaluated? Explain.

6. Interview several school psychologists regarding their data-based decision-making practices. Do they regularly engage in this practice? If not, why? If they do, obtain some examples of how they apply the methods and principles discussed in this chapter.

CHAPTER 13

Moving the Field Forward
Mapping the Future of School Psychology

One of us (KWM) recalls a visit with a prospective school psychologist, a woman who, having completed her undergraduate education several years ago and having worked in the fields of early childhood education and mental health for 10 years, was considering a career change into the field of school psychology. As the conversation progressed past the usual questions regarding application deadlines, selection procedures, financial support, training opportunities, and so forth, she asked some unusual intriguing questions regarding the future of school psychology, questions that surpassed what is typical in these kinds of interviews. Understandably, she was concerned about the employment outlook in school psychology, considering that she would need to invest 3 or more years and change professions in order to gain entry into the field. On this issue, she was assured that the employment outlook for school psychologists was projected to continue to be favorable for the next several years, despite a somewhat questionable economic outlook in general. Then she asked some more complicated questions: "Where is school psychology heading?" "What will the field look like in 10 years?" "What will happen to school psychology if public education undergoes major changes?" These questions led to an interesting discussion but also to some equivocation in providing answers to her questions.

It is easier to project certain aspects of the future of the field (e.g., employment trends, demographics) but much more complicated to predict with great confidence what the future will hold. In fact, what we can predict with the most confidence is that significant changes continue to be ahead of us. From our present standpoint in time and experience, we can quite confidently describe *what we would like to see* as the future of school psychology, and in this volume we have attempted to provide a road map or model for the field. In fact, the title of this book, *School Psychology for the 21st Century: Foundations and Practices,* was developed from our very specific objective of writing a book on school psychology that went beyond merely describing the history and present status of school psychology and actively advocated for what we consider to be models of good practice now and in the future, as the 21st century moves ahead. However, describing *what will be* is a more complicated matter, and we realize that prognosticating regarding the future is inherently risky business. Despite the necessary caveats that must be considered in writing a chapter on moving the field of school psychology forward, we believe that such a focus is a fitting way to conclude this volume. Although we recognize that there is some risk that our emphases and predictions might appear naive or off the mark 20 or 30 years from now, we won't let that fact stop us! We are aware of our lack of control of events that will impact our field's future, but at the same time confident that our views are well considered and based on a solid foundation. That said, we recognize the challenge in promoting a view about the future of school psychology. Fortune-telling and soothsaying may be among the oldest of professions, but even as such, they are probably not held in much esteem. Yogi Berra is credited with saying "Prediction is very hard, especially when it's about the future."

Near the turn of the last century—from about 1997 through about 2002—the future of school psychology was a major focus within the field. Several important publications and conferences were developed to address issues related to school psychology in the 21st century. Foremost among these sources include NASP's *School Psychology: A Blueprint for Training and Practice–II* (Ysseldyke et al., 1997; updated in 2006 by Ysseldyke et al.); the proceedings of the Future of School Psychology Conference, which was held November 14–16, 2002, at several sites and webcast from Indianapolis, Indiana (see *www.indiana. edu/~futures* for more details and presentation summaries, some of which were included as articles in special issues of *School Psychology Quarterly*, vol. 18, no. 4, 2003, and *School Psychology Review*, vol. 33, no. 1, 2004); a special issue of *School Psychology Review* (vol. 29, no. 4, 2000) titled "School Psychology in the 21st Century"; and a chapter by Reschly and Ysseldyke (2002) titled "Paradigm Shift: The Past Is Not the Future" in *Best Practices in School Psychology IV* (a chapter that was later updated by Reschly, 2008, in *Best Practices in School Psychology V*, and retitled "School Psychology Paradigm Shift and Beyond"). These sources are all important efforts to make an early-21st-century statement and vision regarding the future of school psychology. We have collectively been influenced by these efforts and have borrowed liberally from these sources in the preparation of this chapter.

This chapter includes a review of some issues related to the history of school psychology and how our past has shaped the present and future of the field in both positive and negative ways. Some prior efforts to predict the future of school psychology are reviewed. We should note that we owe a special debt to Fagan and Wise (2000, 2007) in developing our discussion of prior prognostication efforts, because their analyses of past attempts to predict the future of school psychology are simply the most comprehensive collections of information we have seen on this topic. Following this brief discussion, this chapter proceeds with our own carefully considered predictions regarding the future of the field. Perhaps most important, this chapter ends with our own analysis of a vision of where school psychology "should be" in the future, a summary of our own attempt in this volume to move the field forward and see it make the impact we know it is capable of making.

From Where We Were to Where We Are: The Evolution of School Psychology

Previous chapters in this volume, especially Chapters 2, 5, and 7, have provided an important historical context from which to understand the evolution of the field of school psychology. From its obscure and relatively recent beginnings within the larger fields of psychology and education, school psychology has struggled, grown, and finally arrived as a viable, strong, and mature profession and scientific discipline. There is no question regarding the arrival and maturation of the field, which has evolved into a large and potent force. Although school psychology is still small in comparison with its larger parent fields, there is no denying that it has made significant inroads in influence and that school psychologists are shaping practice, policy, and science at all levels—from the local school to the highest decision-making bodies.

One of the constants in this professional evolution has been the process of struggle and challenge. It is apparent that school psychology has grown and matured despite—or perhaps because of—both external and internal conflicts. Like a small tree that takes root in the rocky outcrops, the processes of opposition and constantly changing conditions have led to the growth of a stubborn, tough, and resilient organism whose roots have sunk in deep, having weathered a few storms. As the field of school psychology has arrived in the first quarter of the 21st century, it is interesting to consider what the future evolution of the field will bring and where it will be at the close of this century. In this regard, we can begin to think about the future by considering the forces that have brought us to the present, because it is quite likely that these same forces will continue to shape the field well beyond our own participation in it.

With respect to the processes that lead to change, we propose that two forces—changing social conditions or challenges and evolving legal aspects of education and psychology—will continue to have a major impact on the evolution of school psychology, just as they have had on its history. We also expect that the two forces will continue to be integrally connected, with changing social conditions and attitudes spawning new legal conditions, and with both forces having an impact on the practice of school psychology. At the midpoint of the 20th century, who could have predicted that changing social attitudes and conditions regarding people with disabilities would have led to the enactment of the Education for All Handicapped Children Act of 1975 in the United States (now known as IDEIA)? Who could have predicted that this federal law would serve as a major impetus for the field of school psychology, tripling in size in the United States in only two or three decades? Likewise, when the law was originated, who could have predicted that certain minor modifications to it, such as extending services to a younger age range (1987, 1990), mandating the use of functional behavior assessment in certain situations (1997), and no longer mandating the ability–achievement discrepancy model as the primary way in which LDs must be documented (2004) would have such a strong impact in professional practice, training, and research in the field?

In a similar vein, it is notable that changing economic and family conditions and social attitudes in the United States and Canada have had a dramatic impact on the demographics, status, and plight of children and that these conditions would result in major initiatives within the field of school psychology. For example, consider the major efforts within the field in recent years regarding providing services to at-risk children and youth, predicting and reducing school violence, and providing appropriate conditions and support for gay and lesbian youth in school settings. Although important aspects of each of these concerns were evident in the 1960s and 1970s, they were certainly not considered to be central issues within school psychology at that time, a statement that can be supported by a quick perusal of the focus and titles of journal articles and books from that era. Thus, we propose that the major changes or evolutions in the field of school psychology during the remainder of the 21st century will not occur in isolation or in a social vacuum. Rather, we believe that the major changes over the next several decades will develop in response to the ever-changing social, demographic, and legal conditions that affect the lives of children and their families and the delivery of school psychology services. It is also important to consider that change in professional practice often precedes changes in educational policy (Grimes & Tilly, 1996). In other words, although the field of school psychology must sometimes adapt practice to fit new policies, the reverse is also true. If practitioners, trainers, and researchers promote best practice in a reflective and proactive manner, it is quite possible that such practices will become codified into policy.

The Challenges of Prognostication: Previous Attempts to Predict the Future of the Field

Before we discuss our own views on the possible future of the field of school psychology, it is important to recognize the challenges and limits of such efforts at prognostication. Ever since school psychology emerged as a distinct field, there have been attempts to look forward and predict what the future might hold for the field. It is worth reviewing some of these earlier predictions in order to put the present state of the field within some context and to develop a lens through which our own views regarding the future of the field might be viewed.

Without question, the most detailed and comprehensive single compendium of prior efforts to provide viewpoints on the future of school psychology is "Perspectives on the Future of School Psychology," a chapter in Fagan and Wise (2000, 2007) in which they reviewed in depth the views of some of the most prominent writers in school psychology regarding the future of the field. This analysis considers prior predictions that proved to be accurate, as well as those predictions that did not come to pass, and discusses them within the context of ever-changing conditions the field has faced, which have made such prognostication difficult. A very brief review of a few of the more interesting viewpoints and predictions from this source is a useful addition to the current chapter.

The first well-known viewpoint or prediction regarding the future of school psychology was published in the 1930s, at a point when the field really did not even have a clear identity. Leta Hollingworth (1933), one of the pioneers of school psychology, promoted her predictions regarding the future of psychological services in public schools in an article in a professional journal. Her predictions were more specifically aimed at the upcoming 25 years, or the period from 1933 to 1958. Hollingworth saw a future in which educational practice and the delivery of psychological services in schools would be informed by science and rational thinking, in which psychological services in schools would become commonplace, and in which the combination of these variables would eliminate many of the problems of the time. In her own words: "The school will be fitted to the child. Suicide of pupils, in despair at failure, will be unknown. Truancy will become a thing of the past.... Special talents and defects will be considered in school placements" (Hollingworth, 1933, p. 379). Her predictions proved to be both accurate and inaccurate, given that school psychology ultimately did emerge as a major player in public education but also that its influence obviously did not eliminate most of the major ills faced by children and youth in school settings.

With the advent of APA's Division of School Psychology (Division 16) in 1945, and with the convening of the historic Thayer Conference on the future of school psychology in 1954, the period surrounding the midpoint of the 20th century provided new opportunities for those engaged in leadership within the burgeoning field to reflect on its progress to date and to consider what the future might bring. The general view regarding the development of the field during that time period was that school psychologists should be firmly grounded in clinical psychology and group testing but that in the future they would rely more heavily on specialized, individualized assessment and intervention techniques (Luckey, 1951). Certainly, the role of school psychologists as skilled individual assessment specialists came to pass, although the specialized interventionist role has been accomplished with mixed success. At the Thayer conference, new initiatives for the young Division 16 included establishing credentialing guidelines for school psychologists in the various U.S. states and differentiating doctoral from master's- (or specialist-) level training in credentialing (Fagan & Wise, 2000, 2007). Division 16 was successful in promoting important developments in state department of education credentialing patterns, although the differentiating of doctoral and nondoctoral school psychologists never gained significant or widespread influence. In addition, prominent participants at this conference correctly anticipated the future growth opportunities in the field, although it is doubtful that they could have possibly predicted the explosive growth that occurred in response to the changing educational landscape in the United States after the original IDEIA law was enacted.

As the field of school psychology began to come into its own in the 1960s and 1970s, the volume of professional literature increased substantially, and some of these writings addressed viewpoints regarding the future of the field. In our view, one of the most insightful efforts in this regard was Susan Gray's (1963) book, *The Psychologist in the Schools.* This volume was developed to provide a broad overview of the nascent field of school psychology and to provide a template for best practice. Perhaps the single greatest contribution of this work was the inclusion of two comprehensive chapters on the school psychologist as a *data-oriented problem solver.* Gray's work predated the current movement in data-based decision making and problem solving by two decades and established an important foundation for what in our view is one of the most significant roles that school psychologists can play. She foresaw a field in which school psychologists, armed with solid training in effective assessment, diagnosis, intervention, and scientific inquiry methods, would continually use these skills within a scientist-practitioner framework to propose testable hypotheses regarding learning and behavioral problems and would evaluate these hypotheses through carefully selecting and continually monitoring intervention efforts. Some other important future views during this era included Hirst's (1963) almost prescient prediction that there would be a strong increase in the professional workforce over the next two decades; Magary's (1967) discussion of the future emergence of the primary importance of the consultation role for school psychologists and the need for increased collaboration and cooperation on school teams and within professional organizations; Bardon and Bennet's (1974) call for more sophisticated and extensive training of school psychologists; and Tindall's (1979) comments regarding the emergence of increasing conflict between NASP and APA and the emerging problems of professional role constriction.

In the first edition of this volume, we cautiously made a few predictions of our own regarding the future of school psychology, some of which we have included and updated in this next section of this chapter. How did we do in this brief interval of time (about 5 years)? Overall, pretty well. Of course, some of these predictions were fairly easy to make. We prognosticated that that *school psychologists would serve an increasingly diverse population,* and that the *diversity of school psychologists would continue to lag behind that of the populations we serve.* Even in this short time span, both of these predictions have proven to be more true today than they were when we made them. Another on-target prediction we made was that *public sector financial stress will further inhibit growth and will require innovative service delivery approaches*. As we wrote the first edition, we had no way of knowing that this prediction would prove to be more true than we could have possibly imagined. The great worldwide recession that started with the near collapse of the financial and real estate industries in 2007 has indeed created a situation where public institutions—especially schools—have been hard hit. Increasing caseloads and shrinking budgets have been the order of the day within many systems during the past 4 years, which has forced many school psychologists—and all varieties of education professionals for that matter—to rethink how we provide effective services. We also predicted that *school psychologists will have increased access to new and effective technologies and tools*. This prediction has certainly shown some fruition as we have witnessed advances in the development of innovative new practices (RTI, for example) and an increase in dissemination of evidence-based interventions. We also think that the financial stresses on public education the past few years have slowed down what is possible in this regard. In the first edition, we prognosticated that *significant new federal initiatives will continue to affect the practice of school psychology*. The previous edition was written prior to knowing the impact of the reauthorization of IDEIA-2004 and its allowance of RTI practices instead of the traditional achievement–ability discrepancy model for assessing LDs. We probably underestimated the truth of that prediction, given that the speed and fervor with which RTI has been adopted and embraced have been truly stunning, something we might have hoped for but did not really anticipate. Regarding our prior prediction that *an increasing percentage of children and youth in schools will be at risk*, we see this assessment as truly being the case, mostly because the worldwide economic downturn has continued to increase the percentage of families with children who are living in financial distress or poverty. We also missed the mark to some extent (at least in the short term) by predicting in the first edition that *public schools will become increasingly specialized, unique, focused, and individualized*. In the relatively short period of time since we originally made this prognostication, we don't think that much has changed in this vein, partly because the time lag is still relatively brief and partly because of increased financial stresses in public education during the past few years. In short, we did pretty well with our prior predictions, but we also acknowledge that we didn't put ourselves "out on a limb" with any wild guesses or extremely long-term views of what might happen.

As we look retrospectively at the best known previous attempts to predict the future of school psychology, including our own predictions in the first edition of this volume, it is obvious that their accuracy and impact have been mixed. Some of these prior attempts ended up being far off the mark, whereas others were right on target. With the trepidation that comes from treading these well-traveled waters of prognostication, we now move our focus of this chapter to our own current predictions regarding the future of school psychology.

School Psychology in the 21st Century: Our Predictions

The predictions offered in this section have not simply been pulled out of the proverbial hat. Rather, our views regarding the future of school psychology are implicit within the previous chapters of this volume and, in some cases, serve as an important foundation for these chapters. Some of these predictions are quite easy to make, and we are confident enough in them to consider them as continuing to fall in the "no-brainer" category. Others are more complicated and stem from a confluence of where we think the evidence is pointing and where we think it "ought" to point. As we acknowledge the limitations in any prognostication process, we also believe that the following prognostications, which are mostly consistent with or even a continuation of our predictions from the first edition of this volume, represent the future of the field of school psychology.

- *School psychologists will serve an increasingly diverse population.* This prediction continues to fall into the "no-brainer" category. As we have shown in Chapter 3, the population of students and families who are served by school psychologists will continue to reflect increased diversity with regard to race or ethnicity, language, cultural background, and familial composition. The state of California is often considered to be a cultural barometer for future social trends in the United States. Presently, no single racial/ethnic group constitutes more than 50% of the population of the schools in that state. The website for the *Languages of Los Angeles* project at UCLA (*www.humnet.ucla.edu/languagesofla/default. htm*) indicates that more than 56 major primary languages are spoken by residents of Los Angeles (up from 50 languages in our 2006 edition of this volume), and there have been some estimates that the students served by the Los Angeles Unified School District speak an even greater number of primary or native languages. We believe that these figures represent unmistakable trends that will ultimately spread to some extent to all regions of the United States and Canada. Stated simply, school psychologists in the future will be expected to have the skills and technology to provide educational and mental health services to an increasingly diverse population.

- *The diversity of school psychologists will increasingly lag behind that of the populations they serve.* Although the population of students and their families served by school psychologists will continue to increase in the 21st century, the diversity of school psychologists will continue to lag behind that of the general population and is destined to become even more disparate in this regard, at least for the next quarter century. At the 2002 Futures Conference, a presentation by Curtis, Grier, and Hunley (2003, 2004) demonstrated convincingly that, despite some overall increases in ethnic/racial diversity of school psychologists in recent years (and a generally strong desire for more diversity within the field), school psychology has become distinctly "Caucasian and female." Expected increases in racial/ethnic diversity among school psychologists will be more than offset by larger increases in all forms of diversity among constituent populations served, causing even greater disparity between typical practitioners and clients. We believe that a major challenge in this regard is that the increased disparity in diversity representation between school psychologists and the populations they serve may foster increased perceptions of a "credibility gap," to borrow a well-known phrase from American politics in the 1960s.

- *School psychologists will continue to be in short supply.* At least through the first quarter of the 21st century, and even with some hiring slowdowns or freezes resulting from continued financial stresses on public education systems, all indications are that there will continue to be a strong demand for school psychologists in the United States, and that this demand will outstrip the supply to some extent. These personnel shortages will continue to be especially problematic in rural and urban school systems and in selected regions. As a result, employment prospects for school psychologists will continue to be favorable. The NASP-recommended ratio of one school psychologist per 1,000 students in a school system will be unattainable in many school systems, particularly in poorer districts and in regions in which shortages are most notable. Our prognostication on this issue has been tempered somewhat since the publication of our first edition of this volume in 2006 by the "great recession" that began with the financial crisis of 2007 and, as of 2011, continues to have a negative effect on public sector and private sector hiring. That said, we note that graduates of our respective training programs, particularly those who were willing to relocate geographically for professional opportunities, had few troubles getting hired (and often had multiple job offers), even during the peak periods of national unemployment. Related to this issue, we foresee a continued strong need not only for school psychology practitioners but ultimately also for school psychology educators or trainers. We believe that it is likely that the recession-related freezes on hiring for university faculty positions in school psychology and other fields will ultimately subside, and that it will be accompanied by a pent-up demand for new school psychology faculty. The emerging generation of school psychology educators will need to develop increasingly responsive and innovative ways to make school psychology training available to graduate students, sometimes in nontraditional ways.

• *Public sector financial stress will further inhibit growth and will require innovative service delivery approaches.* Even in the relatively strong economic times during which we wrote the first edition of this volume, this particular prediction also fell within the "no-brainer" category. Since about 1980, public services in the United States, especially public education and mental health services, have been operating under increasing economic and political duress, a complicated result of unfunded federal and state mandates, tax cuts at the federal level shifting financial burdens to local governments, changes in social and economic conditions, and the advent of a political climate in which many politicians and citizens have fostered a distrust in the public sector and a great desire to reduce its size and increase its efficiency. The great worldwide economic crisis and recession that began in 2007 absolutely strengthened the position of this unfortunate prognostication. School psychology services have traditionally been almost exclusively connected to the public sector, and the larger political and economic trends have and will continue to greatly shape and affect the field. On the negative side, many school psychologists will be asked to do "more with less" and will experience higher caseloads and less availability of internal and external support services for the students they serve. On the positive side, these trends will necessitate a climate in which many school psychologists will seize the challenge as an opportunity to deliver services in nontraditional ways, such as moving away from a model of solving one student problem at a time and toward developing systems-level orientations and preventive approaches (Shapiro, 2000) as well as changing the way we do business to conform to a culture of "what works" (see Reschly, 2008). We believe that a move away from targeting services exclusively at the individual student level is inevitable and that the 21st century will see a significant expansion in efforts by school psychologists to engage in prevention activities and to affect entire classrooms, schools, and systems through their services, including both direct and consultative services.

• *Role expansion in school psychology will increase.* Despite (or perhaps because of) the staffing shortages and economic challenges that will be faced by the field, many school psychologists will continue to advocate effectively for role expansion and will increasingly distance themselves from the traditional gatekeeper or sorter roles in which static psychometric classification activities are *de rigueur.* Although some educational systems (and, frustratingly, some school psychology practitioners) will refuse to extricate the school psychologist from the traditional test-and-place role, innovative school psychologists will successfully negotiate ways to provide meaningful solutions to educational, social, and behavioral problems, and the successes of these efforts will spawn support for role expansion by administrators and teachers who recognize what their school psychologist can do for them. Furthermore, a growing number of school psychology training programs will develop innovative curricula and mission statements that will facilitate such continued role expansion and intervention and problem-solving orientations. We have already witnessed some of this transition taking place. Although it is true that some systems are highly resistant to progressive changes, educational systems that historically have used the psychologist almost exclusively in the sorter role are often more than willing to modify their expectations and place the psychologist in a consultation, training, and intervention role once they see how well a progressively trained practitioner can help them solve big problems within the system. To borrow a phrase, once the genie is out of the bottle, it's hard to get it back in.

• *School psychologists will have increased access to new and effective technologies and tools.* As we have witnessed in recent years with the advent of new models for effective behavioral and academic supports in schools, school psychologists in the 21st century will continue to have increasing access to exciting new tools for providing effective services. In fact, we believe that there will be a dramatic increase in the availability of such effective new tools. The often repeated proverb "necessity is the mother of invention" will certainly come into play here, because the very big and very real problems faced by children and their families in this century will absolutely necessitate better solutions. Furthermore, the maturing research base in the fields of psychology and education and the increasingly innovative technology by which this information is accessed (e.g., instant Internet-based access) will make the availability of new information and tools almost immediate. We anticipate that exciting innovations such as these will continue to shape the practice of school psychology and the fields of education and psychology in general as we move increasingly in the direction of being a science-based profession.

• *Significant new federal initiatives will continue to affect the practice of school psychology.* This prediction also continues to fit in the "no-brainer" category of prediction. Looking forward to the middle and end of the 21st century, none of us can possibly imagine the specific social, political, and economic conditions that will result in changes to federal education laws, but if the past is a guide, we can be assured that such changes will indeed happen. In fact, if you are smart, you can safely bet your paycheck on this prediction (not that we are advocating gambling ...). The 20th-century federal legislation in the United States that most clearly affected school psychology was the passage of the original IDEIA in 1975. The 1990, 1997, and 2004 reauthorizations of this law also resulted in immediate responses in some aspects of school psychology practice and training. As we have previously noted, we anticipated the inclusion of the RTI method for assessing student LDs in the 2004 reauthorization, but were surprised—no, stunned is a better word—by how rapidly this new and unmandated provision took off to become a *tour de force* with a life of its own. Expect further modifications to IDEIA to have similar effects over time. And it takes no stretch of the imagination to believe that some new federal law, similar or greater in impact on school psychology as IDEIA, will become reality later in the 21st century. Although the U.S. federal government does not have the primary responsibility for public education (it is considered a "creature of the states"), presidential administrations have increasingly used federal education initiatives (many of them unfunded or only partially funded) to shape or mandate state policies, and the U.S. Congress has likewise demonstrated similar propensities. As the documentary film *Waiting for Superman* has noted, it seems as though every newly elected U.S. president publicly states that he wants to be "the education president," and that usually means far-reaching new federal initiatives. It is quite possible that a future 21st-century federal law will dwarf IDEIA and the current No Child Left Behind Act in terms of impact on education and the practice of school psychology. Will publicly funded tuition vouchers for private education become a widespread reality? (Don't think it can't happen—there is an increasing groundswell of interest in this idea.) Will new federal laws bring the special education census to 25% of the student population nationally? Will IEPs become an entitlement of all students, and not just those identified as having disabilities? Will IDEIA be abolished or replaced by something entirely different? These are only a handful of examples of possible future legislation that would affect education, and school psychology, in a dramatic way.

• *An increasing percentage of children and youth in schools will be at risk.* This prediction is one that we wish we didn't feel compelled to continue to make, but it nonetheless is on the horizon. According to varied social, economic, and health indicators, children born in the United States during the 21st century will face unprecedented new challenges and opportunities. For a growing percentage of these children, the result will be increased exposure to circumstances that place them at risk for academic, social, behavioral, health, or economic problems, which are often intertwined (Children's Defense Fund, 2001, 2010; Crockett, 2003, 2004). We see these probable developments as having a clear impact on the field of school psychology. As these risk factors continue, more students will need to become the focus of concern for school teams, and the result will be more opportunities for school psychologists to play a role in developing appropriate, effective programs to support these children. This eventuality not only will require more involvement from school psychologists but will also further enhance the need for practitioners to focus their services in a manner that moves increasingly farther away from the "one child at a time'" model of solving educational and social problems.

• *Public schools will become increasingly specialized, unique, focused, and individualized.* Although some individuals may yearn for the perceived "golden age" of public education of the 1950s and early 1960s, when baby boomers nationwide experienced a great deal of perceived similarity or homogeneity among their public schooling curricula and socialization experiences, we believe that the future of public schools may possibly be in the direction of less, not more, uniformity and homogeneity in the schooling experience. Despite some recent federal, state, and provincial initiatives to exert greater control and impose greater accountability among public schools, an interesting social dynamic is evolving that may make the future increasingly diverse, despite financial stresses on public education. Families in the 21st century want and expect more choice and more control over their children's education than was typical in past decades. We anticipate that some of the current fringe or experimental educational innovations may become more common as the 21st century progresses. As a result, a small but increasing percentage of students will receive public education in schools that today represent only a small, experimental component of public schooling. Examples of some of these emerging experimental education innovations include charter schools, smaller and more individualized secondary schools (currently being promoted and funded by the Bill and Melinda Gates Foundation), alternative school offerings, magnet schools, non-English language immersion schools, same-gender classrooms and schools, and highly focused specialized schools that emphasize themes such as Afrocentric education, performing arts, science and technology, and international/global education. The continued popularity and growth of the charter school movement in the United States (also popularized in the documentary film *Waiting for Superman*) is an example of this type of specialization of which we are talking. Although not all charter schools are in strong demand or produce the outcomes that are desired, many are so popular that entrance into these publicly funded entities is by application and lottery drawings. These trends should not be a surprise—they simply reflect the reality of an increasingly pluralistic society within North America. As a result of this trend away from homogeneity, school psychologists of the 21st century will increasingly be expected to provide more individualized services, assist in making more individual accommodations within mainstream educational environments, and work with school teams that operate under increasingly unique and diverse mission statements.

• *Assessment will continue to be important and will become more useful for intervention.* In reading this volume, you likely have sensed two somewhat contrasting themes: that we view psychological and educational assessment of students to be a critically important activity for school psychologists and that we exceedingly dislike the models of school psychology that are rigidly focused on a gatekeeper or sorter role, or a test-and-place paradigm. We don't actually see a contradiction here. The problem, in our view, is not that school psychologists focus much of their work on assessment but rather that so much of the traditional assessment enterprise is not particularly helpful for solving children's educational and mental health concerns and so many of these tasks have kept school psychologists out of the intervention planning and delivery role. We believe that assessment will continue to be an important role for school psychologists throughout the 21st century, although this role will become increasingly expanded beyond the assessment and classification niche. Moreover, we believe that over time there will continue to be improvements in the quality and usefulness of assessment methods and tools, both for classification and intervention planning purposes. The 21st century will see the much-discussed but seldom implemented notion of effectively linking assessment to intervention become more a part of routine practice for school psychologists. In addition, if the field moves increasingly toward prevention and systems change, perhaps assessment will include more formative measures for all students. It is feasible that school psychologists might have a role in the development, management, and implementation of such formative or schoolwide assessments.

• *The 21st century includes a bright future for school psychologists.* Although some of our prognostications may be frightening—they certainly are premised on the idea that changes are inevitable and not always desirable—we are "bullish" (to borrow a phrase from the stock market) on the future of the field of school psychology. In fact, we are more bullish on the future of school psychology than we are on the future of the stock market. We believe that the 21st century will see the fruits of the maturation of school psychology and that school psychologists will become increasingly important players in the education and mental health fields. The 20th century witnessed the maturation of the field of school psychology, with its symbolic move from adolescence to adulthood. We have no reservations recommending a career in school psychology to prospective professionals who possess the requisite skills, personal resiliency, commitment, and adaptability to be successful and who are motivated by a desire to help shape the future of children and their families through innovative education and mental health service delivery.

Mapping Our Future: A Vision for School Psychology

We see the 21st century as being ripe for a major positive impact from the field of school psychology if the field sees and seizes the opportunity in a proactive manner. As Sheridan and D'Amato stated in the parallel special issues of *School Psychology Review* and *School*

Psychology Quarterly devoted to the proceedings of the 2002 Future of School Psychology Conference:

> Although many visionaries have offered frameworks to advance a new identity for school psychology, one thing is very clear.... To realize even the smallest dream for the future of school psychology, it is absolutely essential that all major players—professional organizations, trainers, practitioners—take active steps to make it happen. These steps must be taken proactively, strategically, and assertively. They must be taken with confidence in one's own skill and expertise but more importantly, they must be taken in cooperation and coordination with others in related fields and disciplines. (2003, p. 354; 2004, p. 8)

The 21st century is no longer in its infancy, and this quote is now about a decade old, but we think it still fits. We agree that steps toward positive change in the field of school psychology must be taken in cooperation and coordination with our partners in other fields and disciplines. We also believe that the necessity for such coordinated efforts and partnerships should not discourage individual school psychologists from taking small positive steps on their own. As we have stated previously, changes in practice can precede changes in policy. Although top-down change that results from strong and coordinated leadership efforts at the national and state or provincial levels is certainly a model with substantial precedent, bottom-up efforts at the grassroots level is also a viable pattern for change. It has been our observation—something we have tried to emphasize within this volume—that individual initiative and efforts of school psychology practitioners, researchers, and trainers, particularly those efforts that are firmly grounded in good theory, science, and practice, are likely to make a significant impact. The "power of one" should not be underestimated.

Although grassroots efforts of individuals and groups can have an enormous positive impact, they also frequently fall by the wayside. Why is this? There are several possible explanations. One possibility we have tried to emphasize is that our efforts to solve problems through the framework of school psychology must be grounded in good theory and science. Efforts that are not built on this solid framework are bound to eventually fail, because no matter how much popularity they attain, they lack the substance to sustain themselves. A somewhat contrasting explanation for failure of efforts within the field of school psychology to make the positive impact that is sought is that, although the scientific base behind our efforts may be solid, these efforts may be misguided in other ways. In other words, we sometimes have situations in which we enlist our considerable scientific, technological, and theoretical resources but focus on unimportant, irrelevant, or ill-considered problems and issues. As Conoley and Gutkin (1995) stated in a widely cited article on the failure of school psychology to realize its potential: "School psychology does not suffer from a lack of good science. It suffers from a science that is devoted almost exclusively to answering the wrong sets of questions. It is a science that is preoccupied with the problems of individuals rather than understanding the ecologies in which people function" (p. 210).

We emphatically agree with this criticism. Even if our efforts to enact positive change in delivering educational and mental health services to children and youth are girded by strong theory and scientific rigor, they will ultimately fail if they are focused on the wrong questions, issues, or focal points. An almost obsessive search for within-child psychopathology, preoccupation with descriptive assessment tools that do not inform intervention, and failure to take into account the complex environments and ecological systems in which children exist are but three examples of using theory and science to focus on the wrong issues. For the record, we acknowledge that within-child deficits or dysfunctions do exist and that individually focused assessment and intervention efforts are often necessary and useful. Our concern is that these realities have become the only truth for many practitioners and researchers in our field and that this focus has obscured the more expansive, context-driven view of helping children succeed. For the field of school psychology to move forward in an effective and powerful manner, the major interests and inquiry points of our practitioners, researchers, and trainers must focus on the important issues that are most likely to result in our services influencing positively and in a major way the educational and mental health needs of children and youth.

Priority Goals and Outcomes from the 2002 Futures Conference

Clearly, efforts to move the field of school psychology forward in achieving its full potential to help serve the educational and mental health needs of children, adolescents, their families, and learning environments must be guided by a strong scientific foundation and must focus on the most critical and functional variables. Successful efforts in this regard must also be guided by a cohesive vision or action plan that articulates clearly the essential goals, outcomes, and domains that will result in the quantity and quality of positive impact we seek. In this regard, we are enthusiastic about the priority goals that emerged from the 2002 Future of School Psychology Conference. Although these goals cannot take into consideration every possible concern, situation, or solution that we must seek in the 21st century, they provide a cohesive road map for moving the field forward over the next several decades. Table 13.1 lists the five general outcome goals identified as critical by conference participants and work group leaders broken down by subgoals and various types of efforts needed. These outcome goals include improved academic competence for all children (Outcome 1), improved social–emotional functioning for all children (Outcome 2), enhanced family–school partnerships and parental involvement in schools (Outcome 3), more effective education and instruction for all learners (Outcome 4), and increased child and family services in schools that promote health and mental health and are integrated with community services (Outcome 5). According to Dawson, Cummings, Harrison, Short, Gorin, and Palomares (2003, 2004), the 15 priority strategies outlined in Table 13.1 resulted from analyses by work group chairs at the Futures conference and were later tied to action plans (which are available on the Futures conference website at *www.indiana.edu/~futures*). We believe that priority goals and strategies are an example of using a solid scientific-theoretical base to focus on the right issues and that this template can serve as a positive guide to helping the field of school psychology more fully achieve its promise.

Concluding Comments: Another Look at the "Triangle of Support"

In reviewing the priority goals and outcomes from the 2002 Futures conference (presented in Table 13.1 and in the previous section of this chapter), it is striking to note the strong focus on prevention and early intervention as well as the explicit emphasis on public health models of service delivery. Each of the five outcome areas includes some emphasis on the need for primary prevention of academic or social–emotional problems, the necessity of early intervention, and/or the importance of using public health models in school psychology service delivery. We emphatically agree that these emphasis areas must be an essential part of the future of school psychology. In several previous

TABLE 13.1. Priority Goals and Outcomes from the 2002 Future of School Psychology Conference

Outcome	Goal
Outcome 1: Improved academic competence for all children	
Advocacy and public policy	Goal A: Advocate for universal early prevention and intervention programs that emphasize language, cognitive, and social–emotional development and are placed in the context of ethnicity, socioeconomic status, gender, and language.
Practice	Goal B: Ensure that assessment practices of school psychologists are linked to strategies to improve academic performance and that those assessment practices account for the influence of ethnicity, SES, gender, and language on learning outcomes.
Preservice and inservice	Goal C: Develop and implement preservice and inservice training for school psychologists related to universal early prevention and intervention programs.
Outcome 2: Improved social–emotional functioning for all children	
Advocacy and public policy	Goal A: Promote the availability of a comprehensive range of services, from supportive and inclusive placements through interim alternative placements, for students with severe emotional and behavioral disorders.
Collaboration and communication	Goal B: Educate all stakeholders about the importance of social–emotional competencies for children.
Practice	Goal C: Ensure that school psychologists develop a systematic plan in all schools to reduce social–emotional barriers to learning.
Outcome 3: Enhanced family–school partnerships and parental involvement in schools	
Research and knowledge base	Goal A: Identify evidence-based models of effective family–school partnerships.
Practice	Goal B: Ensure that school psychologists engage in activities to change the culture of schooling by making families integral partners in the educational process of children.
Preservice training	Goal C: Change preservice education and training of school psychologists candidates to infuse a focus on families as integral partners in the educational process.
Outcome 4: More effective education and instruction for all learners	
Research and knowledge base	Goal A: Identify key components of effective instruction for all learners, including evidence-based approaches to prevention and early intervention for learning problems.
Inservice training	Goal B: Provide inservice training for school psychologists in the use of a data-based problem-solving model to implement evidence-based instruction and interventions.
Preservice and inservice training	Goal C: Implement a national preservice and inservice training initiative for school psychologists regarding effective instruction.
Outcome 5: Increased child and family services in schools that promote health and mental health and that are integrated with community services	
Practice	Goal A: Define and promote population-based service delivery in schools and school psychology.
Inservice training	Goal B: Prepare current practitioners to implement a public health model.
Preservice training	Goal C: Prepare future practitioners to implement a public health model.

Note. From Dawson et al. (2003). Copyright 2003 by the American Psychological Association. Reprinted by permission.

chapters of this volume, we have strongly emphasized prevention and early intervention and the need for affecting whole systems as well as individual children and adolescents. That said, we believe it is appropriate to conclude this final chapter of *School Psychology for the 21st Century* with some additional comments regarding the necessity of moving school psychology practice in this direction.

Figure 13.1 provides another look at the triangle of academic and behavior support model for delivery of school psychology services that has been discussed in prior chapters of this volume. This model is built on the premise that school psychology services should reach all students at all levels of an educational or mental health system. It is also based on the public health model of disease prevention, in which prevention efforts are divided into three distinct areas reflected in the three levels of the triangle (see Adams et al., 1997; Cowen et al., 1996; Edelstein & Mickelson, 1986; Merrell & Buchanan, 2006, for more information on public health prevention models). This model is very consistent with the recent trend toward emphasizing positive behavioral and academic supports for students, as illustrated by the work that has been promoted by the U.S. Department of Education's OSEP Technical Assistance Center on Positive Behavior Supports (see *www.pbis.org* for more information) and the work of researchers and school systems that is highlighted through this center.

To conclude this final chapter, it is useful to once again consider this triangle model of tiered prevention and intervention efforts and its implications for the practice of school psychology. The bottom of the triangle represents *primary prevention*, the prevention of the occurrence or expression of a particular problem or promotion of universal supports designed to enable, strengthen, or increase likelihood of success. In this model, primary prevention efforts are directed at the approximately 80% of "typical" students, but in reality addressing all students, with the understanding that some students will need additional supports. Such efforts are systems and group based and involve brief

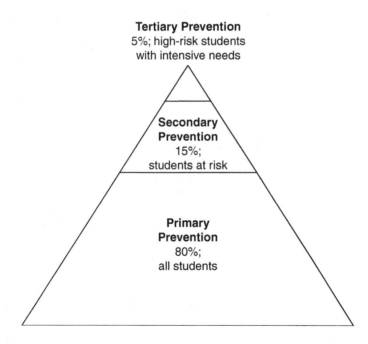

Tertiary Prevention
5%; high-risk students
with intensive needs

Secondary Prevention
15%;
students at risk

Primary Prevention
80%;
all students

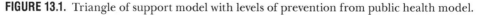

FIGURE 13.1. Triangle of support model with levels of prevention from public health model.

universal screening procedures and the delivery of educational and mental health services within entire classrooms or schools. The middle of the triangle represents *secondary prevention*, or the prevention of side effects or a worsening of an existing problem. Secondary prevention is also conceptualized as early intervention—identifying the early onset of a problem and taking proactive steps to keep the problem from worsening. In the triangle model, secondary prevention services are directed at approximately 15% of students in typical school systems who are beginning to show signs of academic, behavioral, and/or social–emotional problems or who have significant risk factors that make them vulnerable to such problems. Secondary prevention efforts may involve brief, individual screening and assessment procedures and services delivered within classrooms, within small pull-out groups, and, to a limited extent, with individual students identified as at risk. The top of the triangle represents *tertiary prevention*, a concept similar to *rehabilitation*—specific efforts are needed to reduce the serious problem symptoms and to increase the assets of individuals who have severe academic, behavioral, and social–emotional problems with very intense needs. Such services should typically be limited to a small percentage of the entire school population—approximately 5% of students whose problems are so serious that they require high-intensity efforts. At this level, assessment efforts are individualized, based on a multimethod design, and comprehensive. Interventions are often delivered individually (such as intense academic tutoring, individual skill training, or mental health counseling). However, in some cases, interventions at the top of the triangle may be delivered in small groups or in classrooms. Special program participation is a given for individual children and youth who require tertiary prevention services to help alleviate their intensive problems. Finally, those students whose intensive needs place them at the very top of the triangle must often receive educational and mental health services in a coordinated manner across school and community settings, using a *wrap-around* model of service in which services are complementary and coordinated and address the full spectrum of needs.

Our view is that the best models of school psychology practice take into account each of the three levels of the tiered triangle, based on the underlying premises of public health models. In most situations, school psychologists should devote a portion of their time to providing services at each level, thus reaching all students. The desired or optimum distribution of services across each of the three levels will vary with specific assignments and with specific populations, but in general, progressive school psychology services should address all areas, not just the "top of the triangle," as has so often been the case in typical practice. By distributing their expertise across all levels of service delivery needs, school psychologists will ultimately make a larger impact on systems and will prevent many students from "moving up" to a higher level of the triangle.

Public health models of prevention and systems-based triangle models of service delivery are nothing new (Merrell & Buchanan, 2006). These models have existed in various stages of refinement within the fields of public health, disease prevention, and community psychology for many years. What is new is the explicit application of these models to the fields of education and children's mental health services in recent years. More specifically, the articulation of these models as a guide to providing effective school psychology services is a new and innovative development. Given the challenges that appear to be looming in the 21st century for children and their families, educational systems, the field of school psychology, and society and culture in general, we believe that these models represent the best hope for the practice of school psychology in the next several decades. *Status quo* models of school psychology practice that continue the obsession with seeking and identifying pathology, within-child etiologies for learning and social–emotional problems, solving problems exclusively "one child at a time," and providing interventions without considering systemic or ecological contexts are doomed to hinder the progress of the field. We believe that such models, which are unfortunately still very prevalent within school psychology, are ultimately futile and will be consigned to the junkyard of our professional history. Or at least we hope so. Our optimistic view of the field of school psychology in the 21st century is that it will reach its full promise for positively affecting the educational and mental health needs of children and adolescents. The 20th century evidenced the development and maturation of the field. In the 21st century, school psychologists have a tremendous opportunity and obligation to fulfill the promises that are now within reach.

DISCUSSION QUESTIONS AND ACTIVITIES

1. Some previous efforts to prognosticate or predict the future of school psychology have been wildly incorrect. Why is the task of prognostication regarding this field so difficult, and what are some of the events that have moved the field in ways that were never previously envisioned?

2. Go the Future of School Psychology website at *www.indiana.edu/~futures* and review some of the essays, presentation outlines, and conference summary information. After doing so, list what you believe are the two or three most compelling or important things to come out of the Futures conference and why you see these as so important.

3. We have made some projections or predictions regarding what we believe will be important trends and developments in the near future of the field of school psychology. After reviewing our list of predictions, what would you add to or delete from this list based on your own experiences and conditions in your own area?

4. One of the predictions we have reluctantly made is that the diversity of school psychologists (in terms of gender, ethnicity, and language orientation) will increasingly lag behind the diversity of American society in general. Although numerous efforts have been made to increase the diversity of the field, these efforts have not resulted in making the field more like the population it serves, because the increases in diversity in the field are continually lagging behind the stronger increases in diversity of the general population. Discuss some of the challenges to diversifying the field of school psychology. Brainstorm to develop some innovative ideas to more successfully address this issue.

American Psychological Association Ethical Principles of Psychologists and Code of Conduct (Revised 2010)

Introduction and Applicability

The American Psychological Association's (APA) Ethical Principles of Psychologists and Code of Conduct (hereinafter referred to as the Ethics Code) consists of an Introduction, a Preamble, five General Principles, and specific Ethical Standards. The Introduction discusses the intent, organization, procedural considerations, and scope of application of the Ethics Code. The Preamble and General Principles are aspirational goals to guide psychologists toward the highest ideals of psychology. Although the Preamble and General Principles are not themselves enforceable rules, they should be considered by psychologists in arriving at an ethical course of action. The Ethical Standards set forth enforceable rules for conduct as psychologists. Most of the Ethical Standards are written broadly, in order to apply to psychologists in varied roles, although the application of an Ethical Standard may vary depending on the context. The Ethical Standards are not exhaustive. The fact that a given conduct is not specifically addressed by an Ethical Standard does not mean that it is necessarily either ethical or unethical.

This Ethics Code applies only to psychologists' activities that are part of their scientific, educational, or professional roles as psychologists. Areas covered include but are not limited to the clinical, counseling, and school practice of psychology; research; teaching; supervision of trainees; public service; policy development; social intervention; development of assessment instruments; conducting assessments; educational counseling; organizational consulting; forensic activities; program design and evaluation; and administration. This Ethics Code applies to these activities across a variety of contexts, such as in person, postal, telephone, Internet, and other electronic transmissions. These activities shall be distinguished from the purely private conduct of psychologists, which is not within the purview of the Ethics Code.

Membership in the APA commits members and student affiliates to comply with the standards of the APA Ethics Code and to the rules and procedures used to enforce them. Lack of awareness or misunderstanding of an Ethical Standard is not itself a defense to a charge of unethical conduct.

The procedures for filing, investigating, and resolving complaints of unethical conduct are described in the current Rules and Procedures of the APA Ethics Committee. APA may impose sanctions on its members for violations of the standards of the Ethics Code, including termination of APA membership, and may notify other bodies and individuals of its actions. Actions that violate the standards of the Ethics Code may also lead to the imposition of sanctions on psychologists or students whether or not they are APA members by bodies other than APA, including state psychological associations, other professional groups, psychology boards, other state or federal agencies, and payors for health services. In addition, APA may take action against a member after his or her conviction of a felony, expulsion or suspension from an affiliated state psychological association, or suspension or loss of licensure. When the sanction to be imposed by APA is less than expulsion, the 2001 Rules and Procedures do not guarantee an opportunity for an in-person hearing, but generally provide that complaints will be resolved only on the basis of a submitted record.

The Ethics Code is intended to provide guidance for psychologists and standards of professional conduct that can be applied by the APA and by other bodies that choose to adopt them. The Ethics Code is not intended to be a basis of civil liability. Whether a psychologist has violated the Ethics Code standards does not by itself determine whether the psychologist is legally liable in a court action, whether a contract is enforceable, or whether other legal consequences occur.

The modifiers used in some of the standards of this Ethics Code (e.g., reasonably, appropriate, potentially) are included in the standards when they would (1) allow professional judgment on the part of psychologists, (2) eliminate injustice or inequality that would occur without the modifier, (3) ensure applicability across the broad range of activities conducted by psychologists, or (4) guard against a set of rigid rules that might be quickly outdated. As used in this Ethics Code, the term reasonable means the prevailing professional judgment of psychologists engaged in similar activities in similar circumstances, given the knowledge the psychologist had or should have had at the time.

In the process of making decisions regarding their professional behavior, psychologists must consider this Ethics Code in addition to applicable laws and psychology board regulations. In applying the Ethics Code to their professional work, psychologists may consider other materials and guidelines that have been adopted or endorsed by scientific and professional psychological organizations and the dictates of their own conscience, as well as consult with others within the field. If this Ethics Code establishes a higher standard of conduct than is required by law, psychologists must meet the higher ethical standard. If psychologists' ethical responsibilities conflict with law, regulations, or other governing legal authority, psychologists make known their commitment to this Ethics Code and take steps to resolve the conflict in a responsible manner in keeping with basic principles of human rights.

Preamble

Psychologists are committed to increasing scientific and professional knowledge of behavior and people's understanding of themselves and others and to the use of such knowledge to improve the condition of individuals, organizations, and society. Psychologists respect and protect civil and human rights and the central importance of freedom of inquiry and expression in research, teaching, and publication. They strive to help the public in developing informed judgments and choices concerning human behavior. In doing so, they perform many roles, such as researcher, educator, diagnostician, therapist, supervisor, consultant, administrator, social interventionist, and expert witness. This Ethics Code provides a common set of principles and standards upon which psychologists build their professional and scientific work.

This Ethics Code is intended to provide specific standards to cover most situations encountered by psychologists. It has as its goals the welfare and protection of the individuals and groups with whom psychologists work and the education of members, students, and the public regarding ethical standards of the discipline.

The development of a dynamic set of ethical standards for psychologists' work-related conduct requires a personal commitment and lifelong effort to act ethically; to encourage ethical behavior by students, supervisees, employees, and colleagues; and to consult with others concerning ethical problems.

General Principles

This section consists of General Principles. General Principles, as opposed to Ethical Standards, are aspirational in nature. Their intent is to guide and inspire psychologists toward the very highest ethical ideals of the profession. General Principles, in contrast to Ethical Standards, do not represent obligations and should not form the basis for imposing sanctions. Relying upon General Principles for either of these reasons distorts both their meaning and purpose.

Principle A: Beneficence and Nonmaleficence

Psychologists strive to benefit those with whom they work and take care to do no harm. In their professional actions, psychologists seek to safeguard the welfare and rights of those with whom they interact professionally and other affected persons, and the welfare of animal subjects of research. When conflicts occur among psychologists' obligations or concerns, they attempt to resolve these conflicts in a responsible fashion that avoids or minimizes harm. Because psychologists' scientific and professional judgments and actions may affect the lives of others, they are alert to and guard against personal, financial, social, organizational, or political factors that might lead to misuse of their influence. Psychologists strive to be aware of the possible effect of their own physical and mental health on their ability to help those with whom they work.

Principle B: Fidelity and Responsibility

Psychologists establish relationships of trust with those with whom they work. They are aware of their professional and scientific responsibilities to society and to the specific communities in which they work. Psychologists uphold professional standards of conduct, clarify their professional roles and obligations, accept appropriate responsibility for their behavior, and seek to manage conflicts of interest that could lead to exploitation or harm. Psychologists consult with, refer to, or cooperate with other professionals and institutions to the extent needed to serve the best interests of those with whom they work. They are concerned about the ethical compliance of their colleagues' scientific and professional conduct. Psychologists strive to contribute a portion of their professional time for little or no compensation or personal advantage.

Principle C: Integrity

Psychologists seek to promote accuracy, honesty, and truthfulness in the science, teaching, and practice of psychology. In these activities psychologists do not steal, cheat, or engage in fraud, subterfuge, or intentional misrepresentation of fact. Psychologists strive to keep their promises and to avoid unwise or unclear commitments. In situations in which deception may be ethically justifiable to maximize benefits and minimize harm, psychologists have a serious obligation to consider the need for, the possible consequences of, and their responsibility to correct any resulting mistrust or other harmful effects that arise from the use of such techniques.

Principle D: Justice

Psychologists recognize that fairness and justice entitle all persons to access to and benefit from the contributions of psychology and to equal quality in the processes, procedures, and services being conducted by psychologists. Psychologists exercise reasonable judgment and take precautions to ensure that their potential biases, the boundaries of their competence, and the limitations of their expertise do not lead to or condone unjust practices.

Principle E: Respect for People's Rights and Dignity

Psychologists respect the dignity and worth of all people, and the rights of individuals to privacy, confidentiality, and self-determination. Psychologists are aware that special safeguards may be necessary to protect the rights and welfare of persons or communities whose vulnerabilities impair autonomous decision making. Psychologists are aware of and respect cultural, individual, and role differences, including those based on age, gender, gender identity, race, ethnicity, culture, national origin, religion, sexual orientation, disability, language, and socioeconomic status and consider these factors when working with members of such groups. Psychologists try to eliminate the effect on their work of biases based on those factors, and they do not knowingly participate in or condone activities of others based upon such prejudices.

Standard 1: Resolving Ethical Issues

1.01 Misuse of Psychologists' Work

If psychologists learn of misuse or misrepresentation of their work, they take reasonable steps to correct or minimize the misuse or misrepresentation.

1.02 Conflicts Between Ethics and Law, Regulations, or Other Governing Legal Authority

If psychologists' ethical responsibilities conflict with law, regulations, or other governing legal authority, psychologists clarify the nature of the conflict, make known their commitment to the Ethics Code, and take reasonable steps to resolve the conflict consistent with the General Principles and Ethical Standards of the Ethics Code. Under no circumstances may this standard be used to justify or defend violating human rights.

1.03 Conflicts Between Ethics and Organizational Demands

If the demands of an organization with which psychologists are affiliated or for whom they are working are in conflict with this Ethics Code, psychologists clarify the nature of the conflict, make known their commitment to the Ethics Code, and take reasonable steps to resolve the conflict consistent with the General Principles and Ethical Standards of the Ethics Code. Under no circumstances may this standard be used to justify or defend violating human rights.

1.04 Informal Resolution of Ethical Violations

When psychologists believe that there may have been an ethical violation by another psychologist, they attempt to resolve the issue by bringing it to the attention of that individual, if an informal resolution appears appropriate and the intervention does not violate any confidentiality rights that may be involved. (See also Standards 1.02, Conflicts Between Ethics and Law, Regulations, or Other Governing Legal Authority, and 1.03, Conflicts Between Ethics and Organizational Demands.)

1.05 Reporting Ethical Violations

If an apparent ethical violation has substantially harmed or is likely to substantially harm a person or organization and is not appropriate for informal resolution under Standard 1.04, Informal Resolution of Ethical Violations, or is not resolved properly in that fashion, psychologists take further action appropriate to the situation. Such action might include referral to state or national committees on professional ethics, to state licensing boards, or to the appropriate institutional authorities. This standard does not apply when an intervention would violate confidentiality rights or when psychologists have been retained to review the work of another psychologist whose professional conduct is in question. (See also Standard 1.02, Conflicts Between Ethics and Law, Regulations, or Other Governing Legal Authority.)

1.06 Cooperating with Ethics Committees

Psychologists cooperate in ethics investigations, proceedings, and resulting requirements of the APA or any affiliated state psychological association to which they belong. In doing so, they address any confidentiality issues. Failure to cooperate is itself an ethics violation. However, making a request for deferment of adjudication of an ethics complaint pending the outcome of litigation does not alone constitute noncooperation.

1.07 Improper Complaints

Psychologists do not file or encourage the filing of ethics complaints that are made with reckless disregard for or willful ignorance of facts that would disprove the allegation.

1.08 Unfair Discrimination Against Complainants and Respondents

Psychologists do not deny persons employment, advancement, admissions to academic or other programs, tenure, or promotion, based solely upon their having made or their being the subject of an ethics complaint. This does not preclude taking action based upon the outcome of such proceedings or considering other appropriate information.

Standard 2: Competence

2.01 Boundaries of Competence

(a) Psychologists provide services, teach, and conduct research with populations and in areas only within the boundaries of their competence, based on their education, training, supervised experience, consultation, study, or professional experience.

(b) Where scientific or professional knowledge in the discipline of psychology establishes that an understanding of factors associated with age, gender, gender identity, race, ethnicity, culture, national origin, religion, sexual orientation, disability, language, or socioeconomic status is essential for effective implementation of their services or research, psychologists have or obtain the training, experience, consultation, or supervision necessary to ensure the competence of their services, or they make appropriate referrals, except as provided in Standard 2.02, Providing Services in Emergencies.

(c) Psychologists planning to provide services, teach, or conduct research involving populations, areas, techniques, or technologies new to them undertake relevant education, training, supervised experience, consultation, or study.

(d) When psychologists are asked to provide services to individuals for whom appropriate mental health services are not available and for which psychologists have not obtained the competence necessary, psychologists with closely related prior training or experience may provide such services in order to ensure that services are not denied if they make a reasonable effort to obtain the competence required by using relevant research, training, consultation, or study.

(e) In those emerging areas in which generally recognized standards for preparatory training do not yet exist, psychologists nevertheless take reasonable steps to ensure the competence of their work and to protect clients/patients, students, supervisees, research participants, organizational clients, and others from harm.

(f) When assuming forensic roles, psychologists are or become reasonably familiar with the judicial or administrative rules governing their roles.

2.02 Providing Services in Emergencies

In emergencies, when psychologists provide services to individuals for whom other mental health services are not available and for which psychologists have not obtained the necessary training, psychologists may provide such services in order to ensure that services are not denied. The services are discontinued as soon as the emergency has ended or appropriate services are available.

2.03 Maintaining Competence

Psychologists undertake ongoing efforts to develop and maintain their competence.

2.04 Bases for Scientific and Professional Judgments

Psychologists' work is based upon established scientific and professional knowledge of the discipline. (See also Standards 2.01e, Boundaries of Competence, and 10.01b, Informed Consent to Therapy.)

2.05 Delegation of Work to Others

Psychologists who delegate work to employees, supervisees, or research or teaching assistants or who use the services of others, such as interpreters, take reasonable steps to (1) avoid delegating such work to persons who have a multiple relationship with those being served that would likely lead to exploitation or loss of objectivity; (2) authorize only those responsibilities that such persons can be expected to perform competently on the basis of their education, training, or experience, either independently or with the level of supervision being provided; and (3) see that such persons perform these services competently. (See also Standards 2.02, Providing Services in Emergencies; 3.05, Multiple Relationships; 4.01, Maintaining Confidentiality; 9.01, Bases for Assessments; 9.02, Use of Assessments; 9.03, Informed Consent in Assessments; and 9.07, Assessment by Unqualified Persons.)

2.06 Personal Problems and Conflicts

(a) Psychologists refrain from initiating an activity when they know or should know that there is a substantial likelihood that their personal problems will prevent them from performing their work-related activities in a competent manner.

(b) When psychologists become aware of personal problems that may interfere with their performing work-related duties adequately, they take appropriate measures, such as obtaining professional consultation or assistance, and determine whether they should limit, suspend, or terminate their work-related duties. (See also Standard 10.10, Terminating Therapy.)

Standard 3: Human Relations

3.01 Unfair Discrimination

In their work-related activities, psychologists do not engage in unfair discrimination based on age, gender, gender identity, race, ethnicity, culture, national origin, religion, sexual orientation, disability, socioeconomic status, or any basis proscribed by law.

3.02 Sexual Harassment

Psychologists do not engage in sexual harassment. Sexual harassment is sexual solicitation, physical advances, or verbal or nonverbal conduct that is sexual in nature, that occurs in connection with the psychologist's activities or roles as a psychologist, and that either (1) is unwelcome, is offensive, or creates a hostile workplace or educational environment, and the psychologist knows or is told this or (2) is sufficiently severe or intense to be abusive to a reasonable person in the context. Sexual harassment can consist of a single intense or severe act or of multiple persistent or pervasive acts. (See also Standard 1.08, Unfair Discrimination Against Complainants and Respondents.)

3.03 Other Harassment

Psychologists do not knowingly engage in behavior that is harassing or demeaning to persons with whom they interact in their work based on factors such as those persons' age, gender, gender identity, race, ethnicity, culture, national origin, religion, sexual orientation, disability, language, or socioeconomic status.

3.04 Avoiding Harm

Psychologists take reasonable steps to avoid harming their clients/patients, students, supervisees, research participants, organizational clients, and others with whom they work, and to minimize harm where it is foreseeable and unavoidable.

3.05 Multiple Relationships

(a) A multiple relationship occurs when a psychologist is in a professional role with a person and (1) at the same time is in another role with the same person, (2) at the same time is in a relationship with a person closely associated with or related to the person with whom the psychologist has the professional relationship, or (3) promises to enter into another relationship in the future with the person or a person closely associated with or related to the person.

A psychologist refrains from entering into a multiple relationship if the multiple relationship could reasonably be expected to impair the psychologist's objectivity, competence, or effectiveness in performing his or her functions as a psychologist, or otherwise risks exploitation or harm to the person with whom the professional relationship exists.

Multiple relationships that would not reasonably be expected to cause impairment or risk exploitation or harm are not unethical.

(b) If a psychologist finds that, due to unforeseen factors, a potentially harmful multiple relationship has arisen, the psychologist takes reasonable steps to resolve it with due regard for the best interests of the affected person and maximal compliance with the Ethics Code.

(c) When psychologists are required by law, institutional policy, or extraordinary circumstances to serve in more than one role in judicial or administrative proceedings, at the outset they clarify role expectations and the extent of confidentiality and thereafter as changes occur. (See also Standards 3.04, Avoiding Harm, and 3.07, Third-Party Requests for Services.)

3.06 Conflict of Interest

Psychologists refrain from taking on a professional role when personal, scientific, professional, legal, financial, or other interests or relationships could reasonably be expected to (1) impair their objectivity, competence, or effectiveness in performing their functions as psychologists or (2) expose the person or organization with whom the professional relationship exists to harm or exploitation.

3.07 Third-Party Requests for Services

When psychologists agree to provide services to a person or entity at the request of a third party, psychologists attempt to clarify at the outset of the service the nature of the relationship with all individuals or organizations involved. This clarification includes the role of the psychologist (e.g., therapist, consultant, diagnostician, or expert witness), an identification of who is the client, the probable uses of the services provided or the information obtained, and the fact that there may be limits to confidentiality. (See also Standards 3.05, Multiple Relationships, and 4.02, Discussing the Limits of Confidentiality.)

3.08 Exploitative Relationships

Psychologists do not exploit persons over whom they have supervisory, evaluative, or other authority such as clients/patients, students, supervisees, research participants, and employees. (See also Standards 3.05, Multiple Relationships; 6.04, Fees and Financial Arrangements; 6.05, Barter with Clients/Patients; 7.07, Sexual Relationships with Students and Supervisees; 10.05, Sexual Intimacies with Current Therapy Clients/Patients; 10.06, Sexual Intimacies with Relatives or Significant Others of Current Therapy Clients/Patients; 10.07, Therapy with Former Sexual Partners; and 10.08, Sexual Intimacies with Former Therapy Clients/Patients.)

3.09 Cooperation with Other Professionals

When indicated and professionally appropriate, psychologists cooperate with other professionals in order to serve their clients/patients effectively and appropriately. (See also Standard 4.05, Disclosures.)

3.10 Informed Consent

(a) When psychologists conduct research or provide assessment, therapy, counseling, or consulting services in person or via electronic transmission or other forms of communication, they obtain the informed consent of the individual or individuals using language that is reasonably understandable to that person or persons except when conducting such activities without consent is mandated by law or governmental regulation or as otherwise provided in this Ethics Code. (See also Standards 8.02, Informed Consent to Research; 9.03, Informed Consent in Assessments; and 10.01, Informed Consent to Therapy.)

(b) For persons who are legally incapable of giving informed consent, psychologists nevertheless (1) provide an appropriate explanation, (2) seek the individual's assent, (3) consider such persons' preferences and best interests, and (4) obtain appropriate permission from a legally authorized person, if such substitute consent is permitted or required by law. When consent by a legally authorized person is not permitted or required by law, psychologists take reasonable steps to protect the individual's rights and welfare.

(c) When psychological services are court ordered or otherwise mandated, psychologists inform the individual of the nature of the anticipated services, including whether the services are court ordered or mandated and any limits of confidentiality, before proceeding.

(d) Psychologists appropriately document written or oral consent, permission, and assent. (See also Standards 8.02, Informed Consent to Research; 9.03, Informed Consent in Assessments; and 10.01, Informed Consent to Therapy.)

3.11 Psychological Services Delivered to or Through Organizations

(a) Psychologists delivering services to or through organizations provide information beforehand to clients and when appropriate those directly affected by the services about (1) the nature and objectives of the services, (2) the intended recipients, (3) which of the individuals are clients, (4) the relationship the psychologist will have with each person and the organization, (5) the probable uses of services provided and information obtained, (6) who will have access to the information, and (7) limits of confidentiality. As soon as feasible, they provide information about the results and conclusions of such services to appropriate persons.

(b) If psychologists will be precluded by law or by organizational roles from providing such information to particular individuals or groups, they so inform those individuals or groups at the outset of the service.

3.12 Interruption of Psychological Services

Unless otherwise covered by contract, psychologists make reasonable efforts to plan for facilitating services in the event that psychological services are interrupted by factors such as the psychologist's illness, death, unavailability, relocation, or retirement or by the client's/patient's relocation or financial limitations. (See also Standard 6.02c, Maintenance, Dissemination, and Disposal of Confidential Records of Professional and Scientific Work.)

Standard 4: Privacy and Confidentiality

4.01 Maintaining Confidentiality

Psychologists have a primary obligation and take reasonable precautions to protect confidential information obtained through or stored in any medium, recognizing that the extent and limits of confidentiality may be regulated by law or established by institutional rules or professional or scientific relationship. (See also Standard 2.05, Delegation of Work to Others.)

4.02 Discussing the Limits of Confidentiality

(a) Psychologists discuss with persons (including, to the extent feasible, persons who are legally incapable of giving informed consent and their legal representatives) and organizations with whom they establish a scientific or professional relationship (1) the relevant limits of confidentiality and (2) the foreseeable uses of the information generated through their psychological activities. (See also Standard 3.10, Informed Consent.)

(b) Unless it is not feasible or is contraindicated, the discussion of confidentiality occurs at the outset of the relationship and thereafter as new circumstances may warrant.

(c) Psychologists who offer services, products, or information via electronic transmission inform clients/patients of the risks to privacy and limits of confidentiality.

4.03 Recording

Before recording the voices or images of individuals to whom they provide services, psychologists obtain permission from all such persons or their legal representatives. (See also Standards 8.03, Informed Consent for Recording Voices and Images in Research; 8.05, Dispensing with Informed Consent for Research; and 8.07, Deception in Research.)

4.04 Minimizing Intrusions on Privacy

(a) Psychologists include in written and oral reports and consultations, only information germane to the purpose for which the communication is made.

(b) Psychologists discuss confidential information obtained in their work only for appropriate scientific or professional purposes and only with persons clearly concerned with such matters.

4.05 Disclosures

(a) Psychologists may disclose confidential information with the appropriate consent of the organizational client, the individual client/patient, or another legally authorized person on behalf of the client/patient unless prohibited by law.

(b) Psychologists disclose confidential information without the consent of the individual only as mandated by law, or where permitted by law for a valid purpose such as to (1) provide needed professional services; (2) obtain appropriate professional consultations; (3) protect the client/patient, psychologist, or others from harm; or (4) obtain payment for services from a client/patient, in which instance disclosure is limited to the minimum that is necessary to achieve the purpose. (See also Standard 6.04e, Fees and Financial Arrangements.)

4.06 Consultations

When consulting with colleagues, (1) psychologists do not disclose confidential information that reasonably could lead to the identification of a client/patient, research participant, or other person or organization with whom they have a confidential relationship unless they have obtained the prior consent of the person or organization or the disclosure cannot be avoided, and (2) they disclose information only to the extent necessary to achieve the purposes of the consultation. (See also Standard 4.01, Maintaining Confidentiality.)

4.07 Use of Confidential Information for Didactic or Other Purposes

Psychologists do not disclose in their writings, lectures, or other public media, confidential, personally identifiable information concerning their clients/patients, students, research participants, organizational clients, or other recipients of their services that they obtained during the course of their work, unless (1) they take reasonable steps to disguise the person or organization, (2) the person or organization has consented in writing, or (3) there is legal authorization for doing so.

Standard 5: Advertising and Other Public Statements

5.01 Avoidance of False or Deceptive Statements

(a) Public statements include but are not limited to paid or unpaid advertising, product endorsements, grant applications, licensing applications, other credentialing applications, brochures, printed matter, directory listings, personal resumes or curricula vitae, or comments for use in media such as print or electronic transmission, statements in legal proceedings, lectures and public oral presentations, and published materials. Psychologists do not knowingly make public statements that are false, deceptive, or fraudulent concerning their research, practice, or other work activities or those of persons or organizations with which they are affiliated.

(b) Psychologists do not make false, deceptive, or fraudulent statements concerning (1) their training, experience, or competence; (2) their academic degrees; (3) their credentials; (4) their institutional or association affiliations; (5) their services; (6) the scientific or clinical basis for, or results or degree of success of, their services; (7) their fees; or (8) their publications or research findings.

(c) Psychologists claim degrees as credentials for their health services only if those degrees (1) were earned from a regionally accredited educational institution or (2) were the basis for psychology licensure by the state in which they practice.

5.02 Statements by Others

(a) Psychologists who engage others to create or place public statements that promote their professional practice, products, or activities retain professional responsibility for such statements.

(b) Psychologists do not compensate employees of press, radio, television, or other communication media in return for publicity in a news item. (See also Standard 1.01, Misuse of Psychologists' Work.)

(c) A paid advertisement relating to psychologists' activities must be identified or clearly recognizable as such.

5.03 Descriptions of Workshops and Non-Degree-Granting Educational Programs

To the degree to which they exercise control, psychologists responsible for announcements, catalogs, brochures, or advertisements describing workshops, seminars, or other non-degree-granting educational programs ensure that they accurately describe the audience for which the program is intended, the educational objectives, the presenters, and the fees involved.

5.04 Media Presentations

When psychologists provide public advice or comment via print, Internet, or other electronic transmission, they take precautions to ensure that statements (1) are based on their professional knowledge, training, or experience in accord with appropriate psychological literature and practice; (2) are otherwise consistent with this Ethics Code; and (3) do not indicate that a professional relationship has been established with the recipient. (See also Standard 2.04, Bases for Scientific and Professional Judgments.)

5.05 Testimonials

Psychologists do not solicit testimonials from current therapy clients/patients or other persons who because of their particular circumstances are vulnerable to undue influence.

5.06 In-Person Solicitation

Psychologists do not engage, directly or through agents, in uninvited in-person solicitation of business from actual or potential therapy clients/patients or other persons who because of their particular circumstances are vulnerable to undue influence. However, this prohibition does not preclude (1) attempting to implement appropriate collateral contacts for the purpose of benefiting an already engaged therapy client/patient or (2) providing disaster or community outreach services.

Standard 6: Record Keeping and Fees

6.01 Documentation of Professional and Scientific Work and Maintenance of Records

Psychologists create, and to the extent the records are under their control, maintain, disseminate, store, retain, and dispose of records and data relating to their professional and scientific work in order to (1) facilitate provision of services later by them or by other professionals, (2) allow for replication of research design and analyses, (3) meet institutional requirements, (4) ensure accuracy of billing and payments, and (5) ensure compliance with law. (See also Standard 4.01, Maintaining Confidentiality.)

6.02 Maintenance, Dissemination, and Disposal of Confidential Records of Professional and Scientific Work

(a) Psychologists maintain confidentiality in creating, storing, accessing, transferring, and disposing of records under their control, whether these are written, automated, or in any other medium. (See also Standards 4.01, Maintaining Confidentiality, and 6.01, Documentation of Professional and Scientific Work and Maintenance of Records.)

(b) If confidential information concerning recipients of psychological services is entered into databases or systems of records available to persons whose access has not been consented to by the recipient, psychologists use coding or other techniques to avoid the inclusion of personal identifiers.

(c) Psychologists make plans in advance to facilitate the appropriate transfer and to protect the confidentiality of records and data in the event of psychologists' withdrawal from positions or practice. (See also Standards 3.12, Interruption of Psychological Services, and 10.09, Interruption of Therapy.)

6.03 Withholding Records for Nonpayment

Psychologists may not withhold records under their control that are requested and needed for a client's/patient's emergency treatment solely because payment has not been received.

6.04 Fees and Financial Arrangements

(a) As early as is feasible in a professional or scientific relationship, psychologists and recipients of psychological services reach an agreement specifying compensation and billing arrangements.

(b) Psychologists' fee practices are consistent with law.

(c) Psychologists do not misrepresent their fees.

(d) If limitations to services can be anticipated because of limitations in financing, this is discussed with the recipient of services as early as is feasible. (See also Standards 10.09, Interruption of Therapy, and 10.10, Terminating Therapy.)

(e) If the recipient of services does not pay for services as agreed, and if psychologists intend to use collection agencies or legal measures to collect the fees, psychologists first inform the person that such measures will be taken and provide that person an opportunity to make prompt payment. (See also Standards 4.05, Disclosures; 6.03, Withholding Records for Nonpayment; and 10.01, Informed Consent to Therapy.)

6.05 Barter with Clients/Patients

Barter is the acceptance of goods, services, or other nonmonetary remuneration from clients/patients in return for psychological services. Psychologists may barter only if (1) it is not clinically contraindicated, and (2) the resulting arrangement is not exploitative. (See also Standards 3.05, Multiple Relationships, and 6.04, Fees and Financial Arrangements.)

6.06 Accuracy in Reports to Payors and Funding Sources

In their reports to payors for services or sources of research funding, psychologists take reasonable steps to ensure the accurate reporting of the nature of the service provided or research conducted, the fees, charges, or payments, and where applicable, the identity of the provider, the findings, and the diagnosis. (See also Standards 4.01, Maintaining Confidentiality; 4.04, Minimizing Intrusions on Privacy; and 4.05, Disclosures.)

6.07 Referrals and Fees

When psychologists pay, receive payment from, or divide fees with another professional, other than in an employer-employee relationship, the payment to each is based on the services provided (clinical, consultative, administrative, or other) and is not based on the referral itself. (See also Standard 3.09, Cooperation with Other Professionals.)

Standard 7: Education and Training

7.01 Design of Education and Training Programs

Psychologists responsible for education and training programs take reasonable steps to ensure that the programs are designed to provide the appropriate knowledge and proper experiences, and to meet the requirements for licensure, certification, or other goals for which claims are made by the program. (See also Standard 5.03, Descriptions of Workshops and Non-Degree-Granting Educational Programs.)

7.02 Descriptions of Education and Training Programs

Psychologists responsible for education and training programs take reasonable steps to ensure that there is a current and accurate description of the program content (including participation in required course- or program-related counseling, psychotherapy, experiential groups, consulting projects, or community service), training goals and objectives, stipends and benefits, and requirements that must be met for satisfactory completion of the program. This information must be made readily available to all interested parties.

7.03 Accuracy in Teaching

(a) Psychologists take reasonable steps to ensure that course syllabi are accurate regarding the subject matter to be covered, bases for evaluating progress, and the nature of course experiences. This standard does not preclude an instructor from modifying course content or requirements when the instructor considers it pedagogically necessary or desirable, so long as students are made aware of these modifications in a manner that enables them to fulfill course requirements. (See also Standard 5.01, Avoidance of False or Deceptive Statements.)

(b) When engaged in teaching or training, psychologists present psychological information accurately. (See also Standard 2.03, Maintaining Competence.)

7.04 Student Disclosure of Personal Information

Psychologists do not require students or supervisees to disclose personal information in course- or program-related activities, either orally or in writing, regarding sexual history, history of abuse and neglect, psychological treatment, and relationships with parents, peers, and spouses or significant others except if (1) the program or training facility has clearly identified this requirement in its admissions and program materials or (2) the information is necessary to evaluate or obtain assistance for students whose personal problems could reasonably be judged to be preventing them from performing their training- or professionally related activities in a competent manner or posing a threat to the students or others.

7.05 Mandatory Individual or Group Therapy

(a) When individual or group therapy is a program or course requirement, psychologists responsible for that program allow students in undergraduate and graduate programs the option of selecting such therapy from practitioners unaffiliated with the program. (See also Standard 7.02, Descriptions of Education and Training Programs.)

(b) Faculty who are or are likely to be responsible for evaluating students' academic performance do not themselves provide that therapy. (See also Standard 3.05, Multiple Relationships.)

7.06 Assessing Student and Supervisee Performance

(a) In academic and supervisory relationships, psychologists establish a timely and specific process for providing feedback to students and supervisees. Information regarding the process is provided to the student at the beginning of supervision.

(b) Psychologists evaluate students and supervisees on the basis of their actual performance on relevant and established program requirements.

7.07 Sexual Relationships with Students and Supervisees

Psychologists do not engage in sexual relationships with students or supervisees who are in their department, agency, or training center or over whom psychologists have or are likely to have evaluative authority. (See also Standard 3.05, Multiple Relationships.)

Standard 8: Research and Publication

8.01 Institutional Approval

When institutional approval is required, psychologists provide accurate information about their research proposals and obtain approval prior to conducting the research. They conduct the research in accordance with the approved research protocol.

8.02 Informed Consent to Research

(a) When obtaining informed consent as required in Standard 3.10, Informed Consent, psychologists inform participants about (1) the purpose of the research, expected duration, and procedures; (2) their right to decline to participate and to withdraw from the research once participation has begun; (3) the foreseeable consequences of declining or withdrawing; (4) reasonably foreseeable factors that may be expected to influence their willingness to participate such as potential risks, discomfort, or adverse effects; (5) any prospective research benefits; (6) limits of confidentiality; (7) incentives for participation; and (8) whom to contact for questions about the research and research participants' rights. They provide opportunity for the prospective participants to ask questions and receive answers. (See also Standards 8.03, Informed Consent for Recording Voices and Images in Research; 8.05, Dispensing with Informed Consent for Research; and 8.07, Deception in Research.)

(b) Psychologists conducting intervention research involving the use of experimental treatments clarify to participants at the outset of the research (1) the experimental nature of the treatment; (2) the services that will or will not be available to the control group(s) if appropriate; (3) the means by which assignment to treatment and control groups will be made; (4) available treatment alternatives if an individual does not wish to participate in the research or wishes to withdraw once a study has begun; and (5) compensation for or monetary costs of participating including, if appropriate, whether reimbursement from the participant or a third-party payor will be sought. (See also Standard 8.02a, Informed Consent to Research.)

8.03 Informed Consent for Recording Voices and Images in Research

Psychologists obtain informed consent from research participants prior to recording their voices or images for data collection unless (1) the research consists solely of naturalistic observations in public places, and it is not anticipated that the recording will be used in a manner that could cause personal identification or harm, or (2) the research design includes deception, and consent for the use of the recording is obtained during debriefing. (See also Standard 8.07, Deception in Research.)

8.04 Client/Patient, Student, and Subordinate Research Participants

(a) When psychologists conduct research with clients/patients, students, or subordinates as participants, psychologists take steps to protect the prospective participants from adverse consequences of declining or withdrawing from participation.

(b) When research participation is a course requirement or an opportunity for extra credit, the prospective participant is given the choice of equitable alternative activities.

8.05 Dispensing with Informed Consent for Research

Psychologists may dispense with informed consent only (1) where research would not reasonably be assumed to create distress or harm and involves (a) the study of normal educational practices, curricula, or classroom management methods conducted in educational settings; (b) only anonymous questionnaires, naturalistic observations, or archival research for which disclosure of responses would not place participants at risk of criminal or civil liability or damage their financial standing, employability, or reputation, and confidentiality is protected; or (c) the study of factors related to job or organization effectiveness conducted in organizational settings for which there is no risk to participants' employability, and confidentiality is protected or (2) where otherwise permitted by law or federal or institutional regulations.

8.06 Offering Inducements for Research Participation

(a) Psychologists make reasonable efforts to avoid offering excessive or inappropriate financial or other inducements for research participation when such inducements are likely to coerce participation.

(b) When offering professional services as an inducement for research participation, psychologists clarify the nature of the services, as well as the risks, obligations, and limitations. (See also Standard 6.05, Barter with Clients/Patients.)

8.07 Deception in Research

(a) Psychologists do not conduct a study involving deception unless they have determined that the use of deceptive techniques is justified by the study's significant prospective scientific, educational, or applied value and that effective nondeceptive alternative procedures are not feasible.

(b) Psychologists do not deceive prospective participants about research that is reasonably expected to cause physical pain or severe emotional distress.

(c) Psychologists explain any deception that is an integral feature of the design and conduct of an experiment to participants as early as is feasible, preferably at the conclusion of their participation, but no later than at the conclusion of the data collection, and permit participants to withdraw their data. (See also Standard 8.08, Debriefing.)

8.08 Debriefing

(a) Psychologists provide a prompt opportunity for participants to obtain appropriate information about the nature, results, and conclusions of the research, and they take reasonable steps to correct any misconceptions that participants may have of which the psychologists are aware.

(b) If scientific or humane values justify delaying or withholding this information, psychologists take reasonable measures to reduce the risk of harm.

(c) When psychologists become aware that research procedures have harmed a participant, they take reasonable steps to minimize the harm.

8.09 Humane Care and Use of Animals in Research

(a) Psychologists acquire, care for, use, and dispose of animals in compliance with current federal, state, and local laws and regulations, and with professional standards.

(b) Psychologists trained in research methods and experienced in the care of laboratory animals supervise all procedures involving animals and are responsible for ensuring appropriate consideration of their comfort, health, and humane treatment.

(c) Psychologists ensure that all individuals under their supervision who are using animals have received instruction in research methods and in the care, maintenance, and handling of the species being used, to the extent appropriate to their role. (See also Standard 2.05, Delegation of Work to Others.)

(d) Psychologists make reasonable efforts to minimize the discomfort, infection, illness, and pain of animal subjects.

(e) Psychologists use a procedure subjecting animals to pain, stress, or privation only when an alternative procedure is unavailable and the goal is justified by its prospective scientific, educational, or applied value.

(f) Psychologists perform surgical procedures under appropriate anesthesia and follow techniques to avoid infection and minimize pain during and after surgery.

(g) When it is appropriate that an animal's life be terminated, psychologists proceed rapidly, with an effort to minimize pain and in accordance with accepted procedures.

8.10 Reporting Research Results

(a) Psychologists do not fabricate data. (See also Standard 5.01a, Avoidance of False or Deceptive Statements.)

(b) If psychologists discover significant errors in their published data, they take reasonable steps to correct such errors in a correction, retraction, erratum, or other appropriate publication means.

8.11 Plagiarism

Psychologists do not present portions of another's work or data as their own, even if the other work or data source is cited occasionally.

8.12 Publication Credit

(a) Psychologists take responsibility and credit, including authorship credit, only for work they have actually performed or to which they have substantially contributed. (See also Standard 8.12b, Publication Credit.)

(b) Principal authorship and other publication credits accurately reflect the relative scientific or professional contributions of the individuals involved, regardless of their relative status. Mere possession of an institutional position, such as department chair, does not justify authorship credit. Minor contributions to the research or to the writing for publications are acknowledged appropriately, such as in footnotes or in an introductory statement.

(c) Except under exceptional circumstances, a student is listed as principal author on any multiple-authored article that is substantially based on the student's doctoral dissertation. Faculty advisors discuss publication credit with students as early as feasible and throughout the research and publication process as appropriate. (See also Standard 8.12b, Publication Credit.)

8.13 Duplicate Publication of Data

Psychologists do not publish, as original data, data that have been previously published. This does not preclude republishing data when they are accompanied by proper acknowledgment.

8.14 Sharing Research Data for Verification

(a) After research results are published, psychologists do not withhold the data on which their conclusions are based from other competent professionals who seek to verify the substantive claims through reanalysis and who intend to use such data only for that purpose, provided that the confidentiality of the participants can be protected and unless legal rights concerning proprietary data preclude their release. This does not preclude psychologists from requiring that such individuals or groups be responsible for costs associated with the provision of such information.

(b) Psychologists who request data from other psychologists to verify the substantive claims through reanalysis may use shared data only for the declared purpose. Requesting psychologists obtain prior written agreement for all other uses of the data.

8.15 Reviewers

Psychologists who review material submitted for presentation, publication, grant, or research proposal review respect the confidentiality of and the proprietary rights in such information of those who submitted it.

Standard 9: Assessment

9.01 Bases for Assessments

(a) Psychologists base the opinions contained in their recommendations, reports, and diagnostic or evaluative statements, including forensic testimony, on information and techniques sufficient to substantiate their findings. (See also Standard 2.04, Bases for Scientific and Professional Judgments.)

(b) Except as noted in 9.01c, psychologists provide opinions of the psychological characteristics of individuals only after they have conducted an examination of the individuals adequate to support their statements or conclusions. When, despite reasonable efforts, such an examination is not practical, psychologists document the efforts they made and the result of those efforts, clarify the probable impact of their limited information on the reliability and validity of their opinions, and appropriately limit the nature and extent of their conclusions or recommendations. (See also Standards 2.01, Boundaries of Competence, and 9.06, Interpreting Assessment Results.)

(c) When psychologists conduct a record review or provide consultation or supervision and an individual examination is not warranted or necessary for the opinion, psychologists explain this and the sources of information on which they based their conclusions and recommendations.

9.02 Use of Assessments

(a) Psychologists administer, adapt, score, interpret, or use assessment techniques, interviews, tests, or instruments in a manner and for purposes that are appropriate in light of the research on or evidence of the usefulness and proper application of the techniques.

(b) Psychologists use assessment instruments whose validity and reliability have been established for use with members of the population tested. When such validity or reliability has not been established, psychologists describe the strengths and limitations of test results and interpretation.

(c) Psychologists use assessment methods that are appropriate to an individual's language preference and competence, unless the use of an alternative language is relevant to the assessment issues.

9.03 Informed Consent in Assessments

(a) Psychologists obtain informed consent for assessments, evaluations, or diagnostic services, as described in Standard 3.10, Informed Consent, except when (1) testing is mandated by law or governmental regulations; (2) informed consent is implied because testing is conducted as a routine educational, institutional, or organizational activity (e.g., when participants voluntarily agree to assessment when applying for a job); or (3) one purpose of the testing is to evaluate decisional capacity. Informed consent includes an explanation of the nature and purpose of the assessment, fees, involvement of third parties, and limits of confidentiality and sufficient opportunity for the client/patient to ask questions and receive answers.

(b) Psychologists inform persons with questionable capacity to consent or for whom testing is mandated by law or governmental regulations about the nature and purpose of the proposed assessment services, using language that is reasonably understandable to the person being assessed.

(c) Psychologists using the services of an interpreter obtain informed consent from the client/patient to use that interpreter, ensure that confidentiality of test results and test security are maintained, and include in their recommendations, reports, and diagnostic or evaluative statements, including forensic testimony, discussion of any limitations on the data obtained. (See also Standards 2.05, Delegation of Work to Others; 4.01, Maintaining Confidentiality; 9.01, Bases for Assessments; 9.06, Interpreting Assessment Results; and 9.07, Assessment by Unqualified Persons.)

9.04 Release of Test Data

(a) The term test data refers to raw and scaled scores, client/patient responses to test questions or stimuli, and psychologists' notes and recordings concerning client/patient statements and behavior during an examination. Those portions of test materials that include client/patient responses are included in the definition of test data. Pursuant to a client/patient release, psychologists provide test data to the client/patient or other persons identified in the release. Psychologists may refrain from releasing test data to protect a client/patient or others from substantial harm or misuse or misrepresentation of the data or the test, recognizing that in many instances release of confidential information under these circumstances is regulated by law. (See also Standard 9.11, Maintaining Test Security.)

(b) In the absence of a client/patient release, psychologists provide test data only as required by law or court order.

9.05 Test Construction

Psychologists who develop tests and other assessment techniques use appropriate psychometric procedures and current scientific or professional knowledge for test design, standardization, validation, reduction or elimination of bias, and recommendations for use.

9.06 Interpreting Assessment Results

When interpreting assessment results, including automated interpretations, psychologists take into account the purpose of the assessment as well as the various test factors, test-taking abilities, and other characteristics of the person being assessed, such as situational, personal, linguistic, and cultural differences, that might affect psychologists' judgments or reduce the accuracy of their interpretations. They indicate any significant limitations of their interpretations. (See also Standards 2.01b and c, Boundaries of Competence, and 3.01, Unfair Discrimination.)

9.07 Assessment by Unqualified Persons

Psychologists do not promote the use of psychological assessment techniques by unqualified persons, except when such use is conducted for training purposes with appropriate supervision. (See also Standard 2.05, Delegation of Work to Others.)

9.08 Obsolete Tests and Outdated Test Results

(a) Psychologists do not base their assessment or intervention decisions or recommendations on data or test results that are outdated for the current purpose.

(b) Psychologists do not base such decisions or recommendations on tests and measures that are obsolete and not useful for the current purpose.

9.09 Test Scoring and Interpretation Services

(a) Psychologists who offer assessment or scoring services to other professionals accurately describe the purpose, norms, validity, reliability, and applications of the procedures and any special qualifications applicable to their use.

(b) Psychologists select scoring and interpretation services (including automated services) on the basis of evidence of the validity of the program and procedures as well as on other appropriate considerations. (See also Standard 2.01b and c, Boundaries of Competence.)

(c) Psychologists retain responsibility for the appropriate application, interpretation, and use of assessment instruments, whether they score and interpret such tests themselves or use automated or other services.

9.10 Explaining Assessment Results

Regardless of whether the scoring and interpretation are done by psychologists, by employees or assistants, or by automated or other outside services, psychologists take reasonable steps to ensure that explanations of results are given to the individual or designated representative unless the nature of the relationship precludes provision of an explanation of results (such as in some organizational consulting, preemployment or security screenings, and forensic evaluations), and this fact has been clearly explained to the person being assessed in advance.

9.11 Maintaining Test Security

The term test materials refers to manuals, instruments, protocols, and test questions or stimuli and does not include test data as defined in Standard 9.04, Release of Test Data. Psychologists make reasonable efforts to maintain the integrity and security of test materials and other assessment techniques consistent with law and contractual obligations, and in a manner that permits adherence to this Ethics Code.

Standard 10: Therapy

10.01 Informed Consent to Therapy

(a) When obtaining informed consent to therapy as required in Standard 3.10, Informed Consent, psychologists inform clients/patients as early as is feasible in the therapeutic relationship about the nature and anticipated course of therapy, fees, involvement of third parties, and limits of confidentiality and provide sufficient opportunity for the client/patient to ask questions and receive answers. (See also Standards 4.02, Discussing the Limits of Confidentiality, and 6.04, Fees and Financial Arrangements.)

(b) When obtaining informed consent for treatment for which generally recognized techniques and procedures have not been established, psychologists inform their clients/patients of the developing nature of the treatment, the potential risks involved, alternative treatments that may be available, and the voluntary nature of their participation. (See also Standards 2.01e, Boundaries of Competence, and 3.10, Informed Consent.)

(c) When the therapist is a trainee and the legal responsibility for the treatment provided resides with the supervisor, the client/patient, as part of the informed consent procedure, is informed that the therapist is in training and is being supervised and is given the name of the supervisor.

10.02 Therapy Involving Couples or Families

(a) When psychologists agree to provide services to several persons who have a relationship (such as spouses, significant others, or parents and children), they take reasonable steps to clarify at the outset (1) which of the individuals are clients/patients and (2) the relationship the psychologist will have with each person. This clarification includes the psychologist's role and the probable uses of the services provided or the information obtained. (See also Standard 4.02, Discussing the Limits of Confidentiality.)

(b) If it becomes apparent that psychologists may be called on to perform potentially conflicting roles (such as family therapist and then witness for one party in divorce proceedings), psychologists take reasonable steps to clarify and modify, or withdraw from, roles appropriately. (See also Standard 3.05c, Multiple Relationships.)

10.03 Group Therapy

When psychologists provide services to several persons in a group setting, they describe at the outset the roles and responsibilities of all parties and the limits of confidentiality.

10.04 Providing Therapy to Those Served by Others

In deciding whether to offer or provide services to those already receiving mental health services elsewhere, psychologists carefully consider the treatment issues and the potential client's/patient's welfare. Psychologists discuss these issues with the client/patient or another legally authorized person on behalf of the client/patient in order to minimize the risk of confusion and conflict, consult with the other service providers when appropriate, and proceed with caution and sensitivity to the therapeutic issues.

10.05 Sexual Intimacies with Current Therapy Clients/Patients

Psychologists do not engage in sexual intimacies with current therapy clients/patients.

10.06 Sexual Intimacies with Relatives or Significant Others of Current Therapy Clients/Patients

Psychologists do not engage in sexual intimacies with individuals they know to be close relatives, guardians, or significant others of current clients/patients. Psychologists do not terminate therapy to circumvent this standard.

10.07 Therapy with Former Sexual Partners

Psychologists do not accept as therapy clients/patients persons with whom they have engaged in sexual intimacies.

10.08 Sexual Intimacies with Former Therapy Clients/Patients

(a) Psychologists do not engage in sexual intimacies with former clients/patients for at least two years after cessation or termination of therapy.

(b) Psychologists do not engage in sexual intimacies with former clients/patients even after a two-year interval except in the most unusual circumstances. Psychologists who engage in such activity after the two years following cessation or termination of therapy and of having no sexual contact with the former client/patient bear the burden of demonstrating that there has been no exploitation, in light of all relevant factors, including (1) the amount of time that has passed since therapy terminated; (2) the nature, duration, and intensity of the therapy; (3) the circumstances of termination; (4) the client's/patient's personal history; (5) the client's/patient's current mental status; (6) the likelihood of adverse impact on the client/patient; and (7) any statements or actions made by the therapist during the course of therapy suggesting or inviting the possibility of a posttermination sexual or romantic relationship with the client/patient. (See also Standard 3.05, Multiple Relationships.)

10.09 Interruption of Therapy

When entering into employment or contractual relationships, psychologists make reasonable efforts to provide for orderly and appropriate resolution of responsibility for client/patient care in the event that the employment or contractual relationship ends, with paramount consideration given to the welfare of the client/patient. (See also Standard 3.12, Interruption of Psychological Services.)

10.10 Terminating Therapy

(a) Psychologists terminate therapy when it becomes reasonably clear that the client/patient no longer needs the service, is not likely to benefit, or is being harmed by continued service.

(b) Psychologists may terminate therapy when threatened or otherwise endangered by the client/patient or another person with whom the client/patient has a relationship.

(c) Except where precluded by the actions of clients/patients or third-party payors, prior to termination psychologists provide pretermination counseling and suggest alternative service providers as appropriate.

History and Effective Date

The American Psychological Association's Council of Representatives adopted this version of the APA Ethics Code during its meeting on August 21, 2002. The Code became effective on June 1, 2003. The Council of Representatives amended this version of the Ethics Code on February 20, 2010. The amendments became effective on June 1, 2010. Inquiries concerning the substance or interpretation of the APA Ethics Code should be addressed to the Director, Office of Ethics, American Psychological Association, 750 First St. NE, Washington, DC 20002-4242. The standards in this Ethics Code will be used to adjudicate complaints brought concerning alleged conduct occurring on or after the effective date. Complaints will be adjudicated on the basis of the version of the Ethics Code that was in effect at the time the conduct occurred.

The APA has previously published its Ethics Code as follows:

American Psychological Association. (1953). *Ethical standards of psychologists.* Washington, DC: Author.

American Psychological Association. (1959). Ethical standards of psychologists. *American Psychologist, 14,* 279–282.

American Psychological Association. (1963). Ethical standards of psychologists. *American Psychologist, 18,* 56–60.

American Psychological Association. (1968). Ethical standards of psychologists. *American Psychologist, 23,* 357–361.

American Psychological Association. (1977, March). Ethical standards of psychologists. APA *Monitor,* 22–23.

American Psychological Association. (1979). *Ethical standards of psychologists.* Washington, DC: Author.

American Psychological Association. (1981). Ethical principles of psychologists. *American Psychologist, 36,* 633–638.

American Psychological Association. (1990). Ethical principles of psychologists (Amended June 2, 1989). *American Psychologist, 45,* 390–395.

American Psychological Association. (1992). Ethical principles of psychologists and code of conduct. *American Psychologist, 47,* 1597–1611.

American Psychological Association. (2002). Ethical principles of psychologists and code of conduct. *American Psychologist, 57,* 1060–1073.

Request copies of the APA's Ethical Principles of Psychologists and Code of Conduct from the APA Order Department, 750 First St. NE, Washington, DC 20002-4242, or phone (202) 336-5510

National Association of School Psychologists Principles for Professional Ethics (Revised 2010)

TABLE OF CONTENTS

Introduction

The mission of the National Association of School Psychologists (NASP) is to represent school psychology and support school psychologists to enhance the learning and mental health of all children and youth. NASP's mission is accomplished through identification of appropriate evidence-based education and mental health services for all children; implementation of professional practices that are empirically supported, data driven, and culturally competent; promotion of professional competence of school psychologists; recognition of the essential components of high-quality graduate education and professional development in school psychology; preparation of school psychologists to deliver a continuum of services for children, youth, families, and schools; and advocacy for the value of school psychological services, among other important initiatives.

School psychologists provide effective services to help children and youth succeed academically, socially, behaviorally, and emotionally. School psychologists provide direct educational and mental health services for children and youth, as well as work with parents, educators, and other professionals to create supportive learning and social environments for all children. School psychologists apply their knowledge of both psychology and education during consultation and collaboration with others. They conduct effective decision making using a foundation of assessment and data collection. School psychologists engage in specific services for students, such as direct and indirect interventions that focus on academic skills, learning, socialization, and mental health. School psychologists provide services to schools and families that enhance the competence and well-being of children, including promotion of effective and safe learning environments, prevention of academic and behavior problems, response to crises, and improvement of family–school collaboration. The key foundations for all services by school psychologists are understanding of diversity in development and learning; research and program evaluation; and legal, ethical, and professional practice. All of these components and their relationships are depicted in Appendix A, a graphic representation of a national model for comprehensive and integrated services by school psychologists. School psychologists are credentialed by state education agencies or other similar state entities that have the statutory authority to regulate and establish credentialing requirements for professional practice within a state. School psychologists typically work in public or private schools or other educational contexts.

The NASP *Principles for Professional Ethics* is designed to be used in conjunction with the NASP *Standards for Graduate Preparation of School Psychologists, Standards for the Credentialing of School Psychologists,* and *Model for Comprehensive and Integrated School Psychological Services* to provide a unified set of national principles that guide graduate education, credentialing, professional practices, and ethical behavior of effective school psychologists. These NASP policy documents are intended to define contemporary school psychology; promote school psychologists' services for children, families, and schools; and provide a foundation for the future of school psychology. These NASP policy documents are used to communicate NASP's positions and advocate for qualifications and practices of school psychologists with stakeholders, policy makers, and other professional groups at the national, state, and local levels.

The formal principles that elucidate the proper conduct of a professional school psychologist are known as *ethics*. In 1974, NASP adopted its first code of ethics, the *Principles for Professional Ethics (Principles)*, and revisions were made in 1984, 1992, 1997, and 2000. The purpose of the Principles is to protect the public and those who receive school psychological services by sensitizing school psychologists to the ethical aspects of their work, educating them about appropriate conduct, helping them monitor their own behavior, and providing standards to be used in the resolution of complaints of unethical conduct.[1] NASP members and school psychologists who are certified by the National School Psychologist Certification System are bound to abide by NASP's code of ethics.[2]

The NASP *Principles for Professional Ethics* were developed to address the unique circumstances associated with providing school psychological services. The duty to educate children and the legal authority to do so rests with state governments. When school psychologists employed by a school board make decisions in their official roles, such acts are seen as actions by state government. As state actors, school-based practitioners have special obligations to all students. They must know and respect the rights of students under the U.S. Constitution and federal and state statutory law. They must balance the authority of parents to make decisions about their children with the needs and rights of those children, and the purposes and authority of schools. Furthermore, as school employees, school psychologists have a legal as well as an ethical obligation to take steps to protect all students from reasonably foreseeable risk of harm. Finally, school-based practitioners work in a context that emphasizes multidisciplinary problem solving and intervention.[3] For these reasons, psychologists employed by the schools may have less control over aspects of service delivery than practitioners in private practice. However, within this framework, it is expected that school psychologists will make careful, reasoned, and principled ethical choices[4] based on knowledge of this code, recognizing that responsibility for ethical conduct rests with the individual practitioner.

School psychologists are committed to the application of their professional expertise for the purpose of promoting improvement in the quality of life for students, families, and school communities. This objective is pursued in ways that protect the dignity and rights of those involved. School psychologists consider the interests and rights of children and youth to be their highest priority in decision making, and act as advocates for all students. These assumptions necessitate that school psychologists "speak up" for the needs and rights of students even when it may be difficult to do so.

The *Principles for Professional Ethics*, like all codes of ethics, provide only limited guidance in making ethical choices. Individual judgment is necessary to apply the code to situations that arise in professional practice. Ethical dilemmas may be created by situations involving competing ethical principles, conflicts between ethics and law, the conflicting interests of multiple parties, the dual roles of employee and pupil advocate, or because it is difficult to decide how statements in the ethics code apply to a particular situation.[5] Such situations are often complicated and may require a nuanced application of these *Principles* to effect a resolution that results in the greatest benefit for the student and concerned others. When difficult situations arise, school psychologists are advised to use a systematic problem-solving process to identify the best course of action. This process should include identifying the ethical issues involved, consulting these *Principles*, consulting colleagues with greater expertise, evaluating the rights and welfare of all affected parties, considering alternative solutions and their consequences, and accepting responsibility for the decisions made.[6][7]

The NASP *Principles for Professional Ethics* may require a more stringent standard of conduct than law, and in those situations in which both apply, school psychologists are expected to adhere to the Principles. When conflicts between ethics and law occur, school psychologists are expected to take steps to resolve conflicts by problem solving with others and through positive, respected, and legal channels. If not able to resolve the conflict in this manner, they may abide by the law, as long as the resulting actions do not violate basic human rights.[8]

In addition to providing services to public and private schools, school psychologists may be employed in a variety of other settings, including juvenile justice institutions, colleges and universities, mental health clinics, hospitals, and private practice. The principles in this code should be considered by school psychologists in their ethical decision making regardless of employment setting. However, this revision of the code, like its precursors, focuses on the special challenges associated with providing school psychological services in schools and to students. School psychologists who provide services directly to children, parents, and other clients as private practitioners, and those who work in health and mental health settings, are encouraged to be knowledgeable of federal and state law regulating mental health providers, and to consult the American Psychological Association's (2002) *Ethical Principles of Psychologists and Code of Conduct* for guidance on issues not directly addressed in this code.

Four broad ethical themes[9] provide the organizational framework for the 2010 *Principles for Professional Ethics*. The four broad ethical themes subsume 17 ethical principles. Each principle is then further articulated by multiple specific standards of conduct. The broad themes, corollary principles, and ethical standards are to be considered in decision making. NASP will seek to enforce the 17 ethical principles and corollary standards that appear in the *Principles for Professional Ethics* with its members and school psychologists who hold the Nationally Certified School Psychologist (NCSP) credential in accordance with NASP's *Ethical and Professional Practices Committee Procedures* (2008). Regardless of role, clientele, or setting, school psychologists should reflect on the theme and intent of each ethical principle and standard to determine its application to his or her individual situation.

The decisions made by school psychologists affect the welfare of children and families and can enhance their schools and communities. For this reason, school psychologists are encouraged to strive for excellence rather than simply meeting the minimum obligations outlined in the NASP *Principles for Professional Ethics*,[10] and to engage in the lifelong learning that is necessary to achieve and maintain expertise in applied professional ethics.

Definition of Terms as Used in the *Principles for Professional Ethics*

Client: The *client* is the person or persons with whom the school psychologist establishes a professional relationship for the purpose of providing school psychological services. A school psychologist–client professional relationship is established by an informed agreement with client(s) about the school psychologist's ethical and other duties to each party.[11] While not clients per se, classrooms, schools, and school systems also may be recipients of school psychological services and often are parties with an interest in the actions of school psychologists.

Child: A *child*, as defined in law, generally refers to a minor, a person younger than the age of majority. Although this term may be regarded as demeaning when applied to teenagers, it is used in this document when necessary to denote minor status. The term *student* is used when a less precise term is adequate.

Informed Consent: Informed consent means that the person giving consent has the legal authority to make a consent decision, a clear understanding of what it is he or she is consenting to, and that his or her consent is freely given and may be withdrawn without prejudice.[12]

Assent: The term *assent* refers to a minor's affirmative agreement to participate in psychological services or research.

Parent: The term *parent* may be defined in law or district policy, and can include the birth or adoptive parent, an individual acting in the place of a natural or adoptive parent (a grandparent or other relative, stepparent, or domestic partner), and/or an individual who is legally responsible for the child's welfare.

Advocacy: School psychologists have a special obligation to speak up for the rights and welfare of students and families, and to provide a voice to clients who cannot or do not wish to speak for themselves. *Advocacy* also occurs when school psychologists use their expertise in psychology and education to promote changes in schools, systems, and laws that will benefit schoolchildren, other students, and families.[13] Nothing in this code of ethics, however, should be construed as requiring school psychologists to engage in insubordination (willful disregard of an employer's lawful instructions) or to file a complaint about school district practices with a federal or state regulatory agency as part of their advocacy efforts.

School-Based Versus Private Practice: School-based practice refers to the provision of school psychological services under the authority of a state, regional, or local educational agency. School-based practice occurs if the school psychologist is an employee of the schools or contracted by the schools on a per case or consultative basis. *Private practice* occurs when a school psychologist enters into an agreement with a client(s) rather than an educational agency to provide school psychological services and the school psychologist's fee for services is the responsibility of the client or his or her representative.

I. Respecting the Dignity and Rights of All Persons

School psychologists engage only in professional practices that maintain the dignity of all with whom they work. In their words and actions, school psychologists demonstrate respect for the autonomy of persons and their right to self-determination, respect for privacy, and a commitment to just and fair treatment of all persons.

Principle I.1. Autonomy and Self-Determination (Consent and Assent)

School psychologists respect the right of persons to participate in decisions affecting their own welfare.

Standard I.1.1

School psychologists encourage and promote parental participation in school decisions affecting their children (see Standard II.3.10). However, where school psychologists are members of the school's educational support staff, not all of their services require informed parent consent. It is ethically permissible to provide school-based consultation services regarding a child or adolescent to a student assistance team or teacher without informed parent consent as long as the resulting interventions are under the authority of the teacher and within the scope of typical classroom interventions.[14] Parent consent is not ethically required for a school-based school psychologist to review a student's educational records, conduct classroom observations, assist in within-classroom interventions and progress monitoring, or to participate in educational screenings conducted as part of a regular program of instruction. Parent consent is required if the consultation about a particular child or adolescent is likely to be extensive and ongoing and/or if school actions may result in a significant intrusion on student or family privacy beyond what might be expected in the course of ordinary school activities.[15] Parents must be notified prior to the administration of school-or classroom-wide screenings for mental health problems and given the opportunity to remove their child or adolescent from participation in such screenings.

Standard I.1.2

Except for urgent situations or self-referrals by a minor student, school psychologists seek parent consent (or the consent of an adult student) prior to establishing a school psychologist–client relationship for the purpose of psychological diagnosis, assessment of eligibility for special education or disability accommodations, or to provide ongoing individual or group counseling or other nonclassroom therapeutic intervention.*

- It is ethically permissible to provide psychological assistance without parent notice or consent in emergency situations or if there is reason to believe a student may pose a danger to others; is at risk for self-harm; or is in danger of injury, exploitation, or maltreatment.

- When a student who is a minor self-refers for assistance, it is ethically permissible to provide psychological assistance without parent notice or consent for one or several meetings to establish the nature and degree of the need for services and assure the child is safe and not in danger. It is

---

*It is recommended that school district parent handbooks and websites advise parents that a minor student may be seen by school health or mental health professionals (e.g., school nurse, counselor, social worker, school psychologist) without parent notice or consent to ensure that the student is safe or is not a danger to others. Parents should also be advised that district school psychologists routinely assist teachers in planning classroom instruction and monitoring its effectiveness and do not need to notify parents of, or seek consent for, such involvement in student support.

ethically permissible to provide services to mature minors without parent consent where allowed by state law and school district policy. However, if the student is not old enough to receive school psychological assistance independent of parent consent, the school psychologist obtains parent consent to provide continuing assistance to the student beyond the preliminary meetings or refers the student to alternative sources of assistance that do not require parent notice or consent.

Standard I.1.3

School psychologists ensure that an individual providing consent for school psychological services is fully informed about the nature and scope of services offered, assessment/intervention goals and procedures, any foreseeable risks, the cost of services to the parent or student (if any), and the benefits that reasonably can be expected. The explanation includes discussion of the limits of confidentiality, who will receive information about assessment or intervention outcomes, and the possible consequences of the assessment/intervention services being offered. Available alternative services are identified, if appropriate. This explanation takes into account language and cultural differences, cognitive capabilities, developmental level, age, and other relevant factors so that it may be understood by the individual providing consent. School psychologists appropriately document written or oral consent. Any service provision by interns, practicum students, or other trainees is explained and agreed to in advance, and the identity and responsibilities of the supervising school psychologist are explained prior to the provision of services.[16]

Standard I.1.4

School psychologists encourage a minor student's voluntary participation in decision making about school psychological services as much as feasible. Ordinarily, school psychologists seek the student's assent to services; however, it is ethically permissible to bypass student assent to services if the service is considered to be of direct benefit to the student and/or is required by law.[17]

- If a student's assent for services is not solicited, school psychologists nevertheless honor the student's right to be informed about the services provided.

- When a student is given a choice regarding whether to accept or refuse services, the school psychologist ensures the student understands what is being offered, honors the student's stated choice, and guards against overwhelming the student with choices he or she does not wish or is not able to make.[18]

Standard I.1.5

School psychologists respect the wishes of parents who object to school psychological services and attempt to guide parents to alternative resources.

Principle I.2. Privacy and Confidentiality

School psychologists respect the right of persons to choose for themselves whether to disclose their private thoughts, feelings, beliefs, and behaviors.

Standard I.2.1

School psychologists respect the right of persons to self-determine whether to disclose private information.

Standard I.2.2

School psychologists minimize intrusions on privacy. They do not seek or store private information about clients that is not needed in the provision of services. School psychologists recognize that client–school psychologist communications are privileged in most jurisdictions and do not disclose information that would put the student or family at legal, social, or other risk if shared with third parties, except as permitted by the mental health provider–client privilege laws in their state.[19]

Standard I.2.3

School psychologists inform students and other clients of the boundaries of confidentiality at the outset of establishing a professional relationship. They seek a shared understanding with clients regarding the types of information that will and will not be shared with third parties. However, if a child or adolescent is in immediate need of assistance, it is permissible to delay the discussion of confidentiality until the immediate crisis is resolved. School psychologists recognize that it may be necessary to discuss confidentiality at multiple points in a professional relationship to ensure client understanding and agreement regarding how sensitive disclosures will be handled.

Standard I.2.4

School psychologists respect the confidentiality of information obtained during their professional work. Information is not revealed to third parties without the agreement of a minor child's parent or legal guardian (or an adult student), except in those situations in which failure to release information would result in danger to the student or others, or where otherwise required by law. Whenever feasible, student assent is obtained prior to disclosure of his or her confidences to third parties, including disclosures to the student's parents.

Standard I.2.5

School psychologists discuss and/or release confidential information only for professional purposes and only with persons who have a legitimate need to know. They do so within the strict boundaries of relevant privacy statutes.

Standard I.2.6

School psychologists respect the right of privacy of students, parents, and colleagues with regard to sexual orientation, gender identity, or transgender status. They do not share information about the sexual orientation, gender identity, or transgender status of a student (including minors), parent, or school employee with anyone without that individual's permission.[20]

Standard I.2.7

School psychologists respect the right of privacy of students, their parents and other family members, and colleagues with regard to sensitive health information (e.g., presence of a communicable disease). They do not share sensitive health information about a student, parent, or school employee with others without that individual's permission (or the permission of a parent or guardian in the case of a minor). School psychologists consult their state laws and department of public health for guidance if they believe a client poses a health risk to others.[21]

Principle I.3. Fairness and Justice

In their words and actions, school psychologists promote fairness and justice. They use their expertise to cultivate school climates that are safe and welcoming to all persons regardless of actual or perceived characteristics, including race, ethnicity, color, religion, ancestry, national origin, immigration status, socioeconomic status, primary language, gender, sexual orientation, gender identity, gender expression, disability, or any other distinguishing characteristics.

Standard I.3.1

School psychologists do not engage in or condone actions or policies that discriminate against persons, including students and their families, other recipients of service, supervisees, and colleagues based on actual or perceived characteristics including race; ethnicity; color; religion; ancestry; national origin; immigration status; socioeconomic status; primary language; gender; sexual orientation, gender identity, or gender expression; mental, physical, or sensory disability; or any other distinguishing characteristics.

Standard I.3.2

School psychologists pursue awareness and knowledge of how diversity factors may influence child development, behavior, and school learning. In conducting psychological, educational, or behavioral evaluations or in providing interventions, therapy, counseling, or consultation services, the school psychologist takes into account individual characteristics as enumerated in Standard I.3.1 so as to provide effective services.[22]

Standard I.3.3

School psychologists work to correct school practices that are unjustly discriminatory or that deny students, parents, or others their legal rights. They take steps to foster a school climate that is safe, accepting, and respectful of all persons.

Standard I.3.4

School psychologists strive to ensure that all children have equal opportunity to participate in and benefit from school programs and that all students and families have access to and can benefit from school psychological services.[23]

II. Professional Competence and Responsibility

Beneficence, or responsible caring, means that the school psychologist acts to benefit others. To do this, school psychologists must practice within the boundaries of their competence, use scientific knowledge from psychology and education to help clients and others make informed choices, and accept responsibility for their work.[24]

Principle II.1. Competence

To benefit clients, school psychologists engage only in practices for which they are qualified and competent.

Standard II.1.1

School psychologists recognize the strengths and limitations of their training and experience, engaging only in practices for which they are qualified. They enlist the assistance of other specialists in supervisory, consultative, or referral roles as appropriate in providing effective services.

Standard II.1.2

Practitioners are obligated to pursue knowledge and understanding of the diverse cultural, linguistic, and experiential backgrounds of students, families, and other clients. When knowledge and understanding of diversity characteristics are essential to ensure competent assessment, intervention, or consultation, school psychologists have or obtain the training or supervision necessary to provide effective services, or they make appropriate referrals.

Standard II.1.3

School psychologists refrain from any activity in which their personal problems may interfere with professional effectiveness. They seek assistance when personal problems threaten to compromise their professional effectiveness (also see III.4.2).

Standard II.1.4

School psychologists engage in continuing professional development. They remain current regarding developments in research, training, and professional practices that benefit children, families, and schools. They also understand that professional skill development beyond that of the novice practitioner requires well-planned continuing professional development and professional supervision.

Principle II.2. Accepting Responsibility for Actions

School psychologists accept responsibility for their professional work, monitor the effectiveness of their services, and work to correct ineffective recommendations.

Standard II.2.1

School psychologists review all of their written documents for accuracy, signing them only when correct. They may add an addendum, dated and signed, to a previously submitted report if information is found to be inaccurate or incomplete.

Standard II.2.2

School psychologists actively monitor the impact of their recommendations and intervention plans. They revise a recommendation, or modify or terminate an intervention plan, when data indicate the desired outcomes are not being attained. School psychologists seek the assistance of others in supervisory, consultative, or referral roles when progress monitoring indicates that their recommendations and interventions are not effective in assisting a client.

Standard II.2.3

School psychologists accept responsibility for the appropriateness of their professional practices, decisions, and recommendations. They correct misunderstandings resulting from their recommendations, advice, or information and take affirmative steps to offset any harmful consequences of ineffective or inappropriate recommendations.

Standard II.2.4

When supervising graduate students' field experiences or internships, school psychologists are responsible for the work of their supervisees.

Principle II.3. Responsible Assessment and Intervention Practices

School psychologists maintain the highest standard for responsible professional practices in educational and psychological assessment and direct and indirect interventions.

Standard II.3.1

Prior to the consideration of a disability label or category, the effects of current behavior management and/or instructional practices on the student's school performance are considered.

Standard II.3.2

School psychologists use assessment techniques and practices that the profession considers to be responsible, research-based practice.

- School psychologists select assessment instruments and strategies that are reliable and valid for the child and the purpose of the assessment. When using standardized measures, school psychologists adhere to the procedures for administration of the instrument that are provided by the author or publisher or the instrument. If modifications are made in the administration procedures for standardized tests or other instruments, such modifications are identified and discussed in the interpretation of the results.

- If using norm-referenced measures, school psychologists choose instruments with up-to-date normative data.

- When using computer-administered assessments, computer-assisted scoring, and/or interpretation programs, school psychologists choose programs that meet professional standards for accuracy and validity. School psychologists use professional judgment in evaluating the accuracy of computer-assisted assessment findings for the examinee.

Standard II.3.3

A psychological or psychoeducational assessment is based on a variety of different types of information from different sources.

Standard II.3.4

Consistent with education law and sound professional practice, children with suspected disabilities are assessed in all areas related to the suspected disability

Standard II.3.5

School psychologists conduct valid and fair assessments. They actively pursue knowledge of the student's disabilities and developmental, cultural, linguistic, and experiential background and then select, administer, and interpret assessment instruments and procedures in light of those characteristics (see Standard I.3.1. and I.3.2).

Standard II.3.6

When interpreters are used to facilitate the provision of assessment and intervention services, school psychologists take steps to ensure that the interpreters are appropriately trained and are acceptable to clients.[25]

Standard II.3.7

It is permissible for school psychologists to make recommendations based solely on a review of existing records. However, they should utilize a representative sample of records and explain the basis for, and the limitations of, their recommendations.[26]

Standard II.3.8

School psychologists adequately interpret findings and present results in clear, understandable terms so that the recipient can make informed choices.

Standard II.3.9

School psychologists use intervention, counseling and therapy procedures, consultation techniques, and other direct and indirect service methods that the profession considers to be responsible, research-based practice:

- School psychologists use a problem-solving process to develop interventions appropriate to the presenting problems and that are consistent with data collected.

- Preference is given to interventions described in the peer-reviewed professional research literature and found to be efficacious.

Standard II.3.10

School psychologists encourage and promote parental participation in designing interventions for their children. When appropriate, this includes linking interventions between the school and the home, tailoring parental involvement to the skills of the family, and helping parents gain the skills needed to help their children.

- School psychologists discuss with parents the recommendations and plans for assisting their children. This discussion takes into account the ethnic/cultural values of the family and includes alternatives that may be available. Subsequent recommendations for program changes or additional services are discussed with parents, including any alternatives that may be available.

- Parents are informed of sources of support available at school and in the community.

Standard II.3.11

School psychologists discuss with students the recommendations and plans for assisting them. To the maximum extent appropriate, students are invited to participate in selecting and planning interventions.[27]

Principle II.4 Responsible School-Based Record Keeping

School psychologists safeguard the privacy of school psychological records and ensure parent access to the records of their own children.

Standard II.4.1

School psychologists discuss with parents and adult students their rights regarding creation, modification, storage, and disposal of psychological and educational records that result from the provision of services. Parents and adult students are notified of the electronic storage and transmission of personally identifiable school psychological records and the associated risks to privacy.[28]

Standard II.4.2

School psychologists maintain school-based psychological and educational records with sufficient detail to be useful in decision making by another professional and with sufficient detail to withstand scrutiny if challenged in a due process or other legal procedure.[29]

Standard II.4.3

School psychologists include only documented and relevant information from reliable sources in school psychological records.

Standard II.4.4

School psychologists ensure that parents have appropriate access to the psychological and educational records of their child.

- Parents have a right to access any and all information that is used to make educational decisions about their child.
- School psychologists respect the right of parents to inspect, but not necessarily to copy, their child's answers to school psychological test questions, even if those answers are recorded on a test protocol (also see II.5.1).[30]

Standard II.4.5

School psychologists take steps to ensure that information in school psychological records is not released to persons or agencies outside of the school without the consent of the parent except as required and permitted by law.

Standard II.4.6

To the extent that school psychological records are under their control, school psychologists ensure that only those school personnel who have a legitimate educational interest in a student are given access to the student's school psychological records without prior parent permission or the permission of an adult student.

Standard II.4.7

To the extent that school psychological records are under their control, school psychologists protect electronic files from unauthorized release or modification (e.g., by using passwords and encryption), and they take reasonable steps to ensure that school psychological records are not lost due to equipment failure.

Standard II.4.8

It is ethically permissible for school psychologists to keep private notes to use as a memory aid that are not made accessible to others. However, as noted in Standard II.4.4, any and all information that is used to make educational decisions about a student must be accessible to parents and adult students.

Standard II.4.9

School psychologists, in collaboration with administrators and other school staff, work to establish district policies regarding the storage and disposal of school psychological records that are consistent with law and sound professional practice. They advocate for school district policies and practices that:

- safeguard the security of school psychological records while facilitating appropriate parent access to those records
- identify time lines for the periodic review and disposal of outdated school psychological records that are consistent with law and sound professional practice
- seek parent or other appropriate permission prior to the destruction of obsolete school psychological records of current students
- ensure that obsolete school psychology records are destroyed in a way that the information cannot be recovered

Principle II.5 Responsible Use of Materials

School psychologists respect the intellectual property rights of those who produce tests, intervention materials, scholarly works, and other materials.

Standard II.5.1

School psychologists maintain test security, preventing the release of underlying principles and specific content that would undermine or invalidate the use of the instrument. Unless otherwise required by law or district policy, school psychologists provide parents with the opportunity to inspect and review their child's test answers rather than providing them with copies of their child's test protocols. However, on parent request, it is permissible to provide copies of a child's test protocols to a professional who is qualified to interpret them.

Standard II.5.2

School psychologists do not promote or condone the use of restricted psychological and educational tests or other assessment tools or procedures by individuals who are not qualified to use them.

Standard II.5.3

School psychologists recognize the effort and expense involved in the development and publication of psychological and educational tests, intervention materials, and scholarly works. They respect the intellectual property rights and copyright interests of the producers of such materials, whether the materials are published in print or digital formats. They do not duplicate copyright-protected test manuals, testing materials, or unused test protocols without the permission of the producer. However, school psychologists understand that, at times, parents' rights to examine their child's test answers may supersede the interests of test publishers.[31][32]

III. Honesty and Integrity in Professional Relationships

To foster and maintain trust, school psychologists must be faithful to the truth and adhere to their professional promises. They are forthright about their qualifications, competencies, and roles; work in full cooperation with other professional disciplines to meet the needs of students and families; and avoid multiple relationships that diminish their professional effectiveness.

Principle III.1. Accurate Presentation of Professional Qualifications

School psychologists accurately identify their professional qualifications to others.

Standard III.1.1

Competency levels, education, training, experience, and certification and licensing credentials are accurately represented to clients, recipients of services, and others. School psychologists correct any misperceptions of their qualifications. School psychologists do not represent themselves as specialists in a particular domain without verifiable training and supervised experience in the specialty.

Standard III.1.2

School psychologists do not use affiliations with persons, associations, or institutions to imply a level of professional competence that exceeds that which has actually been achieved.

Principle III.2. Forthright Explanation of Professional Services, Roles, and Priorities

School psychologists are candid about the nature and scope of their services.

Standard III.2.1

School psychologists explain their professional competencies, roles, assignments, and working relationships to recipients of services and others in their work setting in a forthright and understandable manner. School psychologists explain all professional services to clients in a clear, understandable manner (see I.1.2).

Standard III.2.2

School psychologists make reasonable efforts to become integral members of the client service systems to which they are assigned. They establish clear roles for themselves within those systems while respecting the various roles of colleagues in other professions.

Standard III.2.3

The school psychologist's commitment to protecting the rights and welfare of children is communicated to the school administration, staff, and others as the highest priority in determining services.

Standard III.2.4

School psychologists who provide services to several different groups (e.g., families, teachers, classrooms) may encounter situations in which loyalties are conflicted. As much as possible, school psychologists make known their priorities and commitments in advance to all parties to prevent misunderstandings.

Standard III.2.5

School psychologists ensure that announcements and advertisements of the availability of their publications, products, and services for sale are factual and professional. They do not misrepresent their degree of responsibility for the development and distribution of publications, products, and services.

Principle III.3. Respecting Other Professionals

To best meet the needs of children, school psychologists cooperate with other professionals in relationships based on mutual respect.

Standard III.3.1

To meet the needs of children and other clients most effectively, school psychologists cooperate with other psychologists and professionals from other disciplines in relationships based on mutual respect. They encourage and support the use of all resources to serve the interests of students. If a child or other client is receiving similar services from another professional, school psychologists promote coordination of services.

Standard III.3.2

If a child or other client is referred to another professional for services, school psychologists ensure that all relevant and appropriate individuals, including the client, are notified of the change and reasons for the change. When referring clients to other professionals, school psychologists provide clients with lists of suitable practitioners from whom the client may seek services.

Standard III.3.3

Except when supervising graduate students, school psychologists do not alter reports completed by another professional without his or her permission to do so.

Principle III.4. Multiple Relationships and Conflicts of Interest

School psychologists avoid multiple relationships and conflicts of interest that diminish their professional effectiveness.

Standard III.4.1

The Principles for Professional Ethics provide standards for professional conduct. School psychologists, in their private lives, are free to pursue their personal interests, except to the degree that those interests compromise professional effectiveness.

Standard III.4.2

School psychologists refrain from any activity in which conflicts of interest or multiple relationships with a client or a client's family may interfere with professional effectiveness. School psychologists attempt to resolve such situations in a manner that provides greatest benefit to the client. School psychologists whose personal or religious beliefs or commitments may influence the nature of their professional services or their willingness to provide certain services inform clients and responsible parties of this fact. When personal beliefs, conflicts of interests, or multiple relationships threaten to diminish professional effectiveness or would be viewed by the public as inappropriate, school psychologists ask their supervisor for reassignment of responsibilities, or they direct the client to alternative services.[33]

Standard III.4.3

School psychologists do not exploit clients, supervisees, or graduate students through professional relationships or condone these actions by their colleagues. They do not participate in or condone sexual harassment of children, parents, other clients, colleagues, employees, trainees, supervisees, or research participants. School psychologists do not engage in sexual relationships with individuals over whom they have evaluation authority, including college students in their classes or program, or any other trainees, or supervisees. School psychologists do not engage in sexual relationships with their current or former pupil-clients; the parents, siblings, or other close family members of current pupil-clients; or current consultees.

Standard III.4.4

School psychologists are cautious about business and other relationships with clients that could interfere with professional judgment and effectiveness or potentially result in exploitation of a client.

Standard III.4.5

NASP requires that any action taken by its officers, members of the Executive Council or Delegate Assembly, or other committee members be free from the appearance of impropriety and free from any conflict of interest. NASP leaders recuse themselves from decisions regarding proposed NASP initiatives if they may gain an economic benefit from the proposed venture.

Standard III.4.6

A school psychologist's financial interests in a product (e.g., tests, computer software, professional materials) or service can influence his or her objectivity or the perception of his or her objectivity regarding that product or service. For this reason, school psychologists are obligated to disclose any significant financial interest in the products or services they discuss in their presentations or writings if that interest is not obvious in the authorship/ownership citations provided.

Standard III.4.7

School psychologists neither give nor receive any remuneration for referring children and other clients for professional services.

Standard III.4.8

School psychologists do not accept any remuneration in exchange for data from their client database without the permission of their employer and a determination of whether the data release ethically requires informed client consent.

Standard III.4.9

School psychologists who provide school-based services and also engage in the provision of private practice services (dual setting practitioners) recognize the potential for conflicts of interests between their two roles and take steps to avoid such conflicts. Dual setting practitioners:

- are obligated to inform parents or other potential clients of any psychological and educational services available at no cost from the schools prior to offering such services for remuneration
- may not offer or provide private practice services to a student of a school or special school program where the practitioner is currently assigned
- may not offer or provide private practice services to the parents or family members of a student eligible to attend a school or special school program where the practitioner is currently assigned
- may not offer or provide an independent evaluation as defined in special education law for a student who attends a local or cooperative school district where the practitioner is employed
- do not use tests, materials, equipment, facilities, secretarial assistance, or other services belonging to the public sector employer unless approved in advance by the employer
- conduct all private practice outside of the hours of contracted public employment
- hold appropriate credentials for practice in both the public and private sectors

IV. Responsibility to Schools, Families, Communities, the Profession, and Society

School psychologists promote healthy school, family, and community environments. They assume a proactive role in identifying social injustices that affect children and schools and strive to reform systems-level patterns of injustice. They maintain the public trust in school psychologists by respecting law and encouraging ethical conduct. School psychologists advance professional excellence by mentoring less experienced practitioners and contributing to the school psychology knowledge base.

Principle IV.1. Promoting Healthy School, Family, and Community Environments

School psychologists use their expertise in psychology and education to promote school, family, and community environments that are safe and healthy for children.

Standard IV.1.1

To provide effective services and systems consultation, school psychologists are knowledgeable about the organization, philosophy, goals, objectives, culture, and methodologies of the settings in which they provide services. In addition, school psychologists develop partnerships and networks with community service providers and agencies to provide seamless services to children and families.

Standard IV.1.2

School psychologists use their professional expertise to promote changes in schools and community service systems that will benefit children and other clients. They advocate for school policies and practices that are in the best interests of children and that respect and protect the legal rights of students and parents.[34]

Principle IV.2. Respect for Law and the Relationship of Law and Ethics

School psychologists are knowledgeable of and respect laws pertinent to the practice of school psychology. In choosing an appropriate course of action, they consider the relationship between law and the Principles for Professional Ethics.

Standard IV.2.1

School psychologists recognize that an understanding of the goals, procedures, and legal requirements of their particular workplace is essential for effective functioning within that setting.

Standard IV.2.2

School psychologists respect the law and the civil and legal rights of students and other clients. The Principles for Professional Ethics may require a more stringent standard of conduct than law, and in those situations school psychologists are expected to adhere to the Principles.

Standard IV.2.3

When conflicts between ethics and law occur, school psychologists take steps to resolve the conflict through positive, respected, and legal channels. If not able to resolve the conflict in this manner, they may abide by the law, as long as the resulting actions do not violate basic human rights.[35]

Standard IV.2.4

School psychologists may act as individual citizens to bring about change in a lawful manner. They identify when they are speaking as private citizens rather than as employees. They also identify when they speak as individual professionals rather than as representatives of a professional association.

Principle IV.3. Maintaining Public Trust by Self-Monitoring and Peer Monitoring

School psychologists accept responsibility to monitor their own conduct and the conduct of other school psychologists to ensure it conforms to ethical standards.

Standard IV.3.1

School psychologists know the Principles for Professional Ethics and thoughtfully apply them to situations within their employment context. In difficult situations, school psychologists consult experienced school psychologists or state associations or NASP.

Standard IV.3.2

When a school psychologist suspects that another school psychologist or another professional has engaged in unethical practices, he or she attempts to resolve the suspected problem through a collegial problem-solving process, if feasible.

Standard IV.3.3

If a collegial problem-solving process is not possible or productive, school psychologists take further action appropriate to the situation, including discussing the situation with a supervisor in the employment setting, consulting state association ethics committees, and, if necessary, filing a formal ethical violation complaint with state associations, state credentialing bodies, or the NASP Ethical and Professional Practices Committee in accordance with their procedures.

Standard IV.3.4

When school psychologists are concerned about unethical practices by professionals who are not NASP members or do not hold the NCSP, informal contact is made to discuss the concern if feasible. If the situation cannot be resolved in this manner, discussing the situation with the professional's supervisor should be considered. If necessary, an appropriate professional organization or state credentialing agency could be contacted to determine the procedures established by that professional association or agency for examining the practices in question.

Principle IV.4. Contributing to the Profession by Mentoring, Teaching, and Supervision

As part of their obligation to students, schools, society, and their profession, school psychologists mentor less experienced practitioners and graduate students to assure high quality services, and they serve as role models for sound ethical and professional practices and decision making.

Standard IV.4.1

School psychologists who serve as directors of graduate education programs provide current and prospective graduate students with accurate information regarding program accreditation, goals and objectives, graduate program policies and requirements, and likely outcomes and benefits.

Standard IV.4.2

School psychologists who supervise practicum students and interns are responsible for all professional practices of the supervisees. They ensure that practicum students and interns are adequately supervised as outlined in the NASP *Graduate Preparation Standards for School Psychologists*. Interns and graduate students are identified as such, and their work is cosigned by the supervising school psychologist.

Standard IV.4.3

School psychologists who employ, supervise, or train professionals provide appropriate working conditions, fair and timely evaluation, constructive supervision, and continuing professional development opportunities.

Standard IV.4.4

School psychologists who are faculty members at universities or who supervise graduate education field experiences apply these ethical principles in all work with school psychology graduate students. In addition, they promote the ethical practice of graduate students by providing specific and comprehensive instruction, feedback, and mentoring.

Principle IV.5. Contributing to the School Psychology Knowledge Base

To improve services to children, families, and schools, and to promote the welfare of children, school psychologists are encouraged to contribute to the school psychology knowledge base by participating in, assisting in, or conducting and disseminating research.

Standard IV.5.1

When designing and conducting research in schools, school psychologists choose topics and employ research methodology, research participant selection procedures, data-gathering methods, and analysis and reporting techniques that are grounded in sound research practice. School psychologists identify their level of training and graduate degree to potential research participants.

Standard IV.5.2

School psychologists respect the rights, and protect the well-being, of research participants. School psychologists obtain appropriate review and approval of proposed research prior to beginning their data collection.

- Prior to initiating research, school psychologists and graduate students affiliated with a university, hospital, or other agency subject to the U.S. Department of Health and Human Services (DHHS) regulation of research first obtain approval for their research from their Institutional Review Board for Research Involving Human Subjects (IRB) as well as the school or other agency in which the research will be conducted. Research proposals that have not been subject to IRB approval should be reviewed by individuals knowledgeable about research methodology and ethics and approved by the school administration or other appropriate authority.

- In planning research, school psychologists are ethically obligated to consider carefully whether the informed consent of research participants is needed for their study, recognizing that research involving more than minimum risk requires informed consent, and that research with students involving activities that are not part of ordinary, typical schooling requires informed consent. Consent and assent protocols provide the information necessary for potential research participants to make an informed and voluntary choice about participation. School psychologists evaluate the potential risks (including risks of physical or psychological harm, intrusions on privacy, breach of confidentiality) and benefits of their research and only conduct studies in which the risks to participants are minimized and acceptable.

Standard IV.5.3

School psychologists who use their assessment, intervention, or consultation cases in lectures, presentations, or publications obtain written prior client consent or they remove and disguise identifying client information.

Standard IV.5.4

School psychologists do not publish or present fabricated or falsified data or results in their publications and presentations.

Standard IV.5.5

School psychologists make available their data or other information that provided the basis for findings and conclusions reported in publications and presentations, if such data are needed to address a legitimate concern or need and under the condition that the confidentiality and other rights of research participants are protected.

Standard IV.5.6

If errors are discovered after the publication or presentation of research or other information, school psychologists make efforts to correct errors by publishing errata, retractions, or corrections.

Standard IV.5.7

School psychologists only publish data or other information that make original contributions to the professional literature. They do not report the same study in a second publication without acknowledging previous publication of the same data. They do not duplicate significant portions of their own or others' previous publications without permission of copyright holders.

Standard IV.5.8

When publishing or presenting research or other work, school psychologists do not plagiarize the works or ideas of others. They appropriately cite and reference all sources, print or digital, and assign credit to those whose ideas are reflected. In inservice or conference presentations, school psychologists give credit to others whose ideas have been used or adapted.

Standard IV.5.9

School psychologists accurately reflect the contributions of authors and other individuals who contributed to presentations and publications. Authorship credit is given only to individuals who have made a substantial professional contribution to the research, publication, or presentation. Authors discuss and resolve issues related to publication credit as early as feasible in the research and publication process.

Standard IV.5.10

School psychologists who participate in reviews of manuscripts, proposals, and other materials respect the confidentiality and proprietary rights of the authors. They limit their use of the materials to the activities relevant to the purposes of the professional review. School psychologists who review professional materials do not communicate the identity of the author, quote from the materials, or duplicate or circulate copies of the materials without the author's permission.

Appendix A.

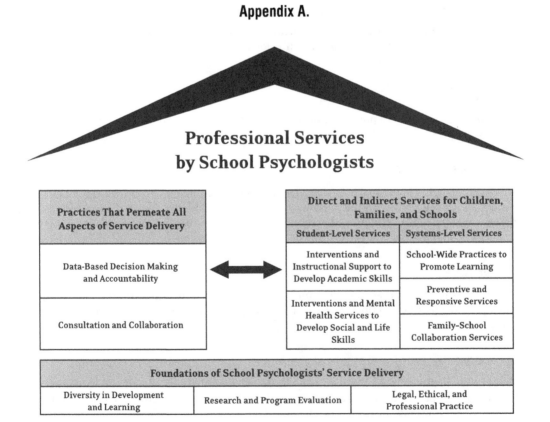

Professional Services by School Psychologists

Practices That Permeate All Aspects of Service Delivery		Direct and Indirect Services for Children, Families, and Schools	
		Student-Level Services	**Systems-Level Services**
Data-Based Decision Making and Accountability		Interventions and Instructional Support to Develop Academic Skills	School-Wide Practices to Promote Learning
		Interventions and Mental Health Services to Develop Social and Life Skills	Preventive and Responsive Services
Consultation and Collaboration			Family-School Collaboration Services

Foundations of School Psychologists' Service Delivery		
Diversity in Development and Learning	Research and Program Evaluation	Legal, Ethical, and Professional Practice

[1]Jacob, S., Decker, D. M., & Hartshorne, T. S. (2011). *Ethics and law for school psychologists* (6th ed.). Hoboken, NJ: Wiley.

[2]National Association of School Psychologists. (2008). *Ethical and Professional Practices Committee Procedures.* Available at *www.nasponline.org.*

[3]Russo, C. J. (2006). *Reutter's the law of public education* (6th ed.). New York: Foundation Press.

[4]Haas, L. J., & Malouf, J. L. (2005). *Keeping up the good work: A practitioner's guide to mental health ethics* (4th ed.). Sarasota, FL: Professional Resource Press.

[5]Jacob-Timm, S. (1999). Ethical dilemmas encountered by members of the National Association of School Psychologists. *Psychology in the Schools, 36,* 205–217.

[6]McNamara, K. (2008). Best practices in the application of professional ethics. In A. Thomas & J. Grimes (Eds.), *Best practices in school psychology V* (pp. 1933–1941). Bethesda, MD: National Association of School Psychologists.

[7]Williams, B., Armistead, L., & Jacob, S. (2008). *Professional ethics for school psychologists: A problem-solving model casebook.* Bethesda, MD: National Association of School Psychologists.

[8]American Psychological Association. (2002). Ethical principles of psychologists and code of conduct. *American Psychologist, 57,* 1060–1073.

[9]Adapted from the Canadian Psychological Association. (2000). *Canadian code of ethics for psychologists* (3rd ed.). Available at *www.cpa.ca.*

[10]Knapp. S., & VandeCreek, L. (2006). *Practical ethics for psychologists: A positive approach.* Washington, DC: American Psychological Association.

[11]Fisher, M. A. (2009). Replacing "who is the client" with a different ethical question. *Professional Psychology: Research and Practice, 40,* 1–7.

[12]Dekraai, M., Sales, B., & Hall, S. (1998). Informed consent, confidentiality, and duty to report laws in the conduct of child therapy. In T. R. Kratochwill & R. J. Morris (Eds.), *The practice of child therapy* (3rd ed., pp. 540–559). Boston: Allyn & Bacon.

[13]Masner, C. M. (2007). *The ethic of advocacy.* Doctoral dissertation, University of Denver. Available at *www.dissertation.com.*

[14]Burns, M. K., Jacob, S., & Wagner, A. (2008). Ethical and legal issues associated with using responsiveness-to-intervention to assess learning disabilities. *Journal of School Psychology, 46,* 263–279.

[15]Corrao, J., & Melton, G. B. (1985). Legal issues in school-based therapy. In J. C. Witt, S. N. Elliot, & F. M. Gresham (Eds.), *Handbook of behavior therapy in education* (pp. 377–399). New York: Plenum Press.

[16]Weithorn, L. A. (1983). Involving children in decisions affecting their own welfare: Guidelines for professionals. In G. B. Melton, G. P. Koocher, & M. J. Saks (Eds.), *Children's competence to consent* (pp. 235–260). New York: Plenum Press.

[17]Weithorn, L. A. (1983). Involving children in decisions affecting their own welfare: Guidelines for professionals. In G. B. Melton, G. P. Koocher, & M. J. Saks (Eds.), *Children's competence to consent* (pp. 235–260). New York: Plenum Press.

[18]Weithorn, L. A. (1983). Involving children in decisions affecting their own welfare: Guidelines for professionals. In G. B. Melton, G. P. Koocher, & M. J. Saks (Eds.), *Children's competence to consent* (pp. 235–260). New York: Plenum Press.

[19]Jacob, S., & Powers, K. E. (2009). Privileged communication in the school psychologist–client relationship. *Psychology in the Schools, 46,* 307–318.

[20]Sterling v. Borough of Minersville, 232 F.3d 190, 2000 U.S. App. LEXIS 27855 (3rd Cir. 2000)

[21]Jacob, S., Decker, D. M., & Hartshorne, T. S. (in press). *Ethics and law for school psychologists* (6th ed.). Hoboken, NJ: Wiley.

[22]Flanagan, R., Miller, J. A., & Jacob, S. (2005). The 2002 revision of APA's ethics code: Implications for school psychologists. *Psychology in the Schools, 42,* 433–444.

[23]Flanagan, R., Miller, J. A., & Jacob, S. (2005). The 2002 revision of APA's ethics code: Implications for school psychologists. *Psychology in the Schools, 42,* 433–445.

[24]Jacob, S., Decker, D. M., & Hartshorne, T. S. (in press). *Ethics and law for school psychologists* (6th ed.). Hoboken, NJ: Wiley.

[25]American Psychological Association. (2002). Ethical principles of psychologists and code of conduct. *American Psychologist, 57,* 1060–1073.

[26]American Psychological Association. (2002). Ethical principles of psychologists and code of conduct. *American Psychologist, 57,* 1060–1073.

[27]Weithorn, L. A. (1983). Involving children in decisions affecting their own welfare: Guidelines for professionals. In G. B. Melton, G. P. Koocher, & M. J. Saks (Eds.), *Children's competence to consent* (pp. 235–260). New York: Plenum Press.

[28]American Psychological Association. (2002). Ethical principles of psychologists and code of conduct. *American Psychologist, 57,* 1060–1073.

[29]Nagy, T. F. (2000). *Ethics in plain English.* Washington, DC: American Psychological Association.

[30]Reschly, D. J., & Bersoff, D. N. (1999). Law and school psychology. In C. R. Reynolds & T. B. Gutkin (Eds.), *Handbook of school psychology* (3rd ed., pp. 1077–1112). New York: Wiley. [Note: this chapter summarizes Department of Education policy letters on the matter of parent inspection of test protocols.]

[31]Reschly, D. J., & Bersoff, D. N. (1999). Law and school psychology. In C. R. Reynolds & T. B. Gutkin (Eds.), *Handbook of school psychology* (3rd ed., pp. 1077–1112). New York: Wiley. [Note: this chapter summarizes Department of Education policy letters on the matter of parent inspection of test protocols.]

[32]Newport-Mesa Unified School District v. State of California Department of Education, 371 F. Supp. 2d 1170; 2005 U.S. Dist. LEXIS 10290 (C.D. Cal. 2005).

[33]American Psychological Association. (2002). Ethical principles of psychologists and code of conduct. American Psychologist, 57, 1060–1073. [34]Prilleltensky, I. (1991). The social ethics of school psychology: A priority for the 1990s. *School Psychology Quarterly, 6,* 200–222.

[35]American Psychological Association. (2002). Ethical principles of psychologists and code of conduct. *American Psychologist, 57,* 1060–1073.

References

Abbott, M., Walton, C., Tapia, Y., & Greenwood, C. R. (1999). Research to practice: A "blueprint" for closing the gap in local schools. *Exceptional Children, 65,* 339–352.

Abramowitz, A. J., O'Leary, S. G., & Futtersak, M. W. (1988). The relative impact of long and short reprimands on children's off-task behavior in the classroom. *Behavior Therapy, 19,* 243–247.

Abramowitz, A. J., O'Leary, S. G., & Rosen, L. A. (1987). Reducing off-task behavior in the classroom: A comparison of encouragement and reprimands. *Journal of Abnormal Child Psychology, 15,* 153–163.

Achenbach, T. M., & Rescorla, L. A. (2001). *Manual for the ASEBA school-age forms and profiles.* Burlington: University of Vermont.

Acker, M. M., & O'Leary, S. G. (1987). Effects of reprimands and praise on appropriate behavior in the classroom. *Journal of Abnormal Child Psychology, 15,* 549–557.

Adams, G., & Carnine, D. (2003). Direct instruction. In H. L. Swanson, K. Harris, & S. Graham (Eds.), *Handbook of learning disabilities* (pp. 403–416). New York: Guilford Press.

Adams, G. R., Hampton, R. L., Gullotta, T. P., Weissberg, R. P., & Ryan, B. A. (Eds.). (1997). *Establishing preventative services.* Thousand Oaks, CA: Sage.

Adams, M. J. (1990). *Beginning to read: Thinking and learning about print.* Cambridge, MA: MIT Press.

Adelman, H. S., & Taylor, L. (1997). Toward a scale-up model for replicating new approaches to schooling. *Journal of Educational and Psychological Consultation, 8,* 197–230.

Alberto, P. A., & Troutman, A. C. (2009). *Applied behavior analysis for teachers* (8th ed.). Upper Saddle River, NJ: Merrill/Prentice Hall.

Alessi, G. (1987). Generative strategies and teaching for generalization. *The Analysis of Verbal Behavior, 5,* 15–27.

Alessi, G. (1988). Diagnosis diagnosed: A systemic reaction. *Professional School Psychology, 3,* 145–151.

American Academy of Pediatrics. (2001). Clinical practice guideline: Treatment of the child with attention-deficit/hyperactivity disorder. *Pediatrics, 105,* 1058–1070.

American Educational Research Association, American Psychological Association, & National Council on Measurement in Education. (1999). *Standards for educational and psychological testing.* Washington, DC: American Educational Research Association.

American Psychiatric Association. (2000). *Diagnostic and statistical manual of mental disorders* (4th ed., text rev.). Washington, DC: Author.

American Psychological Association. (1990). *APA guidelines for providers of psychological services to ethnic, linguistic, and culturally diverse populations.* Retrieved May 3, 2004, from *www.apa.org/pi/oema/resources/policy/provider-guidelines.aspx.*

American Psychological Association. (2002). *Guidelines on multicultural education, training, research, practice, and organizational change for psychologists.* Retrieved May 3, 2004, from *www.apa.org/pi/oema/resources/policy/multicultural-guidelines.aspx.*

American Psychological Association. (2003). *C-18 core faculty in doctoral programs.* Washington, DC: Author.

American Psychological Association. (2007a). *2007 Doctorate employment survey.* Retrieved March 18, 2010, from *www.apa.org/workforce/publications/07–doc-empl/index.aspx.*

American Psychological Association. (2007b). *Guidelines and principles for accreditation of programs in professional psychology.* Washington, DC: Author. Retrieved April 22, 2010, from *www.apa.org/ed/accreditation/about/policies/guiding-principles.pdf.*

American Psychological Association. (2010a). *Ethical principles of psychologists and code of conduct.* Washington, DC: Author. Retrieved August 15, 2010, from *www.apa.org/ethics/code/index.aspx.*

American Psychological Association. (2010b). *Race/ethnicity of doctoral recipients in psychology in the past 10 years: 2010.* Retrieved April 22, 2010, from *www.apa.org/workforce/publications/10–race/index.aspx.*

American Psychological Association Division of School Psychology. (2010). *Archival description of the specialty school psychology.* Retrieved March 18, 2010, from *www.indiana.edu/~div16/goals.html#archival.*

American Psychological Association Presidential Task Force on Evidence-Based Practice. (2006). Evidence-based practice in psychology. *American Psychologist, 61,* 271–285.

American School Counselor Association. (2010). *Student-to-counselor ratio by state 2007–2008.* Retrieved March 19, 2010, from *www.schoolcounselor.org/files/Ratios2007–2008.pdf.*

Angold, A., Costello, E., & Erkanli, A. (1999). Comorbidity. *Journal of Child Psychology and Psychiatry, 40,* 55–87.

Arter, J. A., & Jenkins, J. R. (1977). Examining the benefits and prevalence of modality considerations in special education. *Journal of Special Education, 11,* 281–298.

Arter, J. A., & Jenkins, J. R. (1979). Differential diagnosis-prescriptive teaching: A critical appraisal. *Review of Educational Research, 49,* 517–555.

Atkinson, D. R., Morten, G., & Sue, D. W. (1998). *Counseling American minorities.* Boston: McGraw-Hill.

Baer, D. M., & Bushell, D. (1981). The future of behavior analysis in the schools? Consider its recent past, and then ask a different question. *School Psychology Review, 10,* 259–270.

Baker, S. K., Chard, D. J., Ketterlin-Geller, L. R., Apichatabutra, C., & Doabler, C. (2009). Teaching writing to at-risk students: The quality of evidence for self-regulated strategy development. *Exceptional Children, 75,* 303–318.

Baker, S., Gersten, R., & Scalon, D. (2002). Procedural facilitators and cognitive strategies: Tools for unraveling the mysteries of the writing process, and for providing meaningful access to the general curriculum. *Learning Disabilities Research & Practice, 17,* 65–77.

Bandura, A. (1978). The self-system in reciprocal determination. *American Psychologist, 33,* 344–358.

Barbe, W. B., & Milone, M. N. (1980). Modality. *Instructor, 89,* 44–47.

Bardon, J. I. (1986). Psychology and schooling: The interrelationships among persons, processes, and products. In S. N. Elliott & J. C. Witt (Eds.), *The delivery of psychological services in schools: Concepts, processes, and issues* (pp. 53–79). Hillsdale, NJ: Erlbaum.

Bardon, J. I., & Bennett, V. C. (1974). *School psychology.* Englewood Cliffs, NJ: Prentice Hall.

Barkley, R. A. (1997). *Defiant children: A clinician's manual for assessment and parent training* (2nd ed.). New York: Guilford Press.

Barkley, R. A. (2006). *Attention-deficit/hyperactivity disorder: A handbook for diagnosis and treatment* (3rd ed.). New York: Guilford Press.

Barkely, R. A., Edwards, G. H., Robin, A. L. (1999). *Defiant teens: A clinician's manual for assessment and family intervention.* New York: Guilford Press.

Barkley, R. A., McMurray, M. B., Edelbrock, C. S., & Robbins, K. (1990). Side effects of methylphenidate in children with attention deficit hyperactivity disorder: A systematic, placebo-controlled evaluation. *Pediatrics, 86,* 184–192.

Barnett, D., Ihlo, T., Nichols, A., & Wolsing, L. (2006). Preschool teacher support through class-wide intervention: A description of field-initiated training and evaluation. *Journal of Applied School Psychology, 23,* 77–96.

Barrett, P.M., Farrell, L.J., Ollendick, T.H., & Dadds, M. (2006). Long-term outcomes of an Australian universal prevention trial of anxiety and depression symptoms in children and youth: An evaluation of the FRIENDS program. *Journal of Clinical Child and Adolescent Psychology, 35,* 403–411.

Batsche, G. M., & Curtis, M. J. (2003). The creation of the National School Psychology Certification System. *Communique, 32*(4), 6–7.

Bear, G. G. (2008). Best practices in classroom discipline. In A. Thomas & J. Grimes (Eds.), *Best practices in school psychology V* (pp. 1403–1420). Bethesda, MD: National Association of School Psychologists.

Bellak, L., & Bellak. S. (1949). *The Children's Apperception Test.* Larchmont, NY: CPS.

Bennett, F. C., Brown, R. T., Craver, J., & Anderson, D. (1999). Stimulant medication for the child with attention-deficit/hyperactivity disorder. *Pediatric Clinics of North America, 46,* 929–944.

Bergan, J. R., & Kratochwill, T. R. (1990). *Behavioral consultation and therapy.* New York: Plenum.

Berlin, I. (1974). *Slaves without masters: The free Negro in the antebellum south.* New York: Pantheon.

Berry, J. W., & Annis, R. C. (1974). Acculturative stress: The role of ecology, culture and differentiation. *Journal of Cross-Cultural Psychology, 5,* 382–406.

Bersoff, D. N. (2008). *Ethical conflicts in psychology* (4th ed.). Washington, DC: American Psychological Association.

Best, J. H., & Sidwell, R. T. (1967). *The American legacy of learning: Readings in the history of education.* Philadelphia: Lippincott.

Biglan, A., Mrazek, P. J., Carnine, D., & Flay, B. R. (2003). The integration of research and practice in the prevention of youth problem behaviors. *American Psychologist, 58,* 433–440.

Bijou, S. W. (1993). *Behavior analysis of child development* (rev. ed.). Reno, NV: Context Press.

Board of Education of the Hendrick Hudson Central School District v. Rowley, 458 U.S. 176 (1982).

Board of Education, Sacramento City Unified School District v. Holland, 786 F. Supp. 874 (E.D. Cal. 1992).

Booker, K. (2009). Multicultural considerations in school consultation. In J. M. Jones (Ed.), *The psychology of multiculturalism in the schools: A primer for practice, training, and research* (pp. 173–190). Bethesda, MD: National Association of School Psychologists.

Bracken, B. A., & McCallum, R. S. (1998). *Universal Nonverbal Intelligence Test.* Itasca, IL: Riverside.

Bracken, B. A., & Naglieri, J. A. (2003). Assessing diverse populations with nonverbal tests of general intelligence. In C. R. Reynolds & R. W. Kamphaus (Eds.), *Handbook of psychological and educational assessment of children: Intelligence, aptitude, and achievement* (2nd ed., pp. 243–274). New York: Guilford Press.

Bradley, R., Danielson, L., & Hallahan, D. D. (2002). *Identification of learning disabilities.* Mahwah, NJ: Erlbaum.

Bradley-Johnson, S., & Dean, V. J. (2000). Role change for school psychology: The challenge continues in the new millennium. *Psychology in the Schools, 37*(1), 1–5.

Bramlett, R. K., Murphy, J. J., Johnson, J., Wallingsford, L., & Hall, J. D. (2002). Contemporary practices in school psychology: A national survey of roles and referral problems. *Psychology in the Schools, 39,* 327–335.

Brown v. Board of Education, 347 U.S. 483 (1954).

Brown, J. E., & Doolittle, J. (2008). *A cultural, linguistic, and ecological framework for response to intervention with English language learners.* Retrieved June 23, 2010, from *www.niusileadscape.org/docs/FINAL_PRODUCTS/LearningCarousel/Framework_for_RTI_with_ELLs.pdf.*

Brown, R. T., Freeman, W. S., Perrin, J. M., Stein, M. T., Amler, R. W., & Feldman, H. (2001).

Prevalence and assessment of attention-deficit/hyperactivity disorder in primary care settings. *Pediatrics, 107,* E43.

Brown, M. B., Kissell, S., & Bolen, L. M. (2003). Doctoral school psychology internships in nonschool settings in the United States. *School Psychology International, 24,* 394–404.

Brown, R. T., & Sammons, M. T. (2002). Pediatric psychopharmacology: A review of new developments and recent research. *Professional Psychology: Research and Practice, 33,* 135–147.

Brown-Chidsey, R., & Steege, M. W. (2005). *Response to intervention: Principles and strategies for effective practice.* New York: Guilford Press.

Burns, M. K., & Klingbeil, D. A. (2010). Assessment of academic skills in math within a problem-solving model. In G. Gimpel Peacock, R. A. Ervin, E. J. Daly, & K. W. Merrell (Eds.), *Practical handbook of school psychology: Effective practices for the 21st century* (pp. 86–98). New York: Guilford Press.

Burt, M. K., Dulay, H. C., & Hernandez Chavez, E. (1980). *Bilingual Syntax Measure II.* San Antonio, TX: Harcourt, Brace, Jovanovich.

Butcher, J. N., Williams, C. L., Graham, J. R., Archer, R. P., Tellegen, A., Ben-Porath, Y. S., et al. (1992). *Minnesota Multiphasic Personality Inventory—Adolescent: Manual for administration, scoring, and interpretation.* Minneapolis: University of Minnesota Press.

Butts, R. F. (1978). *Public education in the United States: From revolution to reform.* New York: Holt, Rinehart & Winston.

Calhoun, D. (Ed.). (1969). *The educating of Americans: A documentary history.* Boston: Houghton Mifflin.

Campbell, D. T. (1988). The experimenting society. In S. Overman (Ed.), *Methodology and epistemology for social science* (pp. 290–314). Chicago: University of Chicago Press.

Cangelosi, M. D. (2010). *Identification of specific learning disability: A survey of school psychologists' knowledge and current practice.* Unpublished doctoral dissertation, St. John's University.

Canter, A. (2006). Problem solving and RTI: New roles for school psychologists. *Communiqué, 34*(5). Retrieved July 5, 2010, from: *www.nasponline.org/publications/cq/mocq345rti.aspx.*

Carlberg, C., & Kavale, K. (1980). The efficacy of special versus regular class placement for exceptional children: A meta-analysis. *Journal of Special Education, 14,* 295–309.

Carnine, D. (1989). Designing practice activities. *Journal of Learning Disabilities, 22,* 603–607.

Carnine, D. (1997). Bridging the research-to-practice gap. *Exceptional Children, 63,* 513–521.

Carnine, D. (1999). Campaigns for moving research into practice. *Remedial and Special Education, 20,* 2–6, 35.

Carnine, D. W., Silbert, J., Kame'enui, E. J., & Tarver, S. G. (2004). *Direct instruction reading* (4th ed.). Upper Saddle River, NJ: Merrill/Prentice Hall.

Carroll, J. B. (1963). A model of school learning. *Teachers College Record, 64,* 723–733.

Cedar Rapids Community School District v. Garrett F., 526 U.S. 66 (1999).

Chafouleas, S. M., Riley-Tillman, T. C., & Eckert, T. L. (2003). A comparison of school psychologists' acceptability, training, and use of norm-referenced, curriculum-based, and brief experimental analysis methods to assess reading. *School Psychology Review, 32,* 272–281.

Chambless, D. L., Baker, M. J., Baucom, D. H., Beutler, L. E., Calhoun, K. S., Crits-Christoph, P., et al. (1998). Update on empirically validated therapies, II. *The Clinical Psychologist, 51*(1), 3–16.

Chard, D. J., Vaughn, S., & Tyler, B. J. (2002). A synthesis of research on effective interventions for building reading fluency with elementary students with learning disabilities. *Journal of Learning Disabilities, 35,* 386–406.

Charvat, J. L. (2003). The school psychologist shortage: Evidence for effective advocacy. *Communiqué, 32*(2), 1, 3–4.

Charvat, J. L. (2005). NASP study: How many school psychologists are there? *Communiqué, 33*(6). Retrieved June 25, 2010, from *www.nasponline.org/publications/cq/cq336numsp.aspx.*

Charvat, J. L. (2008). Estimates of the school psychology workforce. Retrieved November 29, 2010, from *www.nasponline.org/advocacy/SP_Workforce_Estimates_9.08.pdf.*

Cherry v. Matthews, 419 F. Supp. 922 (D. D.C. 1976).

Children's Defense Fund. (2001). *The state of America's children yearbook 2001.* Washington, DC: Author.

Children's Defense Fund. (2010). *Priorities for America's children.* Retrieved May 23, 2010, from *www.childrensdefense.org/policy-priorities.*

Chinman, M., Imm, P., & Wandersman, A. (2004). *Getting to outcomes 2004: Promoting accountability through methods and tools for planning, implementation, and evaluation.* Santa Monica, CA: RAND Corporation. Retrieved November 1, 2010, from *www.rand.org/pubs/technical_reports/2004/RAND_TR101.pdf.*

Clark, E. (2002). Working together for a shared vision. *School Psychologist, 57,* 40.

Clopton, K. L., & Haselhuhn, C. W. (2009). School psychology trainer shortage in the USA: Current status and projections for the future. *School Psychology International, 30,* 24–42.

Cohen, J. (1988). *Statistical power analysis for the behavioral sciences* (2nd ed.). Hillsdale, NJ: Erlbaum.

Cohn, M. A., Fredrickson, B. L., Brown, S. L., Mikels, J. A., & Conway, A. M. (2009). Happiness unpacked: Positive emotions increase life satisfaction by building resilience. *Emotion, 9,* 361–368.

Collaborative for Academic, Social, and Emotional Learning. (2003). *Safe and sound: An educational leader's guide to evidence-based social and emotional learning (SEL) programs.* Retrieved from *www.casel.org/downloads/Safe%20and%20Sound/1A_Safe_&_Sound.pdf.*

Compton, S. N. March, J. S. Brent, D. Albano, A. M., et al. (2004). Cognitive-behavioral psychotherapy for anxiety and depressive disorders in children and adolescents: An evidence-based medicine review. *Journal of the American Academy of Child & Adolescent Psychiatry, 43,* 930–959.

Connolly, A. J. (2007). *KeyMath—3: Diagnostic assessment.* San Antonio, TX: Pearson.

Connor, D. F. (2006). Stimulants. In R. A. Barkley, *Attention-deficit/hyperactivity disorder: A handbook for diagnosis and treatment* (3rd ed., pp. 608–647). New York: Guilford Press.

Conoley, J. C., & Gutkin, T. B. (1995). Why didn't—why doesn't—school psychology realize its promise? *Journal of School Psychology, 33,* 209–217.

Cook, T. D., & Campbell, D. T. (1979). *Quasi-experimentation: Design and analysis issues for field settings.* Boston: Houghton Mifflin.

Cooper, J. O., Heron, T. E., & Heward, W. L. (2007). *Applied behavior analysis* (2nd ed.). Upper Saddle River, NJ: Prentice Hall.

Council for Exceptional Children. (2004). *No Child Left Behind Act of 2001: Reauthorization of the Elementary and Secondary Education Act. A technical assistance resource.* Arlington, VA: Author. Retrieved June 10, 2004, from *www.cec.sped.org/content/NavigationMenu/PolicyAdvocacy/CECPolicyResources/overviewNCLB.pdf.*

Cowen, E. L., Hightower, A. D., Pedro-Carroll, J., Work, W. C., Wyman, P. A., & Haffney, W. G. (Eds.). (1996). *School-based prevention for children at risk: The primary mental health project.* Washington, DC: American Psychological Association.

Coyne, M. D., Zipoli, R. P., & Ruby, M. F. (2006). Beginning reading instruction for students at risk for reading disabilities. *Intervention in School and Clinic, 41,* 161–168.

Crockett, D. (2003). Critical issues children face in the 2000s. *School Psychology Quarterly, 18,* 446–453.

Crockett, D. (2004). Critical issues children face in the 2000s. *School Psychology Review, 33,* 78–82.

Cronbach, L. J. (1957). The two disciplines of scientific psychology. *American Psychologist, 1,* 671–684.

Cronbach, L. J. (1975). Beyond the two disciplines of scientific psychology. *American Psychologist, 30,* 116–127.

Cronbach, L. J., & Snow, R. E. (1977). *Aptitudes and instructional methods: A handbook for research on instruction.* New York: Irvington.

Cullinan, D., Lloyd, J., & Epstein, M. H. (1981). Strategy training: A structured approach to arithmetic instruction. *Exceptional Education Quarterly, 2,* 41–49.

Cummins, J. (1984). *Bilingualism and special education: Issues in assessment and pedagogy.* San Diego, CA: College Hill.

346 References

Curtis, M. J. (2002, November). *The changing face of school psychology: Past, present and future.* Webcast presentation at the Future of School Psychology Conference, Indianapolis. Retrieved March 4, 2004, from *www.indiana.edu/~futures/presentations.html.*

Curtis, M. J., Castillo, & Cohen, R. M. (2008). Best practices in system-level change. In A. Thomas & J. Grimes (Eds.), *Best practices in school psychology V* (pp. 887–901). Bethesda, MD: National Association of School Psychologists.

Curtis, M. J., Grier, J. E. C., & Hunley, S. A. (2003). The changing face of school psychology: Trends in data and projections for the future. *School Psychology Quarterly, 18,* 409–430.

Curtis, M. J., Grier, J. E. C., & Hunley, S. A. (2004). The changing face of school psychology: Trends in data and projections for the future. *School Psychology Review, 33,* 49–66.

Curtis, M. J., Hunley, S. A., & Grier, E. C. (2004). The status of school psychology: Implications of a major personnel shortage. *Psychology in the Schools, 41,* 431–442.

Curtis, M. J., Hunley, S. A., Walker, K. J., & Baker, A. C. (1999). Demographic characteristics and professional practices in school psychology. *School Psychology Review, 28,* 104–116.

Curtis, M. J., Lopez, A. D., Batsche, G. M., Minch, D., & Abshier, D. (2007, March). *Status report on school psychology: A national perspective.* Paper presented at the annual convention of the National Association of School Psychologists, New York.

Curtis, M. J., Lopez, A. D., Batsche, G. M., & Smith, J. C. (2006, March). *School psychology 2005: A national perspective.* Paper presented at the annual meeting of the National Association of School Psychologists, Anaheim, CA.

Curtis, M. J., Lopez, A. D., Castillo, J. M., Batsche, G. M., Minch, D., & Smith, J. C. (2008). The status of school psychology: Demographic characteristics, employment conditions, professional practices, and continuing professional development. *Communiqué, 36*(5), 27–29. Retrieved June 25, 2010, from *www.nasponline.org/publications/cq/index_xml.aspx?vol=36&issue=5.*

Curtis, M. J., & Stollar, S. A. (2002). Best practices in system-level change. In A. Thomas & J. Grimes (Eds.), *Best practices in school psychology IV* (pp. 223–234). Bethesda, MD: National Association of School Psychologists.

Daly, B. D. (2007). *Training programs in school psychology and their relation to professional practice.* Unpublished doctoral dissertation, University at Buffalo.

Daly, E. J., Barnett, D. W., Kupzyk, S., Hofstadter, K. L., & Barkley, E. (2010). Summarizing, evaluating, and drawing inferences from intervention data. In G. Gimpel Peacock, R. A. Ervin, E. J. Daly, & K. W. Merrell (Eds.), *Practical handbook of school psychology: Effective practices for the 21st century* (pp. 497–512). New York: Guilford Press.

Daly, E. J., Hofstadter, K. L., Martinez, R. S., & Andersen, M. (2010). Selecting academic interventions for individual students. In G. Gimpel Peacock, R. A. Ervin, E. J. Daly, & K. W. Merrell (Eds.), *Practical handbook of school psychology: Effective practices for the 21st century* (pp. 115–134). New York: Guilford Press.

Daly, E. J., III, Lentz, F. E., & Boyer, J. (1996). The instructional hierarchy: A conceptual model for understanding the effective components of reading interventions. *School Psychology Quarterly, 11,* 369–386.

Daly, E. J., III, Witt, J. C., Martens, B. K., & Dool, E. J. (1997). A model for conducting a functional analysis of academic performance problems. *School Psychology Review, 26,* 554–574.

Dana, R. H. (1993). *Multicultural assessment perspectives for professional psychology.* Boston: Allyn & Bacon.

Daniel R. R. v. State Board of Education, 874 F. 2d 1035 (5th Cir. 1989).

David-Ferdon, C., & Kaslow, N. J. (2008). Evidence-based psychosocial treatments for child and adolescent depression. *Journal of Clinical Child and Adolescent Psychology, 37,* 62–104.

Dawson, M., Cummings, J. A., Harrison, P. L., Short, R. J., Gorin, S., & Palomares, R. (2003). The 2002 multisite conference on the future of school psychology: Next steps. *School Psychology Quarterly, 18,* 497–509.

Dawson, M., Cummings, J. A., Harrison, P. L., Short, R. J., Gorin, S., & Palomares, R. (2004). The 2002 multisite conference on the future of school psychology: Next steps. *School Psychology Review, 33,* 115–125.

DeAvila, E., & Duncan, S. (2005). *Language assessment scales.* New York: McGraw-Hill.

deHirsch, K., Jansky, J. J., & Langford, W. S. (1966). *Predicting reading failure.* New York: Harper & Row.

Demaray, M. K., Carlson, J. S., & Hodgson, K. K. (2003). Assistant professors of school psychology: A national survey of program directors and job applicants. *Psychology in the Schools, 40,* 691–698.

Deno, S. L. (1985). Curriculum-based measurement: The emerging alternative. *Exceptional children, 52,* 219–232.

Deno, S. L. (1986). Formative evaluation of individual student programs: A new role for school psychologists. *School Psychology Review, 15,* 358–374.

Deno, S. L. (2002). Problem-solving as "best practice." In A. Thomas & J. Grimes (Eds.), *Best practices in school psychology IV* (Vol. 1, pp. 37–55). Bethesda, MD: National Association of School Psychologists.

Deno, S. L. (2003). Developments in curriculum-based measurement. *Journal of Special Education, 37,* 184–192.

Deno, S. L., Espin, C. A., & Fuchs, L. S. (2002). Evaluation strategies for preventing and remediating basic skill deficits. In M. R. Shinn, H. M. Walker, & G. Stoner (Eds.), *Interventions for academic and behavior problems: II. Preventive and remedial approaches* (pp. 213–242). Bethesda, MD: National Association of School Psychologists.

Derry, S. J., & Murphy, D. A. (1986). Designing systems that train learning ability: From theory to practice. *Review of Educational Research, 56,* 1–39.

Deshler, D. D., & Schumaker, J. B. (1986). Learning strategies: An instructional alternative for low-achieving adolescents. *Exceptional Children, 52,* 583–590.

Dettmer, P., Thurston, L. P., & Dyck, N. (2005). *Consultation, collaboration, and teamwork for students with special needs* (5th ed.). Boston: Pearson Education.

DeVries v. Fairfax County School Board, 882 F.2d 876 (4th circuit, 1989).

Doll, B., & Lyon, M. A. (1998). Risk and resilience: Implications for the delivery of educational and mental health services in schools. *School Psychology Review, 27,* 348–363.

Dougherty, A. M. (2009). *Psychological consultation and collaboration in school and community settings* (5th ed.). Belmont, CA: Brooks Cole/Cengage Learning.

Dowdy, E., Mays, K. L., Kamphaus, R. W., & Reynolds, C. R. (2009). Roles of diagnosis and classification in school psychology. In C. R. Reynolds & T. B. Gutkin (Eds.), *Handbook of school psychology* (4th ed., pp. 191–209). New York: Wiley.

Drum, D. J., & Figler, H. E. (1973). *Outreach in counselling: Applying the growth and prevention model in schools and colleges.* Oxford, UK: Intext Educational.

Dunn, R. S. (1979). Learning—A matter of style. *Educational Leadership, 36,* 430–432.

DuPaul, G. J., Barkley, R. A., & Connor, D. F. (1998). Stimulants. In R. A. Barkley, *Attention-deficit hyperactivity disorder: A handbook for diagnosis and treatment* (2nd ed., pp. 510–551). New York: Guilford Press.

DuPaul, G. J., & Stoner, G. (2003). *ADHD in the schools: Assessment and intervention strategies* (2nd ed.). New York: Guilford Press.

DuPaul, G. J., Stoner, G., & O'Reilly, M. J. (2008). Best practices in classroom interventions for attention problems. In A. Thomas & J. Grimes (Eds.), *Best practices in school psychology V* (pp. 1421–1438). Bethesda, MD: National Association of School Psychologists.

Durlak, J. A., & Weissberg, R. P. (2007). *The impact of after-school programs that promote personal and social skills.* Chicago: Collaborative for Academic, Social, and Emotional Learning. Retrieved November 17, 2010, from *www.casel.org/downloads/ASP_Full.pdf.*

Durlak, J. A., Weissberg, R. P., Dymnicki, A. B., Taylor, R. D., & Schellinger, K. B. (2011). The impact of enhancing students' social and emotional learning: A meta-analysis of school-based universal interventions. *Child Development, 82,* 405–432.

Earl, L., & Fullan, M. (2002). Using data in leadership for learning. *Cambridge Journal of Education, 33,* 383–394.

Eckert, T. L., Shapiro, E. S., & Lutz, J. G. (1995). Teachers' acceptability of alternative psychoeducational measures: The acceptability of curriculum-based assessment. *School Psychology Review, 24,* 497–511.

Edelstein, B. A., & Michelson, L. (Eds.). (1986). *Handbook of prevention.* New York: Plenum.

Elias, M. J., Zins, J. E., Graczyk, P. A., & Weissberg, R. P. (2003). Implementation, sustainability, and scaling up of social-emotional and academic innovations in public schools. *School Psychology Review, 32,* 303–319.

Elliot, C. D. (2007). *Differential Ability Scales* (2nd ed.). San Antonio, TX: Harcourt Assessment.

Engelman, S. (1997). Theory of mastery and acceleration. In J. W. Lloyd, E. J. Kame'enui, & D. Chard (Eds.), *Issues in educating students with disabilities* (pp. 177–195). Mahwah, NJ: Erlbaum.

Epps, S., Ysseldyke, J., & McGue, M. (1984). Differentiating LD and non-LD students: "I know one when I see one." *Learning Disability Quarterly, 7,* 89–101.

Ern, G. S., Head, K., & Anderson, S. (2009). School psychologists as instructional and behavioral coaches: A natural fit. *Communiqué, 38*(1). Retrieved July 5, 2010, from *www.nasponline.org/publications/cq/mocq381coaches.aspx.*

Ervin, R. A., Gimpel Peacock, G., & Merrell, K. W. (2010). The school psychologist as a problem-solver in the 21st century: Rationale and role definition. In G. Gimpel Peacock, R. A. Ervin, E. J. Daly, & K. W. Merrell (Eds.), *Practical handbook of school psychology: Effective practices for the 21st century* (pp. 3–12). New York: Guilford Press.

Eyberg, S. M., Nelson, M. M., & Boggs, S. R. (2008). Evidence-based psychosocial treatments for children and adolescents with disruptive behavior. *Journal of Clinical Child and Adolescent Psychology, 37,* 215–237.

Ezpeleta, L., Domenech, J. M., & Angold, A. (2006). A comparison of pure and comorbid CD/ODD and depression. *Journal of Child Psychology and Psychiatry, 47,* 704–712.

Fagan, T. K. (1995). Trends in the history of school psychology in the United States. In A. Thomas & J. Grimes (Eds.), *Best practices in school psychology III* (pp. 59–67). Washington, DC: National Association of School Psychologists.

Fagan, T. K. (2002). Trends in the history of school psychology in the United States. In A. Thomas & J. Grimes (Eds.), *Best practices in school psychology IV* (pp. 209–221). Bethesda, MD: National Association of School Psychologists.

Fagan, T. K. (2008). Trends in the history of school psychology in the United States. In A. Thomas & J. Grimes (Eds.), *Best practices in school psychology V* (pp. 2069–2085). Bethesda, MD: National Association of School Psychologists.

Fagan, T. K., & Wells, P. D. (2000). History and status of school psychology accreditation in the United States. *School Psychology Review, 29,* 28–58.

Fagan, T. K., & Wise, P. S. (1994). *School psychology: Past, present, and future.* White Plains, NY: Longman.

Fagan, T. K., & Wise, P. S. (2000). *School psychology: Past, present, and future* (2nd ed.). Bethesda, MA: National Association of School Psychologists.

Fagan, T. K., & Wise, P. S. (2007). *School psychology: Past, present, and future* (3rd ed.). Bethesda, MA: National Association of School Psychologists.

Faraone, S. V., Biederman, J., Morley, C. P., & Spencer, T. J. (2008). Effect of stimulants on height and weight: A review of the literature. *Journal of the American Academy of Child & Adolescent Psychiatry, 47*(9), 994–1009.

Felton, R. H., & Pepper, P. P. (1995). Early identification of phonological deficits in kindergarten and early elementary children at risk for reading disability. *School Psychology Review, 24,* 405–414.

Ferritor, D. C., Buckholt, D., Hamblin, R. L., & Smith, L. (1972). The noneffects of contingent reinforcement for attending behavior on work accomplished. *Journal of Applied Behavior Analysis, 5,* 7–17.

Finger, M. S., & Rand, K. L. (2003). Addressing validity concerns in clinical psychology research. In M. C. Roberts & S. S. Ilardi (Eds.), *Handbook of research methods in clinical psychology* (pp. 13–30). Malden, MA: Blackwell.

Fireoved, R., & Cancelleri, R. (1985). What training programs need to emphasize: Notes from the field. *Trainer's Forum, 5*(1), 4–5.

Fitzpatrick, J. L., Sanders, J. R., & Worthen, B. R. (2004). *Program evaluation: Alternative approaches and practical guidelines* (3rd ed.). Boston: Allyn & Bacon.

Fletcher, J. M., Francis, D. J., Shaywitz, S. E., Lyon, G. R., Foorman, B. R., Stuebing, K. K., et al. (1998). Intelligent testing and the discrepancy model for children with learning disabilities. *Learning Disabilities Research and Practice, 13*, 186–203.

Fletcher, J. M., Shaywitz, S. E., Shankweiler, D. P., Katz, L., Liberman, I. Y., Fowler, A., et al. (1994). Cognitive profiles of reading disability: Comparisons of discrepancy and low achievement definitions. *Journal of Educational Psychology, 85*, 1–23.

Fletcher, J. M., & Vaughn, S. (2009a). Response to intervention: Preventing and remediating academic difficulties. *Child Development Perspectives, 3*, 30–37.

Fletcher, J. M., & Vaughn, S. (2009b). Response to intervention models as alternatives to traditional views of learning disabilities: Response to the commentaries. *Child Development Perspectives, 3*, 48–50.

Florence County School District Four v. Carter 510 U.S. 7 (1993).

Floyd, R. G. (2010). Assessment of cognitive abilities and cognitive processes. In G. Gimpel Peacock, R. A. Ervin, E. J. Daly, & K. W. Merrell (Eds.), *Practical handbook of school psychology: Effective practices for the 21st century* (pp. 48–66). New York: Guilford Press.

Food and Drug Administration. (2009). Communication about an ongoing safety review of stimulant medications used in children with attention-deficit/hyperactivity disorder (ADHD). Retrieved December 21, 2010, from *www.fda.gov/Drugs/DrugSafety/PostmarketDrugSafetyInformationforPatientsandProviders/DrugSafetyInformationforHeathcareProfessionals/ucm165858.htm.*

Forest Grove School District v. T.A.. 129 S.Ct. 2484 (2009),

Forness, S. T. (1970). Educational prescription for the school psychologist. *Journal of School Psychology, 8*, 96–98.

Forness, S. T. (2003a). Barriers to evidence-based treatment: Developmental psychopathology and the interdisciplinary disconnect in school mental health practice. *Journal of School Psychology, 41*, 61–67.

Forness, S. T. (2003b). Parting reflections on education of children with emotional or behavioral disorders. *Education and Treatment of Children, 26*, 320–324.

Forness, S. T., & Kavale, K. A. (2001). Reflections on the future of prevention. *Preventing School Failure, 45*, 75–81.

Francis, D. J., Fletcher, J. M., Stuebing, K. K., Lyon, G. R., Shaywitz, B. A., & Shaywitz, S. E. (2005). Psychometric approaches to the identification of LD: IQ and achievement scores are not sufficient. *Journal of Learning Disabilities, 38*, 98–108.

Frank, G. (1984). The Boulder model: History, rationale, and critique. *Professional Psychology: Research and Practice, 15*, 417–435.

Freeman, K. A. (2003). Single subject designs. In J. C. Thomas & M. Hersen (Eds.), *Understanding research in clinical and counseling psychology* (pp. 181–208). Mahwah, NJ: Erlbaum.

Friedman, R. M. (2003). Improving outcomes for students through the application of a public health model to school psychology: A commentary. *Journal of School Psychology, 41*, 69–75.

Friman, P. C., & Blum, N. (2002). Primary care behavioral pediatrics. In M. Hersen & W. Sledge (Eds.), *Encyclopedia of psychotherapy* (pp. 379–399). New York: Academic Press.

Frisby, C. L. (2009). *Cultural competence in school psychology: Established or elusive construct.* In T. B. Gutkin and C. R. Reynolds (Eds.), *Handbook of school psychology* (4th ed., pp. 855–885). New York: Wiley.

Fuchs, D., Fuchs, L. S., Harris, A. H., & Roberts, P. H. (1996). Bridging the research-to-practice gap with mainstream assistance teams: A cautionary tale. *School Psychology Quarterly, 11*, 244–266.

Fuchs, L. (2003). Assessing intervention responsiveness: Conceptual and technical issues. *Learning Disabilities Research & Practice, 18*, 172–186.

Fuchs, L. S., & Fuchs, D. (2009). On the importance of a unified model of responsiveness to intervention. *Child Development Perspectives, 3*, 41–43.

Fuchs, L. S., Fuchs, D., Hosp, M., & Jenkins, J. (2001). Oral reading fluency as an indicator of reading competence: A theoretical, empirical, and historical analysis. *Scientific Studies in Reading, 5*, 239–256.

Fullan, M. (2000). The three stories of education reform. *Phi Delta Kappan, 8*, 581–584.

Fullan, M., Bertani, A., & Quinn, J. (2004). New lessons for districtwide reform. *Educational Leadership, 4*, 42–46.

Gansle, K. A., & Noell, G. H. (2010). Assessment of skills in written expression within a problem-solving model. In G. Gimpel Peacock, R. A. Ervin, E. J. Daly, & K. W. Merrell (Eds.), *Practical handbook of school psychology: Effective practices for the 21st century* (pp. 99–114). New York: Guilford Press.

Gayer, H. L., Brown, M. B., Gridley, B. E., & Treloar, J. H. (2003). Predoctoral psychology intern selection: Does program type make a difference? *Social Behavior and Personality, 31*, 313–322.

Gersten, R., & Chard, D. (1999). Number sense: Rethinking arithmetic instruction for students with mathematical disabilities. *Journal of Special Education, 33*, 18–28.

Gersten, R., Chard, D., & Baker, S. (2000). Factors enhancing sustained use of research-based instructional practices. *Journal of Learning Disabilities, 33*(5), 445–457.

Gersten, R., Jordan, N. C., & Flojo, J. R. (2005). Early identification and interventions for students with mathematics difficulties. *Journal of Learning Disabilities, 38*, 293–304.

Gersten, R., Vaughn, S., Deshler, D., & Schiller, E. (1997). What we know about using research findings: Implications for improving special education practice. *Journal of Learning Disabilities, 30*, 466–476.

Gettinger, M., & Ball, C. (2008). Best practices in increasing academic engaged time. In A. Thomas & J. Grimes (Eds.), *Best practices in school psychology V* (pp. 1043–1057). Bethesda, MD: National Association of School Psychologists.

Gimpel Peacock, G., Ervin, R. A., Daly, E. J., & Merrell, K. W. (Eds.). (2010). *Practical handbook of school psychology: Effective practices for the 21st century.* New York: Guilford Press.

Glass, G. V. (1983). Effectiveness of special education. *Policy Studies Review, 2*, 65–78.

Glover, T. A., & Vaughn, S. (Eds.). (2010). *The promise of response to intervention: Evaluating current science and practice.* New York: Guilford Press.

Godber, Y. (2008). Best practices in program evaluation. In A. Thomas & J. Grimes (Eds.), *Best practices in school psychology V* (pp. 2193–2205). Bethesda, MD: National Association of School Psychologists.

Gollnick, D., & Chinn, C. (2009). *Multicultural education in a pluralistic society* (8th ed). Upper Saddle River, NJ: Prentice Hall.

Good, R. H., III, Gruba, J., & Kaminski, R. A. (2002). Best practices in using Dynamic Indicators of Basic Early Literacy Skills (DIBELS) in an outcomes-driven model. In A. Thomas & J. Grimes (Eds.), *Best practices in school psychology IV* (Vol. 1, pp. 699–720). Bethesda, MD: National Association of School Psychologists.

Good, R., & Kaminski, R. (1996). Assessment for instructional decisions: Toward a proactive/prevention model of decision-making for early literacy skills. *School Psychology Quarterly, 11*, 326–336.

Good, R. H., Simmons, D. C., & Smith, S. B. (1998). Effective academic interventions in the United States: Evaluating and enhancing the acquisition of early reading skills. *School Psychology Review, 27*, 740–753.

Good, T. L., & Brophy, J. E. (1994). *Looking in classrooms* (6th ed.). New York: HarperCollins.

Good, T. L., & Brophy, J. E. (2007). *Looking into classrooms* (10th ed.). Boston: Allyn & Bacon.

Gopaul-McNicol, S. A. (1997). A theoretical framework for training monolingual school psychologists to work with multilingual/multicultural children: An exploration of the major competencies. *Psychology in the Schools, 34*, 17–29.

Gould, M. S., Walsh, B., Munfakh, J., Kleinman, M., Duan, N., Olfson, M., et al. (2009). Sudden death and use of stimulant medications in youths. *The American Journal of Psychiatry, 166*(9), 992–1001.

Graham, S., Harris, K. R., MacArthur, C. A., & Schwartz, S. (1991). Writing and writing instruction for students with learning disabilities: Review of a research program. *Learning Disabilities Quarterly, 14*, 89–114.

Gray, S. W. (1963). *The psychologist in the schools.* New York: Holt, Rinehart & Winston.

Greenberg, M. T. (2010). School-based prevention: Current status and future challenges. *Effective Education, 2*, 27–52.

Greenberg, M. T., Weissberg, R. P., O'Brien, M. U., Zins, J. E., Fredericks, L., Resnik, H., et al. (2003). Enhancing school-based prevention and youth development through coordinated social, emotional, and academic learning. *American Psychologist, 58*, 466–474.

Greene, M. M. (2003). Program evaluation. In J. C. Thomas & M. Hersen (Eds.), *Understanding research in clinical and counseling psychology* (pp. 209–242). Mahwah, NJ: Erlbaum.

Greenhill, L. L., Halperin, J. M., & Abikoff, H. (1999). Stimulant medications. *Journal of the American Academy of Child & Adolescent Psychiatry, 38*, 503–512.

Greenhill, L. L., Swanson, J. M., Vitiello, B., Davies, M., Clevenger, W., Wu, M., et al. (2001). Impairment and deportment responses to different methylphenidate doses in children with ADHD: The MTA titration trial. *Journal of the American Academy of Child & Adolescent Psychiatry, 40*, 180–187.

Gresham, F. M., & Noell, G. H. (1999). A functional model of assessment and treatment as a foundation of special education. In D. J. Reschly, W. D. Tilly, & J. Grimes (Eds.), *Special education in transition: Functional assessment and noncategorical programming* (pp. 49–80). Longmont, CO: Sopris West.

Gresham, F. M., Watson, T. S., & Skinner, C. H. (2001). Functional behavioral assessment: Principles, procedures, and future directions. *School Psychology Review, 30*, 156–172.

Grimes, J., & Tilly, D. W. (1996). Policy and process: Means to lasting educational change. *School Psychology Review, 25*(4), 465–476.

Grossen, B., Caros, J., Carnine, D., Davis, B., Deshler, D., Schumaker, J., et al. (2002). Big ideas (plus a little effort) produce big results. *Teaching Exceptional Children, 34*, 70–73.

Guiberson, M. (2009). Hispanic representation in special education: Patterns and implications. *Preventing School Failure, 53*(3), 167–176.

Gutman, L. M., McLoyd, V. C., & Tokoyawa, T. (2005). Financial strain, neighborhood stress, parenting behaviors, and adolescent adjustment in urban African American families. *Journal of Research on Adolescence, 15*, 425–449.

Hale, J. B., Fiorello, C. A., Kavanagh, J. A., Holdnack, J. A., & Aloe, A. M. (2007). Is the demise of IQ interpretation justified? A response to special issue authors. *Applied Neuropsychology, 14*, 37–51.

Hall, G. E., & Hord, S. M. (2006). *Implementing change: Patterns, principles, and potholes.* Boston: Allyn & Bacon.

Hall, R. V., Lund, D. E., & Jackson, D. (1968). Effects of teacher attention on study behavior. *Journal of Applied Behavior Analysis, 1*, 1–12.

Halsell, M. A. (2002). Best practices in increasing cross-cultural competence. In A. Thomas & J. Grimes (Eds.), *Best practices in school psychology IV* (pp. 353–362). Bethesda, MD: National Association of School Psychologists.

Hammill, D. D., Pearson, N. A., & Weiderholt, J. L. (2009). *Comprehensive Test of Nonverbal Intelligence* (2nd ed.). Austin, TX: PRO-ED.

Hanf, C. (1969). *A two-stage program for modifying maternal controlling during mother–child (m-c) interaction.* Paper presented at the annual meeting of the Western Psychological Association, Vancouver, BC.

Haring, N. G., Lovitt, T. C., Eaton, M. D., & Hansen, C. L. (1978). *The fourth R: Research in the classroom.* Columbus, OH: Merrill.

Harris-Murri, N., King, K., & Rostenberg, D. (2006). Reducing disproportionate minority representation in special education programs for students with emotional disturbances: Toward a culturally responsive response to intervention model. *Education and Treatment of Children, 29*(4), 779–799.

Hart, B., & Risley, T. R. (1995). *Meaningful differences in the everyday experience of young American children*. Baltimore, MD: Brookes.

Hartman v. Loudoun County Board of Education 118 F.3d. 996 (4th Cir. 1997).

Harvey, V. (2002). Best practices in teaching study skills. In A. Thomas & J. Grimes (Eds.), *Best practices in school psychology IV* (pp. 831–849). Bethesda, MD: National Association of School Psychologists.

Hawkins, R. O., Barnett, D. W., Morrison, J. Q., & Musti-Rao, S. (2010). Choosing targets for assessment and intervention. In G. Gimpel Peacock, R. A. Ervin, E. J. Daly, & K. W. Merrell (Eds.), *Practical handbook of school psychology: Effective practices for the 21st century* (pp. 13–30). New York: Guilford Press.

Hayes, S. C., & Follette, W. C. (1992). Can functional analysis provide a substitute for syndromal classification? *Behavioral Assessment, 14,* 345–365.

Herrnstein, R. J., & Murray, C. (1994). *The bell curve: Intelligence and class structure in American life.* New York: Free Press.

Hildreth, G. H. (1930). *Psychological service for school problems.* Yonkers-on-Hudson, NY: World Book Co.

Hintze, J. M., & Marcotte, A. M. (2010). Student assessment and data-based decision making. In T. A. Glover & S. Vaughn (Eds.), *The promise of response to intervention: Evaluating current science and practice* (pp. 57–77). New York: Guilford Press.

Hirst, W. E. (1963). Know your school psychologist. *School Psychologist, 33*(4), 1.

History of American Education Web Project. (2010). *Progressive period of American education.* Retrieved April 8, 2010, from *www.nd.edu/~rbarger/www7.*

Hoagwood, K., & Johnson, J. (2003). School psychology: A public health framework: I. From evidence-based practices to evidence-based policies. *Journal of School Psychology, 41,* 3–21.

Hoff, K. E., & Sawka-Miller, K. D. (2010). Self-management interventions. In G. Gimpel Peacock, R. A. Ervin, E. J. Daly, & K. W. Merrell (Eds.), *Practical handbook of school psychology: Effective practices for the 21st century* (pp. 337–352). New York: Guilford Press.

Hojnoski, R., Morrison, R., Brown, M., & Matthews, W. (2006). Projective test use among school psychologists: A survey and critique. *Journal of Psychoeducational Assessment, 24,* 145–159.

Hollingworth, L. S. (1933). Psychological service for public schools. *Teachers College Record, 34,* 368–379.

Hood, K. K., & Eyberg, S. M. (2003). Outcomes of parent-child interaction therapy: Mothers' reports of maintenance three to six years after treatment. *Journal of Clinical Child and Adolescent Psychology, 32,* 419–429.

Hoskyn, M., & Swanson, H. L. (2000). Cognitive processing of low achievers and children with reading disabilities: A selective meta-analytic review of the published literature. *School Psychology Review, 29,* 102–119.

Hosp, M. K., Hosp, J. L., & Howell, K. W. (2007). *The ABCs of CBM: A practical guide to curriculum-base measurement.* New York: Guilford Press.

Hosp, M. K., & MacConnell, K. L. (2008). Best practices in curriculum-based evaluation in early reading. In A. Thomas & J. Grimes (Eds.), *Best practices in school psychology V* (pp. 377–396). Bethesda, MD: National Association of School Psychologists.

Hosp, J. L., & Reschly, D. J. (2002). Regional differences in school psychology practice. *School Psychology Review, 31,* 11–29.

Howell, K. W., & Kelley, B. (2002). Curriculum clarification, lesson design, and delivery. In K. L. Lane, F. M. Gresham, & T. O'Shaughnessy (Eds.), *Academic and social–behavioral interventions for students with or at-risk for emotional and behavioral disorders* (pp. 55–73). Boston: Allyn & Bacon.

Howell, K. W., & Nolet, V. (2000). *Curriculum-based evaluation: Teaching and decision making* (3rd ed.). Belmont, CA: Wadsworth.

Howell, K. W., & Schumann, J. (2010). Proactive strategies for promoting learning. In G. Gimpel Peacock, R. A. Ervin, E. J. Daly, & K. W. Merrell (Eds.), *Practical handbook of school psychology: Effective practices for the 21st century* (pp. 235–253). New York: Guilford Press.

Hughes, J. N., & Baker, D. B. (1990). *The Clinical Child Interview.* New York: Guilford Press.

Hunley, S. (2004). The NCSP challenge. *Communique, 32*(5), 35.

Hunter, L. (2003). School psychology: A public health framework: III. Managing disruptive behavior in schools: The value of a public health and evidence-based perspective. *Journal of School Psychology, 41,* 39–59.

Ibraham, F. A., Roysircar-Sodowsky, G., & Ohnishi, H. (2001). Worldview: Recent developments and needed directions. In J. G. Ponterotto, J. M. Casas, L. A. Suzuki, & C. M. Alexander (Eds.), *Handbook of multicultural counseling* (pp. 425–456). Thousand Oaks, CA: Sage.

Ingraham, C. L. (2000). Consultation through a multicultural lens: Multicultural and cross-cultural consultation in schools. *School Psychology Review, 29,* 320–343.

Irving Independent School District v. Tatro, 468 U.S. 883 (1984).

Jacob, S., & Hartshorne, T. S. (2007). *Ethics and law for school psychologists* (5th ed.). Hoboken, NJ: Wiley.

Jacobson, N. S., & Truax, P. (1991). Clinical significance: A statistical approach to defining meaningful clinical change in psychotherapy research. *Journal of Consulting and Clinical Psychology, 59,* 12–19.

Jacob-Timm, S. (1999). Ethically challenging situations encountered by school psychologists. *Psychology in the Schools, 36,* 205–217.

Jaeger, P. T., & Bowman, C. A. (2002). *Disability matters: Legal and pedagogical issues of disability in education.* Westport, CT: Bergin & Garvey.

Jensen, P. S., Arnold, L., Swanson, J. M., Vitiello, B., Abikoff, H. B., Greenhill, L. L., et al. (2007). 3-year follow-up of the NIMH MTA study. *Journal of the American Academy of Child & Adolescent Psychiatry, 46*(8), 989–1002.

Jensen, P. S., Hinshaw, S. P., Kraemer, H. C., Lenora, N., Newcorn, J. H., Abikoff, H. B., et al. (2001). ADHD comorbidity findings from the MTA study: Comparing comorbid subgroups. *Journal of the American Academy of Child & Adolescent Psychiatry, 40,* 147–158.

Jimerson, S. R., Stewart, K., Skokut, M., Cardenas, S., & Malone, H. (2009). How many school psychologists are there in each country of the world? International estimates of school psychologists and school psychologist-to-student ratios. *School Psychology International, 30,* 555–567.

J. L. and M. L. and their minor daughter K. L. v. Mercer Island School District, WD WA (2006).

J. L., M. L., K. L., their minor daughter, v. Mercer Island School District, 575 F.3d 1025 (9th Cir. 2009).

Johnson, D., & Myklebust, H. (1967). *Learning disabilities: Educational principles and practices.* New York: Grune & Stratton.

Johnson, M. B., Whitman, T. L., & Johnson, M. (1980). Teaching addition and subtraction to mentally retarded children: A self-instructional program. *Applied Research in Mental Retardation, 1,* 141–160.

Joint Committee on Testing Practices. (2004). *Code of fair testing practices in education.* Washington, DC: Author. Retrieved September 16, 2010, from *www.apa.org/science/programs/testing/fair-testing.pdf.*

Jones, K. M., & Wickstrom, K. F. (2010). Using functional assessment to select behavioral interventions. In G. Gimpel Peacock, R. A. Ervin, E. J. Daly, & Merrell, K. W. (Eds.), *Practical handbook of school psychology: Effective practices for the 21st century* (pp. 192–212). New York: Guilford Press.

Jones, K. M., Wickstrom, K. F., & Daly, E. J. (2008). Best practices in the brief assessment of reading concerns. In A. Thomas & J. Grimes (Eds.), *Best practices in school psychology V* (pp. 489–501). Bethesda, MD: National Association of School Psychologists.

Joseph, L. M. (2008). Best practices on interventions for students with reading problems. In A. Thomas & J. Grimes (Eds.), *Best practices in school psychology V* (pp. 1163–1180). Bethesda, MD: National Association of School Psychologists.

Juel, C. (1988). Learning to read and write: A longitudinal study of 54 children from first through fourth grades. *Journal of Educational Psychology, 80,* 437–447.

Kame'enui, E., & Carnine, D. (Eds.). (2001). *Effective teaching strategies that accommodate diverse learners.* Columbus, OH: Merrill.

Kaminski, J. W., Valle, L. A., Filene, J. H., & Boyle, C. L. (2006). A meta-analytic review of components associated with parent training program effectiveness. *Journal of Abnormal Child Psychology, 36,* 567–589.

Kaminski, R., Cummings, K. D., Powell-Smith, K. A., & Good, R. H. (2008). Best practices in using dynamic indicators of basic early literacy skills for formative assessment and evaluation. In A. Thomas & J. Grimes (Eds.), *Best practices in school psychology V* (pp. 1181–1204). Bethesda, MD: National Association of School Psychologists.

Kampwirth, T. J., & Bates, M. (1980). Modality preference and teaching method: A review of research. *Academic Therapy, 15,* 597–605.

Kaufman, A. S., & Kaufman, N. L. (2004a). *Kaufman Assessment Battery for Children–Second edition.* Circle Pines, MN: American Guidance Service.

Kaufman, A. S., & Kaufman, N. L. (2004b). *Kaufman Test of Educational Achievement* (2nd ed.). Circle Pines, MN: American Guidance Service.

Kaufman, J. M. (2010). *The tragicomedy of public education: Laughing, crying, thinking, fixing.* Verona, WI: Attainment.

Kavale, K. A. (2005). Effective intervention for students with specific learning disability: The nature of special education. *Learning Disabilities, 13,* 127–138.

Kavale, K. A., & Forness, S. R. (1987). Substance over style: Assessing the efficacy of modality testing and teaching. *Exceptional Children, 54,* 228–239.

Kavale, K. A., Kauffman, J.M., Bachmeier, & LeFever, G. B. (2008). Response-to-intervention: Separating the rhetoric of self-congratulation from the reality of specific learning disability identification. *Learning Disability Quarterly, 31,* 135–150.

Kavale, K. A., & Spaulding, L. S. (2008). Is response to intervention good policy for specific learning disability? *Learning Disabilities Research & Practice, 23,* 169–179.

Kazdin, A. E. (1997). Parent management training: Evidence, outcomes, and issues. *Journal of the American Academy of Child and Adolescent Psychiatry, 36,* 1349–1356.

Kazdin, A. E. (2003a). Psychotherapy for children and adolescents. *Annual Reviews in Psychology, 54,* 253–276.

Kazdin, A. E. (2003b). *Research design in clinical psychology* (4th ed.). Boston: Allyn & Bacon.

Kazdin, A. E. (1999). The meanings and measurement of clinical significance. *Journal of Consulting and Clinical Psychology, 67,* 332–339.

Kazdin, A. E. (2000). *Psychotherapy for children and adolescents: Directions for research and practice.* New York: Oxford University Press.

Kazdin, A. E. (2001). *Behavior modification in applied settings* (6th ed.). Belmont, CA: Wadsworth.

Kazdin, A. E. (2004). Psychotherapy for children and adolescents. In M. J. Lambert (Ed.), *Bergin and Garfield's handbook of psychotherapy and behavior change* (5th ed., pp. 543–589). New York: Wiley.

Kazdin, A. E. (2008a). Evidence-based treatments and delivery of psychological services: Shifting our emphases to increase impact. *Psychological Services, 5,* 201–215.

Kazdin, A. E. (2008b). *The Kazdin method for parenting the defiant child: With no pills, no therapy, no contest of wills.* Boston: Houghton Mifflin.

Kazdin, A. E., & Whitley, M. K. (2006). Comorbidity, case complexity, and effects of evidence-based treatment for children referred for disruptive behavior. *Journal of Consulting and Clinical Psychology, 74,* 455–467.

Keith, T. Z. (2008). Best practices in using and conducting research in applied settings. In A. Thomas & J. Grimes (Eds.), *Best practices in school psychology V* (pp. 2165–2175). Bethesda, MD: National Association of School Psychologists.

Kendall, P. C., & Hedtke, K. A. (2006a). *Cognitive-behavioral therapy for anxious children: Therapist manual* (3rd ed.). Ardmore, PA: Workbook.

Kendall, P. C., & Hedtke, K. A. (2006b). *The Coping Cat workbook* (2nd ed.). Ardmore, PA: Workbook.

Kendall, P. C., Panichelli-Mindel, S. M., Sugarman, A., & Callahan, S. A. (1997). Exposure to child anxiety: Theory, research, and practice. *Clinical Psychology: Science and Practice, 4,* 724–730.

Kendall, P. C., & Suveg, C. (2006). Treating anxiety disorders in youth. In P. C. Kendall (Ed.) *Child and adolescent therapy: Cognitive behavioral procedures* (3rd ed., pp. 243–294). New York: Guilford Press.

Kenyon, P. (1999). *What would you do? An ethical case workbook for human service professionals.* Pacific Grove, CA: Brooks-Cole.

Kerr, M. M., & Nelson, C. M. (2006). *Strategies for managing behavior problems in the classroom* (5th ed.). Upper Saddle River, NJ: Merrill/Prentice Hall.

Kim, B. S. K., & Abreu, J. M. (2001). Acculturation measurement. In J. G. Ponterotto, J. M. Casas, L. A. Suzuki, & C. M. Alexander (Eds.), *Handbook of multicultural counseling* (pp. 394–424). Thousand Oaks, CA: Sage.

Kimble, G. A. (1984). Psychology's two cultures. *American Psychologist, 39,* 833–839.

Kirk, S. A., McCarthy, J. J., & Kirk, W. D. (1968). *The Illinois Test of Psycholinguistic Abilities* (rev. ed.). Urbana: University of Illinois.

Klinger, J. K., Artiles, A. J., Kosleski, E., Harry, B., Zion, S., Tate, W., et al. (2005). Addressing the disproportionate representation of culturally and linguistically diverse students in special education through culturally responsive educational systems. *Education Policy Analysis Archives, 13*(38), 1–43.

Klinger, J. K., & Edwards, P. A. (2006). Cultural considerations with response to intervention models. *Reading Research Quarterly, 41*(1), 108–117.

Knoff, H. M. (2002). Best practices in facilitating school reform, organizational change, and strategic planning. In A. Thomas & J. Grimes (Eds.), *Best practices in school psychology IV* (Vol. 1, pp. 235–253). Bethesda, MD: National Association of School Psychologists.

Knoff, H. M. (2008). Best practices in strategic planning, organizational development, and school effectiveness. In A. Thomas & J. Grimes (Eds.), *Best practices in school psychology V* (pp. 903–916). Bethesda, MD: National Association of School Psychologists.

Kohn, A. (1993). *Punished by rewards: The trouble with gold stars, incentive plans, A's, praise, and other bribes.* Boston: Houghton Mifflin.

Kounin, J. (1970). *Discipline and group management in classrooms.* New York: Holt, Rinehart, & Winston.

Kovacs, M. (1992). *The Children's Depression Inventory.* North Tonawanda, NY: Multi-Health Systems.

Kratochwill, T. R. (2007). Preparing psychologists for evidence-based school practice: Lessons learned and challenges ahead. *American Psychologist, 62,* 829–843.

Kratochwill, T. R. (2008). Best practices in school-based problem-solving consultation: Applications in prevention and intervention systems. In A. Thomas & J. Grimes (Eds.), *Best practices in school psychology V* (pp. 1673–1686). Bethesda, MD: National Association of School Psychologists.

Kratochwill, T. R., & Bergan, J. R. (1990). *Behavioral consultation in applied settings: An individual guide.* New York: Plenum Press.

Kratochwill, T. R., & Shernoff, E. S. (2004). Evidence-based practice: Promoting evidence based interventions in school psychology. *School Psychology Review, 33,* 34–48.

Kratochwill, T. R., & Stoiber, K. C. (2000a). Diversifying theory and science: Expanding boundaries of empirically supported interventions in schools. *Journal of School Psychology, 38,* 349–358.

Kratochwill, T. R., & Stoiber, K. C. (2000b). Empirically supported interventions and school psychology: Conceptual and practical issues: Part II. *School Psychology Quarterly, 15,* 233–253.

Kratochwill, T. R., & Stoiber, K. C. (2002). Evidence-based interventions in school psychology: Conceptual foundations of the Procedural Coding Manual of Division 16 and the Society for the Study of School Psychology Task Force. *School Psychology Quarterly, 17,* 341–389.

Kryzanowski, J., & Carnine, D. W. (1980). Effects of massed versus spaced formats in teaching sound/symbol correspondences to young children. *Journal of Reading Behavior, 12,* 225–230.

LaBerge, D., & Samuels, S. J. (1974). Toward a theory of automatic information processing in reading. *Cognitive Psychology, 6*, 293–323.

Larson, J. P. (2008). *The impact of university training, national training standards, and educational legislation on the role of school psychologists.* Unpublished doctoral dissertation, University of South Dakota.

Lau, M. Y., & Blatchley, L. A. (2009). A comprehensive, multidimensional approach to assessment of culturally and linguistically diverse students. In J. M. Jones (Ed.), *The psychology of multiculturalism in the schools: A primer for practice, training, and research* (pp. 139–171). Bethesda, MD: National Association of School Psychologists.

L.B., and J.B., on behalf of K. B. v. Nebo School District 379 F. 3d 966 (10th Cir. 2004).

Leahey, T. H. (1987). *A history of modern psychology: Main currents in psychological thought* (2nd ed.). Englewood Cliffs, NJ: Prentice Hall.

Learning Disabilities Association of America. (2010, February). *The Learning Disability Association of America's white paper on evaluation, identification, and eligibility criteria for students with specific learning disabilities.* Pittsburgh, PA: Author.

Lentz, B. K. (1992). Self-managed learning strategy systems for children and youth. *School Psychology Review, 21*, 211–228.

Lentz, F. E., & Shapiro, E. S. (1985). Behavioral school psychology: A conceptual model for the delivery of psychological services. In T. Kratochwill (Ed.), *Advances in school psychology* (Vol. 5, pp. 191–221). Hillsdale, NJ: Erlbaum.

Lewinsohn, P. M., & Clarke, G. N. (1999). Psychosocial treatments for adolescent depression. *Clinical Psychology Review, 19*, 329–342.

Linan-Thompson, S., & Vaughn, S. (2010). Evidence-based reading instruction: Developing and implementing reading programs at the core, supplemental, and intervention levels. In G. Gimpel Peacock, R. A. Ervin, E. J. Daly, & K. W. Merrell (Eds.), *Practical handbook of school psychology: Effective practices for the 21st century* (pp. 274–299). New York: Guilford Press.

Little, S. G., & Akin-Little, K. A. (2004). Academic school psychologists: Addressing the shortage. *Psychology in the Schools, 41*, 451–459.

Lopez, E. C. (2008). Best practices in working with school interpreters. In A. Thomas & J. Grimes (Eds.), *Best practices in school psychology V* (pp. 1751–1769). Bethesda, MD: National Association of School Psychologists.

Luckey, B. M. (1951, May). Duties of the school psychologist: Past, present and future. *Division of School Psychologists Newsletter,* pp. 4–10.

Lund, A. R., Reschly, D. J., & Martin, L. M. C. (1998). School psychology personnel needs: Correlates of current patterns and historical trends. *School Psychology Review, 27*, 106–120.

Luthar, S. S., & Cicchetti, D. (2000). The construct of resilience: Implications for interventions and social policies. *Development and Psychopathology, 12*, 857–885.

Lynam, D. R., Milich, R., Zimmerman, R., Novak, S. P., Logan, T. K., Martin, C., et al. (1999). Project DARE: No effects at 10-year follow-up. *Journal of Consulting and Clinical Psychology, 67*, 590–593.

Maag, J. W. (1990). Social skills training in schools. *Special Services in the Schools, 6*, 1–19.

Machek, G., & Nelson, J. (2010). School psychologists' perceptions regarding the practice of identifying reading disabilities: Cognitive assessment and response to intervention considerations. *Psychology in the Schools, 47*, 230–245.

Magary, J. F. (1967). Emerging viewpoints in school psychological services. In J. F. Magary (Ed.), *School psychological services in theory and practice: A handbook* (pp. 671–755). Englewood Cliffs, NJ: Prentice Hall.

March, J. S. (1997). *Multidimensional Anxiety Scale for Children.* North Tonawanda, NY: Multi-Health Systems.

Marcotte, A. M., & Hintze, J. M. (2010). Assessment of academic skills in reading within a problem-solving model. In G. Gimpel Peacock, R. A. Ervin, E. J. Daly, & K. W. Merrell (Eds.), *Practical handbook of school psychology: Effective practices for the 21st century* (pp. 67–85). New York: Guilford Press.

Markwardt, F. C. (1989). *Peabody Individual Achievement Test—Revised.* Circle Pines, MN: American Guidance Service.

Markwardt, F. C. (1997). *Peabody Individual Achievement Test—Revised: Normative update.* Circle Pines, MN: American Guidance Service.

Martines, D. (2003, Fall). Suggestions for training cross-cultural consultant school psychologists. *Trainer's Forum, 23,* 5–13.

Martines, D. (2008). *Multicultural school psychology competencies: A practical guide.* Thousand Oaks, CA: Sage.

Masten, A. S., & Coatsworth, J. D. (1998). The development of competence in favorable and unfavorable environments: Lessons from research on successful children. *American Psychologist, 53,* 205–220.

Mastropieri, M. A., Leinart, A., & Scruggs, T. E. (1999). Strategies to increase reading fluency. *Interventions in School and Clinic, 34,* 278–283.

Mastropieri, M. A., & Scruggs, T. E. (2009). *The inclusive classroom: Strategies for effective instruction* (4th ed.). Upper Saddle River, NJ: Prentice Hall.

Maughan, D. R., Christiansen, E., Jenson, W. R., Olympia, D., & Clark, E. (2005). Behavioral parent training as a treatment for externalizing behaviors and disruptive behavior disorders: A meta-analysis. *School Psychology Review, 34,* 267–286.

McArthur, D. S., & Roberts, D. E. (1982). *Roberts Apperception Test for Children.* Los Angeles: Western Psychological Services.

McDougal, J. L., Clonan, S. M., & Martens, B. K. (2000). Using organizational change procedures to promote the acceptability of prereferral intervention services: The school-based intervention team project. *School Psychology Quarterly, 15,* 149–171.

McGrew, K. S. (2009). CHC theory and the human cognitive abilities project: Standing on the shoulders of the giants of psychometric intelligence research. *Intelligence, 37,* 1–10.

McGrew, K. S., & Woodcock, R. W. (2001). *Technical manual: Woodcock-Johnson III.* Itasca, IL: Riverside.

McIntosh, K., Reinke, W. M., & Herman, K. C. (2010). Schoolwide analysis of data for social behavior problems: Assessing outcomes, selecting targets for intervention, and identifying need for support. In G. Gimpel Peacock, R. A. Ervin, E. J. Daly, & K. W. Merrell (Eds.), *Practical handbook of school psychology: Effective practices for the 21st century* (pp. 135–156). New York: Guilford Press.

McMahon, R. J., & Forehand, R. L. (2003). *Helping the noncompliant child: Family-based treatment for oppositional disorder* (2nd ed.). New York: Guilford Press.

McNeil, C. B., & Hembree-Kigin, T. L. (2010). *Parent-child interaction therapy* (2nd ed.). New York: Springer.

Meichenbaum, D. H., & Goodman, J. (1971). Training impulsive children to talk to themselves: A means of developing self-control. *Journal of Abnormal Psychology, 77,* 117–126.

Merrell, K. W. (2008). *Behavioral, social, and emotional assessment of children and adolescents* (3rd ed.). New York: Routledge/Taylor & Francis.

Merrell, K. W., & Buchanan, R. (2006). Intervention selection in school-based practice: Using public health models to enhance systems capacity of schools. *School Psychology Review, 35,* 167–180.

Merrell, K. W., & Gueldner, B. A. (2010). *Social and emotional learning in the classroom: Promoting mental health and academic success.* New York: Guilford Press.

Messick, S. (1995). Validity of psychological assessment: Validation inferences from persons' responses and performances as scientific inquiry into score meaning. *American Psychologist, 50,* 741–749.

Miller, D. C. (2008). Appendix VII – School psychology training programs. In A. Thomas & J. Grimes (Eds.), *Best practices in school psychology V* (pp. clv–cxcviii). Bethesda, MD: National Association of School Psychologists.

Miller, G., Giovenco, A., & Rentiers, K. A. (1987). Fostering comprehension monitoring in below average readers through self-instruction training. *Journal of Reading Behavior, 19,* 379–394.

Mills v. Board of Education of the District of Columbia 348 F. Supp. 866 (1972).

Molina, B. G., Hinshaw, S. P., Swanson, J. M., Arnold, L., Vitiello, B., Jensen, P. S., & et al. (2009). The MTA at 8 years: Prospective follow-up of children treated for combined-type ADHD in a multisite study. *Journal of the American Academy of Child & Adolescent Psychiatry, 48*(5), 484–500.

MTA Cooperative Group. (1999a). A 14–month randomized clinical trial of treatment strategies for attention-deficit/hyperactivity disorder. *Archives of General Psychiatry, 56,* 1073–1086.

MTA Cooperative Group. (1999b). Moderators and mediators of treatment response for children with attention-deficit/hyperactivity disorder: The multimodal treatment study of children with attention-deficit/hyperactivity disorder. *Archives of General Psychiatry, 56,* 1088–1096.

Muñoz-Sandoval, A. F., Cummins, J., Alvarado, C. G., & Ruef, M. L. (2000). *Bilingual Verbal Ability Tests (BVAT).* Itasca, IL: Riverside.

Muñoz-Sandoval, A. F., Woodcock, R. W., McGrew, K. S., & Mather. N. (2005). *Bateria III Woodcock-Muñoz.* Itasca, IL: Riverside.

Munsey, C. (2010). Psychology internship shortfall continues. *Monitor on Psychology, 41,* 11.

Nastasi, B. K., Varjas, K., Sarkar, S., & Jayasena, A. (1998). Participatory model of mental health programming: Lessons learned from work in a developing country. *School Psychology Review, 27*(2), 260–276.

National Association of School Psychologists. (2004). *National school psychology certification system.* Retrieved February 3, 2004, from *www.nasponline.org/certification/ncsp_system.html.*

National Association of School Psychologists. (2008). *The importance of school mental health services* (position statement). Bethesda, MD: Author. Retrieved October 6, 2010, from *www.nasponline.org/about_nasp/positionpapers/MentalHealthServices.pdf.*

National Association of School Psychologists. (2009). *Recruitment of culturally and linguistically diverse school psychologists* (position statement). Bethesda, MD: Author.

National Association of School Psychologists. (2010a). *Model for comprehensive and integrated school psychological services.* Retrieved November 1, 2010, from *www.nasponline.org/standards/2010standards/2_PracticeModel.pdf.*

National Association of School Psychologists. (2010b). *Principles for professional ethics.* Retrieved November 1, 2010, from *www.nasponline.org/standards/2010standards/1_%20Ethical%20Principles.pdf.*

National Association of School Psychologists. (2010c). *Standards for graduate preparation of school psychologists.* Retrieved October 19, 2010, from *www.nasponline.org/standards/2010standards/1_Graduate_Preparation.pdf.*

National Association of School Psychologists. (2010d). *What is a school psychologist?* Retrieved November 29, 2010, from *www.nasponline.org/about_sp/whatis.aspx.*

National Center for Education Statistics. (2009). *National assessment of reading progress.* Washington, DC: Author. Retrieved October 24, 2010, from *nces.ed.gov/nationsreportcard/reading.*

National Center for Education Statistics. (2010a). *Fast facts on back to school statistics for 2010.* Retrieved November 28, 2010, from *nces.ed.gov/fastfacts/display.asp?id=372.*

National Center for Education Statistics. (2010b). *Status and trends in the education of racial and ethnic minorities.* Retrieved November 29, 2010, from *nces.ed.gov/pubs2010/2010015/indicator2_8.asp#1.asp.*

National Reading Panel. (2000). *Teaching children to read: An evidence-based assessment of the scientific research literature on reading and its implications for reading instruction: Reports of the subgroups.* Bethesda, MD: National Institute of Child Health and Human Development.

National Research Council. (1998). *Preventing reading difficulties in young children.* Washington, DC: National Academy Press.

National Science Foundation. (2010). *Doctoral recipients from U.S. universities: 2009.* Retrieved April 7, 2011, from *www.nsf.gov/statistics/nsf11306.*

Neisser, U., Boodoo, G., Bouchard, T. J., Boykin, A. W., Broday, N., Ceci, S. J., et al. (1996). Intelligence: Knowns and unknowns. *American Psychologist, 51,* 77–101.

Ninness, H. A. C., & Glenn, S. S. (1988). *Applied behavioral analysis in school psychology: A research guide to principles and procedures.* Westport, CT: Greenwood Press.

Oakland, T. (2007). International school psychology. In T. K. Fagan & P. S. Wise, *School psychology: Past, present, and future* (3rd ed., pp. 339–365). Bethesda, MD: National Association of School Psychologists.

Oakland, T. D., & Cunningham, J. (1992). A survey of school psychology in developed and developing countries. *School Psychology International, 13,* 99–129.

Oakland, T. D., & Jimerson, S. R. (2008). History and current status of school psychology internationally. In In A. Thomas & J. Grimes (Eds.), *Best practices in school psychology V* (pp. 2053–2065). Bethesda, MD: National Association of School Psychologists.

Oberti v. Board of Education of the Borough of Clementon School District, 995 F.2d 1204 (3rd Cir. 1993).

Ochoa, S. H., Rivera, B., & Ford, L. (1997). An investigation of school psychology training pertaining to bilingual psycho-educational assessment of primarily Hispanic students: Twenty-five years after Diana v. California. *Journal of School Psychology, 35,* 329–349.

Office of Special Education Programs, Center on Positive Behavioral Interventions and Supports. (2000). Applying positive behavior support and functional behavioral assessment in schools. *Journal of Positive Behavior Interventions, 2,* 131–143.

O'Neill, R. E., Horner, R. H., Albin, R. W., Sprague, J. R., Storey, K., & Newton, J. S. (1997). *Functional assessment and program development for problem behavior: A practical handbook* (2nd ed.). Pacific Grove, CA: Brooks/Cole.

Ortiz, S. O. (2008). *Best practices in nondiscriminatory assessment.* In A. Thomas & J. Grimes (Eds.), *Best practices in school psychology V,* 661–678. Bethesda, MA: National Association of School Psychologists.

Ortiz, S. O., & Flanagan, D. P. (2002). Best practices in working with culturally diverse children and families. In A. Thomas & J. Grimes (Eds.), *Best practices in school psychology IV* (pp. 337–351). Bethesda, MD: National Association of School Psychologists.

Ortiz, S. O., Flanagan, D. P., & Dynda, A. M. (2008). Best practices in working with culturally diverse children and families. In A. Thomas & J. Grimes (Eds.), *Best practices in school psychology V* (pp. 1721–1738). Bethesda, MD: National Association of School Psychologists.

Padilla, A. (2001). Issues in culturally appropriate assessment. In L. A. Suzuki, J. G. Ponterroto, & P. J. Meller (Eds.), *Handbook of multicultural assessment* (2nd ed., pp. 5–28). San Francisco: Wiley.

Padilla, A. M., & Borsato, G. N. (2008). Issues in culturally appropriate psychoeducational assessment. In L. A. Suzuki & J. G. Ponterroto (Eds.), *Handbook of multicultural assessment* (3rd ed., pp. 5–21). San Francisco: Wiley.

Paine, S. C., Radicchi, J., Rosellini, L. C., Deutchman, L., & Darch, C. B. (1983). *Structuring your classroom for academic success.* Champaign, IL: Research Press.

Patterson, G. R. (1982). *Coercive family process.* Eugene, OR: Castalia.

Patterson, G. R., Reid, J. B., & Dishion, T. J. (1992). *Antisocial boys.* Eugene, OR: Castalia.

Pennsylvania Association for Retarded Children (PARC) v. Commonwealth of Pennsylvania, 334 F. Supp. 1257 (E.D. Pa. 1971), 343 F. Supp. 279 (E.D. Pa. 1972).

Pliszka, S. R. (2007). Pharmacologic treatment of attention-deficit hyperactivity disorder: Efficacy, safety, and mechanisms of action. *Neuropsychology Review, 17,* 61–72.

Polk v. Central Susquehanna Intermediate Unit 16, 853 F. 2d 171 (3rd Cir. 1988).

Power, T. J. (2000). Commentary: The school psychologist as community-focused, public health professional: Emerging challenges and implications for training. *School Psychology Review, 29,* 557–559.

Power, T. J. (2003). Promoting children's mental health: Reform through interdisciplinary and community partnerships. *School Psychology Review, 32,* 3–16.

Power, T. J., DuPaul, G. J., Shapiro, E. S., & Parrish, J. M. (1995). Pediatric school psychology: The emergence of a subspecialty. *School Psychology Review, 24,* 244–257.

Power, T. J., Shapiro, E. S., & DuPaul, G. J. (2003). Preparing psychologists to link systems of care in managing and preventing children's health problems. *Journal of Pediatric Psychology, 28,* 147–155.

Pratt, R., & Rittenhouse, G. (Eds.). (1998). *The condition of education: 1998.* Washington, DC: U.S. Government Printing Office.

Pressley, M. (1996). The challenges of instructional scaffolding: The challenges of instruction that supports student thinking. *Learning Disabilities Research and Practice, 11,* 138–146.

Pressley, M. (2006). *Reading instruction that works: The case for balanced teaching* (3rd ed.). New York: Guilford Press.

Pressley, M., Woloshyn, V., Burkell, J., Cariglia-Bull, T., Lysynchuk, L., McGoldrick, J. A., et al. (1995). *Cognitive strategy instruction that really improves children's academic performance* (2nd ed.). Cambridge, MA: Brookline.

Prevatt, F. F. (1999). Personality assessment in the schools. In C. R. Reynolds & T. B. Gutkin (Eds), *Handbook of school psychology* (3rd ed., pp. 434–451). New York: Wiley.

Pullen, P., & Lloyd, J. (2008). Phonics instruction. In *DDL-DR Current Practice Alerts: Alert 14.* Artlington, VA: Council for Exceptional Children, Division for Learning Disabilities.

Pyrczak, F. (2008). *Evaluating research in academic journals: A practical guide to realistic evaluation* (4th ed.). Glendale, CA: Pyraczak.

Rathvon, N. (2008). *Effective school interventions: Evidence-based strategies for improving student outcomes* (2nd ed). New York: Guilford

Ravitch, D. (1974). *The great school wars: New York City, 1805–1973: A history of the public schools as battlefield of social change.* New York: Basic Books.

Ravitch, D. (2000). *Left back: A century of failed school reforms.* New York: Simon & Schuster.

Reid, R., Maag, J. W., Vasa, S. F., & Wright, G. (1994). Who are the children with attention deficit-hyperactivity disorder? A school-based survey. *Journal of Special Education, 28,* 117–137.

Reinke, W., Lewis-Palmer, T., & Merrell, K. (2008). The classroom check-up: A class wide teacher consultation model for increasing praise and decreasing disruptive behavior. *School Psychology Review, 37,* 315–332.

Reschly, D. J. (1997). Utility of individual ability measures and public policy choices for the 21st century. *School Psychology Review, 26,* 234–241.

Reschly, D. J. (2000). The present and future status of school psychology in the United States. *School Psychology Review, 29,* 507–522.

Reschly, D. J. (2008). School psychology paradigm shift and beyond. In A. Thomas & J. Grimes (Eds.), *Best practices in school psychology V* (pp. 3–16). Bethesda, MD: National Association of School Psychologists.

Reschly, D. J., Tilly, W. D., III, & Grimes, J. P. (Eds.). (1999). *Special education in transition: Functional assessment and noncategorical programming.* Longmont, CO: Sopris West.

Reschly, D. J., & Wilson, M. S. (1995). School psychology practitioners and faculty: 1986 to 1991–92 trends in demographics, roles, satisfaction, and system reform. *School Psychology Review, 24,* 62–80.

Reschly, D., & Wilson, M. (1997). Characteristics of school psychology graduate education: Implications for the entry level discussion and doctoral level specialty definition. *School Psychology Review, 26,* 74–92.

Reschly, D. J., & Ysseldyke, J. E. (2002). Paradigm shift: The past is not the future. In A. Thomas & J. Grimes (Eds.), *Best practices in school psychology IV* (pp. 3–36). Bethesda, MD: National Association of School Psychologists.

Reyno, S. M., & McGrath, P. J. (2006). Predictors of parent training efficacy for child externalizing behavior problems—A meta-analytic review. *Journal of Child Psychology and Psychiatry, 47,* 99–111.

Reynolds, C. R., & Gutkin, T. B. (Eds.). (2009). *Handbook of school psychology* (4th ed.). New York: Wiley.

Reynolds, C. R., & Kamphaus, R. W. (2004). *Behavior Assessment System for Children* (2nd ed.). Circle Pines, MN: American Guidance Service.

Reynolds, C. R., & Shaywitz, S. E. (2009). Response to intervention: Prevention and remediation, perhaps. Diagnosis, no. *Child Development Perspectives, 3,* 44–47.

Rhodes, R. L., Ochoa, S., & Ortiz, S. (2005). *Assessing culturally and linguistically diverse students: A practical guide.* New York: Guilford Press.

Rogers, E. M. (1995). *Diffusion of innovations* (5th ed.). New York: Free Press.

Rogers, M. R. (2000). Examining the cultural context of consultation. *School Psychology Review, 29,* 414–418.

Rogers, M., & Lopez, E. (2002). Identifying critical cross-cultural school psychology competencies. *Journal of School Psychology, 40,* 115–141.

Roid, G. H. (2003). *Stanford-Binet Intelligence Scales—Fifth edition.* Itasca, IL: Riverside.

Roid, G. H., & Miller, L. J. (1997). *Leiter International Performance Scale—Revised.* Wood Dale, IL: Stoelting.

Root, R. W., & Resnick, R. J. (2003). An update on the diagnosis and treatment of attention-deficit/hyperactivity disorder in children. *Professional Psychology: Research and Practice, 34,* 34–41.

Rossi, P. H., Lipsey, M. W., & Freeman, H. E. (2004). *Evaluation: A systemic approach* (7th ed.). Thousand Oaks, CA: Sage.

Rothstein, L. F. (2010). *Special education law* (4th ed.). Thousand Oaks, CA: Sage.

Rummler, G. A., & Brache, A. P. (1995). *Improving performance: How to manage the white space on the organization chart* (2nd ed.). San Francisco: Jossey-Bass.

Sacramento City School District v. Rachel H., 14 F. 3d 1398 (9th Cir. 1994).

Samuels, S. J., & Flor, R. F. (1997). The importance of automaticity for developing expertise in reading. *Reading and Writing Quarterly: Overcoming Learning Difficulties, 13,* 107–121.

Samuels, S. J., LaBerge, D., & Bremer, C. (1978). Units of word recognition: Evidence for developmental change. *Journal of Verbal Learning and Verbal Behavior, 17,* 715–720.

Sanders, M. R. (1999). Triple P-Positive parenting program: Towards an empirically validated multilevel parenting and family support strategy for the prevention of behavior and emotional problems in children. *Clinical Child and Family Psychology Review, 2,* 71–90.

Sanders, M. R. (2008). Triple P-Positive parenting program as a public health approach to strengthening parenting. *Journal of Family Psychology, 22,* 506–517.

Sanders, M. R., Markie-Dadds, C., Tully, L. A., & Bor, W. (2000). The Triple P-Positive Parenting Program: A comparison of enhanced, standard, and self-directed behavioral family intervention for parents of children with early onset conduct problems. *Journal of Consulting and Clinical Psychology, 68,* 624–640.

Sattler, J. M. (2008). *Assessment of children: Cognitive applications* (5th ed.). La Mesa, CA: Author.

Savage, T. A., Prout, H. T., & Chard, K. M. (2004). School psychology and issues of sexual orientation: Attitudes, beliefs, and knowledge. *Psychology in the Schools, 41,* 201–210.

Scotti, J. R., Morris, T. L., & Cohen, S. H. (2003). Validity: Making inferences from research outcomes. In J. C. Thomas & M. Hersen (Eds.), *Understanding research in clinical and counseling psychology* (pp. 97–129). Mahwah, NJ: Erlbaum.

Scotti, J. R., Morris, T. L., McNeil, C. B., & Hawkins, R. P. (1996). DSM-IV and disorders of childhood and adolescence: Can structural criteria be functional? *Journal of Consulting and Clinical Psychology, 64,* 1177–1191.

Seo, S., Brownell, M. T., Bishop, A. G., & Dingle, M. (2008). An examination of beginning and special education teachers' classroom practices that engage elementary students with learning disabilities in reading instruction. *Exceptional Children, 75,* 97–122.

Serna, L., Lambros, K. M., Nielsen, E., & Forness, S. R. (2002). Head Start children at risk for emotional or behavioral disorders: Behavioral profiles and clinical implications of a primary prevention program. *Behavioral Disorders, 27,* 137–141.

Serna, L., Nielson, E., Mattern, N., Schau, C., & Forness, S. R. (2002). Use of different measures to identify preschoolers at risk for emotional or behavioral disorders: Impact on gender and ethnicity. *Education and Treatment of Children, 25,* 243–260.

Shapiro, E. S. (1996). *Academic skill problems: Direct assessment and intervention* (2nd ed.). New York: Guilford Press.

Shapiro, E. S. (2000). School psychology from an instructional perspective: Solving big, not little problems. *School Psychology Review, 29,* 560–572.

Shapiro, E. S. (2004). *Academic skill problems: Direct assessment and intervention* (3rd ed.). New York: Guilford Press.

Shapiro, E. S. (2011). *Academic skill problems: Direct assessment and intervention* (4th ed.). New York: Guilford Press.

Shapiro, E. S., Angello, L. M., & Eckert, T. L. (2004). Has curriculum-based assessment become a staple of school psychology practice? An update and extension of knowledge, use, and attitudes from 1990 to 2000. *School Psychology Review, 33,* 249–257.

Shapiro, E. S., & Cole, C. L. (1994). *Behavior change in the classroom: Self-management interventions.* New York: Guilford Press.

Shapiro, E. S., & Eckert, T. L. (1993). Curriculum-based assessment among school psychologists: Knowledge, attitudes, and use. *Journal of School Psychology, 31,* 375–384.

Shapiro, E. S., & Eckert, T. L. (1994). Acceptability of curriculum-based assessment by school psychologists. *Journal of School Psychology, 32,* 167–184.

Shapiro, E. S., & Heick, P. F. (2004). School psychologist assessment practices in the evaluation of students referred for social/behavioral/emotional problems. *Psychology in the Schools, 41,* 551–561.

Shapiro, E. S., & Kratochwill, T. R. (2000). *Behavioral assessment in schools: Theory, research, and clinical foundations* (2nd ed.). New York: Guilford Press.

Shapiro, E. S., & Kratochwill, T. R. (2002). *Conducting school-based assessment of child and adolescent behavior.* New York: Guilford Press.

Sheridan, S. M. (2000). Considerations of multiculturalism and diversity in behavioral consultation with parents and teachers. *School Psychology Review, 29,* 344–353.

Sheridan, S. M., & D'Amato, R. C. (2003). Partnering to chart our futures. *School Psychology Quarterly, 18,* 352–357.

Sheridan, S. M., & D'Amato, R. C. (2004). Partnering to chart our futures. *School Psychology Review, 33,* 7–11.

Sheridan, S. M., & Gutkin, T. B. (2000). The ecology of school psychology: Examining and changing our paradigm for the 21st century. *School Psychology Review, 29,* 485–502.

Sheridan, S. M., & Kratochwill, T. R. (2008). *Conjoint behavioral consultation: Promoting family-school connections and interventions.* New York: Springer.

Sheridan, S. M., Magee, K. L., Blevins, C. A., & Swanger-Gagne, M. S. (2010). Collaboration across systems to support children and families. In G. Gimpel Peacock, R. A. Ervin, E. J. Daly, & K. W. Merrell (Eds.), *Practical handbook of school psychology: Effective practices for the 21st century* (pp. 531–547). New York: Guilford Press.

Shinn, M. R. (Ed.). (1989). *Curriculum-based measurement: Assessing special populations.* New York: Guilford Press.

Shinn, M. R. (Ed.). (1998). *Advances in curriculum-based measurement.* New York: Guilford Press.

Shinn, M. R. (2008). Best practices in using curriculum-based measurement in a problem-solving model. In A. Thomas & J. Grimes (Eds.), *Best practices in school psychology V* (pp. 243–261). Bethesda, MD: National Association of School Psychologists.

Shinn, M. R., Collins, V. L., & Gallagher, S. (1998). Curriculum-based measurement and its use in a problem-solving model with students from minority backgrounds. In M. Shinn (Ed.), *Advanced applications of curriculum-based measurement* (pp. 143–174). New York: Guilford Press.

Shinn, M. R., & Walker, H. M. (Eds.). (2010). *Interventions for achievement and behavior problems in a three-tier model including RTI.* Bethesda, MD: National Association of School Psychologists.

Short, R. J. (2002). School psychology as a separate profession: An unsupportable direction. *School Psychologist, 56,* 111–117.

Sigurdsson, S. O., & Austin, J. (2006). Institutionalization and response maintenance in organizational behavior management. *Journal of Organizational Behavior Management, 26,* 41–77.

Silverman, W. K., & Hinshaw, S. P. (2008). The second special issue on evidence-based psychological treatments for children and adolescents: A 10-year update. *Journal of Clinical Child and Adolescent Psychology, 37,* 1–7.

Silverman, W. K., Pina, A. A., & Viswesvaran, C. (2008). Evidence-based psychosocial treatments for phobic and anxiety disorders in children and adolescents. *Journal of Clinical Child and Adolescent Psychology, 37,* 105–130.

Simmons, D. C., & Kame'enui, E. J. (Eds.). (1998). *What reading research tells us about children with diverse learning needs: Bases and basics.* Mahwah, NJ: Erlbaum.

Simmons, D. C., Kame'enui, E. J., Good, R. H., III, Harn, B. A., Cole, C., & Braun, D. (2002). Building, implementing, and sustaining a beginning reading improvement model school by school and lessons learned. In M. Shinn, G. Stoner, & H. M. Walker (Eds.), *Interventions for academic and behavior problems: II. Preventative and remedial approaches* (pp. 537–569). Bethesda, MD: National Association of School Psychologists.

Simmons, D. C., Kuykendall, K., King, K., Cornachione, C., & Kame'enui, E. J. (2000). Implementation of a schoolwide reading improvement model: "No one ever told us it would be this hard!" *Learning Disabilities Research and Practice, 15,* 92–100.

Skiba, R. J., & Peterson, R. L. (2000). School discipline at a crossroads: From zero tolerance to early response. *Exceptional Children, 66,* 335–347.

Skinner, C. H., Skinner, A. L., & Sterling-Turner, H. E. (2002). Best practices in contingency management: Application of individual and group contingencies in educational settings. In A. Thomas & J. Grimes (Eds.), *Best practices in school psychology IV* (pp. 817–830). Bethesda, MD: National Association of School Psychologists.

Smith, C. L., & Freeman, R. L. (2002). Using continuous system level assessment to build school capacity. *American Journal of Evaluation, 23*(3), 307–319.

Smith, T. L. (1967). Protestant schooling and American nationality, 1800–1850. *Journal of American History, 53,* 687.

Snider, V. E. (1992). Learning styles and learning to read: A critique. *Remedial and Special Education, 13,* 6–18.

Sodowsky, G. R., Kwan, K. K., & Pannu, R. (1995). Ethnic identity of Asians in the United States. In J. G. Ponterotto, J. M. Casas, L. A. Suzuki, & C. M. Alexander (Eds.), *Handbook of multicultural counseling* (pp. 123–154). Thousand Oaks, CA: Sage.

Spectrum K12 School Solutions (2010). *Response to intervention adoption survey 2010.* Retrieved June 30, 2010, from *www.spectrumk12.com.*

Spencer, T. J., Biederman, J., & Wilens, T. (2000). Pharmacotherapy of attention-deficit hyperactivity disorder. *Child Adolescent Psychiatric Clinics of North America, 9,* 77–97.

Spencer, T. J., Biederman, J., Wilens, T., Harding, M., O'Donnell, D., & Griffen, S. (1996). Pharmacotherapy of attention-deficit hyperactivity disorder across the life cycle. *Journal of the American Academy of Child & Adolescent Psychiatry, 35,* 409–432.

Spivak, G., & Swift, M. (1973). The classroom behavior of children: A critical review of teacher-administered rating scales. *Journal of Special Education, 7,* 55–89.

Stanovich, K. E. (1986). Matthew effects in reading: Some consequences of individual differences in the acquisition of early literacy. *Reading Research Quarterly, 21,* 360–406.

Stanovich, K. E. (2000). *Progress in understanding reading: Scientific foundations and new frontiers.* New York: Guilford Press.

Stecker, P. M., Fuchs, L. S., & Fuchs, D. (2005). Using curriculum-based measurement to improve student achievement: Review of the research. *Psychology in the Schools, 42,* 795–819.

Steege, M. W., & Watson, T. S. (2009). *Conducting school-based functional behavioral assessments: A practitioner's guide* (2nd ed.). New York: Guilford Press.

Stein, M., Carnine, D., & Dixon, R. (1998). Direct instruction: Integrating curriculum design and effective teaching practice. *Intervention in School and Clinic, 33,* 227–234.

Stetson, R., Stetson, E. G., & Sattler, J. M. (2001). Assessment of academic achievement. In J. M. Sattler (Ed.), *Assessment of children: Cognitive applications* (4th ed., pp. 576–609). San Diego, CA: Sattler.

Stoiber, K. C., & DeSmet, J. L. (2010). Guidelines for evidence-based practice in selecting interventions. In G. Gimpel Peacock, R. A. Ervin, E. J. Daly, & K. W. Merrell (Eds.), *Practical handbook of school psychology: Effective practices for the 21st century* (pp. 213–234). New York: Guilford Press.

Stokes, T. F., & Baer, D. M. (1977). An implicit technology of generalization. *Journal of Applied Behavior Analysis, 10,* 349–367.

Stoner, G., Shinn, M. R., & Walker, H. M. (1991). *Interventions for achievement and behavior problems.* Washington, DC: National Association of School Psychologists.

Strein, W., Hoagwood, K., & Cohn, A. (2003). School psychology: A public health perspective: I. Prevention, populations, and systems change. *Journal of School Psychology, 41,* 23–38.

Strein, W., & Koehler, J. (2008). Best practices in developing prevention strategies for school psychology practice. In A. Thomas & J. Grimes (Eds.), *Best practices in school psychology V* (pp. 1309–1322). Bethesda, MD: National Association of School Psychologists.

Stuebing, K. K., Fletcher, J. M., LeDoux, J. M., Lyon, G. R., Shaywitz, S. E., & Shaywitz, B. A. (2002). Validity of IQ-discrepancy classifications of reading disabilities: A meta-analysis. *American Educational Research Journal, 39,* 469–518.

Sue, D. (1981). *Counseling the culturally different: Theory and practice* (2nd ed.). New York: Wiley.

Sue, D. W., & Sue, D. (1999). *Counseling the culturally different: Theory and practice* (3rd ed.). New York: Wiley.

Sue, D. W., & Sue, D. (2008). *Counseling the culturally diverse: Theory and practice* (5th ed.). Hoboken, NJ: Wiley.

Sugai, G. (2003). Commentary: Establishing efficient and durable systems of school-based support. *School Psychology Review, 32*(4), 530–535.

Sugai, G., & Horner, R. H. (2002a). The evolution of discipline practices: School-wide positive behavior supports. *Child and Family Behavior Therapy, 24,* 23–50.

Sugai, G., & Horner, R. H. (2002b). An introduction to the special series on positive behavior support. *Journal of Emotional and Behavioral Disorders, 10*(3), 130–136.

Sugai, G., Horner, R. H., Dunlap, G., Hieneman, M., Lewis, T. J., Nelson, C. M., et al. (2000). Applying positive behavioral support and functional behavioral assessment in schools. *Journal of Positive Behavioral Interventions, 2,* 131–143.

Sugai, G., Sprague, J. R., Horner, R. H., & Walker, H. M. (2000). Preventing school violence: The use of office discipline referrals to assess and monitor schoolwide discipline interventions. *Journal of Emotional and Behavioral Disorders, 8,* 94–101.

Swanson, P. N., & De La Paz, S. (1998). Teaching effective comprehension strategies to students with learning and reading disabilities. *Intervention in School and Clinic, 33,* 209–218.

Szapocznik, J., Kurtines, W. M., & Fernandez, T. (1980a). Acculturation, biculturalism, and adjustment among Cuban Americans. In A. M. Padilla (Ed.), *Acculturation: Theory, models and some new findings* (pp. 139–159). Boulder, CO: Westview.

Szapocznik, J., Kurtines, W. M., & Fernandez, T. (1980b). Bicultural involvement and adjustment in Hispanic-American youths. *International Journal of Intercultural Relations, 4,* 353–365.

TADS Team. (2004). Fluoxetine, cognitive-behavioral therapy, and their combination for adolescents with depression: Treatment for adolescents with depression study (TADS) randomized controlled trial. *Journal of the American Medical Association, 292,* 807–820.

TADS Team. (2007). The treatment for adolescents with depression study (TADS): Long-term effectiveness and safety outcomes. *Archives of General Psychiatry, 64,* 1132–1144.

TADS Team. (2009). The Treatment for Adolescents with Depression Study (TADS): Outcomes over 1 year of naturalistic follow-up. *American Journal of Psychiatry, 166,* 1141–1149.

Takushi, R., & Uomoto, J. M. (2001). The clinical interview from a multicultural perspective. In L. A. Suzuki, J. G. Ponterotto, & P. J. Meller (Eds.), *Handbook of multicultural assessment* (pp. 47–66). San Francisco: Jossey-Bass.

Taras, V. (2008). *Instruments for measuring acculturation.* Retrieved January 9, 2011, from *people. ucalgary.ca/~taras/_private/Acculturation_Survey_Catalogue.pdf.*

Tarasoff v. Regents of the University of California, 529 P.2d 334; 118 Cal. Rptr. 129 (Cal. 1974).

Tarasoff v. Regents of the University of California, 17 Cal. 3d 425, 551 P.2d 334; 131 Cal Rptr. 14 (Cal. 1976).

Tarver, S. G., & Dawson, M. M. (1978). Modality preference and the teaching of reading: A review. *Journal of Learning Disabilities, 11,* 5–17.

Taylor, L., Nelson, P., & Adelman, H. S. (1999). Scaling-up reforms across a school district. *Reading and Writing Quarterly, 15,* 303–325.

Taylor, R. D. (2010). Risk and resilience in low-income African American families: Moderating effects of kinship social support. *Cultural Diversity and Ethnic Minority Psychology, 16,* 344–351.

Tharinger, D. J., & Palomares, R. S. (2004). An APA-informed perspective on the shortage of school psychologists: Welcome licensed psychologists into the schools (and did we mention xeriscape gardening together?). *Psychology in the Schools, 41,* 461–472.

Thomas, A. (1998). *Directory of school psychology graduate programs.* Bethesda, MD: National Association of School Psychologists.

Thomas, A., & Grimes, J. (2002). Appendix: University training programs in school psychology. In A. Thomas & J. Grimes (Eds.), *Best practices in school psychology IV* (p. 1749). Bethesda, MD: National Association of School Psychologists.

Thomas, A., & Grimes. J. (Eds.). (2008). *Best practices in school psychology V.* Bethesda, MD: National Association of School Psychologists.

Thurlow, M. L., & Ysseldyke, J. E. (1982). Instructional planning: Information collected by school psychologists vs. information considered useful by teachers. *Journal of School Psychology, 20,* 3–10.

Tilly, D. W., III (2002). Best practices in school psychology as a problem-solving enterprise. In A. Thomas & J. Grimes (Eds.), *Best practices in school psychology IV* (Vol. 1, pp. 21–36). Bethesda, MD: National Association of School Psychologists.

Tilly, D. W., III. (2008). The evolution of school psychology to science-based practice: Problem-solving and the three-tiered model. In A. Thomas & J. Grimes (Eds.), *Best practices in school psychology V* (pp. 17–36). Bethesda, MD: National Association of School Psychologists.

Tindall, R. H. (1979). School psychology: The development of a profession. In G. Phye & D. J. Reschly (Eds.), *School psychology: Perspectives and issues* (pp. 3–24). New York: Academic Press.

Torgesen, J. K. (2009). The response to intervention instructional model: Some outcomes from a large-scale implementation in Reading First schools. *Child Development Perspectives, 3,* 38–40.

Tornquist, E.H., Mastropieri, M.A., Scruggs, T.E., Berry, H.G., & Halloran, W.D. (2009). The impact of poverty on special education students. In T.E. Scruggs & M.A. Mastropieri (Eds.), *Policy and practice: Advances in learning and behavioral disabilities* (Vol. 22, pp. 169–187). Bingley, UK: Emerald.

Tyack, D. B. (Ed.). (1967). *Turning points in American educational history.* Waltham, MA: Blaisdell.

U.S. Bureau of the Census. (1992). *United States Census, 1992 updated.* Washington, DC: U.S. Government Printing Office.

U.S. Bureau of the Census. (2001, March). *Overview of race and Hispanic origin: 2000 census brief* (publication no. C2KBR/01-1). Washington, DC: U.S. Government Printing Office.

U.S. Bureau of the Census. (2010a). *New census report analyzes nation's linguistic diversity.* Retrieved November 28, 2010, from *www.censu.gov/newsroom/releases/archives/american_survey_acs/cb–0–cn58.html.*

U.S. Bureau of the Census. (2010b). *USA quick facts from the US census bureau.* Retrieved November 28, 2010, from *quickfacts.census.goe/qfd/states.00000.html.*

U.S. Department of Education. (2009). *Twenty-eighth annual report to Congress on the implementation of the Individuals with Disabilities Education Act.* Washington, DC: Author. Retrieved September 23, 2010, from *www2.ed.gov/about/reports/annual/osep/2006/parts-b-c/28th-vol-1.pdf.*

U.S. Department of Education. (2010). *A blueprint for reform: The reauthorization of the Elementary and Secondary Education Act.* Alexandria, VA: ED Pubs, U.S. Department of Education. Retrieved July 29, 2010, at *www2.ed.gov/policy/elsec/leg/blueprint/blueprint.pdf.*

U.S. Department of Labor. (2010–2011). *Occupational outlook handbook, 2010–11 edition.* Retrieved July 5, 2010, from *www.bls.gov/oco/oco2001.htm#projections_data.*

VanDerHeyden, A. M. (2010). Analysis of universal academic data to plan, implement, and evaluate schoolwide improvement. In G. Gimpel Peacock, R. A. Ervin, E. J. Daly, & K. W. Merrell

(Eds.), *Practical handbook of school psychology: Effective practices for the 21st century* (pp. 33–47). New York: Guilford Press.

VanDerHeyden, A. M., & Witt, J. C. (2005). Quantifying the context of assessment: Capturing the effect of base rates on screening accuracy. *School Psychology Review, 34*, 161–183.

VanDerHeyden, A. M., Witt, J. C., & Barnett, D. A. (2005). The emergence and possible futures of response to intervention. *Journal of Psychoeducational Assessment, 23*, 339–361.

Vaughn, S., & Edmonds, M. (2006). Reading comprehension for older readers. *Intervention in School and Clinic, 41*, 131–137.

Vaughn, S., & Linan-Thompson, S. (2003). What is special about special education for students with learning disabilities? *Journal of Special Education, 37*, 140–147.

Vázquez, L. A. (1997). A systematic multicultural curriculum model: The pedagogical process. In D. B. Pope-Davis & H. L. K. Coleman (Eds.), *Multicultural counseling competencies: Assessment, education and training, and supervision* (pp. 159–179). Thousand Oaks, CA: Sage.

Vázquez, L. A. (2003, September). *Use of interpreters and translators.* Paper presented at the meeting of the New Mexico Association of School Psychologists, Las Cruces.

Walker, H., Colvin, G., & Ramsey, E. (1995). *Antisocial behavior in public school: Strategies and best practices.* Pacific Grove, CA: Brooks/Cole.

Walker, H. M. (2001). Invited commentary on "Preventing mental disorders in school-aged children: Current state of the field." *Prevention and Treatment, 4*, Article 2. Retrieved July 19, 2005, from journals.apa.org/prevention/volume4/pre0040002c.html.

Walker, H. M., Horner, R. H., Sugai, G., Bullis, M., Sprague, J. R., Bricker, D., et al. (1996). Integrated approaches to preventing antisocial behavior patterns among school-age children and youth. *Journal of Emotional and Behavioral Disorders, 4*, 193–256.

Walkup, J. T., Albano, A. M., Piacentini, J., Birmaher, B., Compton, S. N., Sherrill, J. T., et al. (2008). Cognitive behavioral therapy, sertaline, or a combination in childhood anxiety. *New England Journal of Medicine, 359*, 2753–2766.

Watson, T. S., & Sterling-Turner, H. (2008). Best practices in direct behavioral consultation. In A. Thomas & J. Grimes (Eds.), *Best practices in school psychology V* (pp. 1661–1672). Bethesda, MD: National Association of School Psychologists.

Webster-Stratton, C., Reid, M. J., & Hammond, M. (2004). Treating children with early-onset conduct problems: Intervention outcomes for parent, child, and teacher training. *Journal of Clinical Child and Adolescent Psychology, 33*, 105–124.

Wechsler, D. (2002). *The Wechsler Preschool and Primary Scales of Intelligence—Third edition.* San Antonio, TX: Psychological Corporation.

Wechsler, D. (2003). *Wechsler Intelligence Scale for Children—Fourth edition.* San Antonio, TX: Psychological Corporation.

Wechsler, D. (2008). *Wechsler Adult Intelligence Scale—Fourth edition.* San Antonio, TX: Psychological Corporation.

Wechsler, D. (2009). *Wechsler Individual Achievement Test–Third edition.* San Antonio, TX: Psychological Corporation.

Wechsler, D., & Naglieri, J. A. (2006). *The Wechsler Nonverbal Scale of Ability.* San Antonio, TX: Pearson.

Weissman, S. A., & Gottfredson, D. C. (2001). Attrition from after school programs: Characteristics of students who drop out. *Prevention Science, 2*, 201–205.

Weisz, J. R., Hawley, K. M., & Doss, A. J. (2004). Empirically tested psychotherapies for youth internalizing and externalizing problems and disorders. *Child and Adolescent Psychiatric Clinics of North America, 13*, 729–815.

Welfel, E. R. (2006). *Ethics in counseling and psychotherapy: Standards, research, and emerging issues* (3rd ed.). Belmost, CA: Thomson Brooks/Cole.

White, M. A., & Harris, M. W. (1961). *The school psychologist.* New York: Harper & Brothers.

Wickman, E. K. (1928). *Children's behavior and teachers' attitudes.* New York: Commonwealth Fund, Division of Publications.

Wiederholt, J. L., & Bryant, B. R. (2001). *Gray Oral Reading Tests—Fourth edition.* Austin, TX: PRO-ED.

Wilkinson, G. S., & Robertson, G. J. (2006). *Wide Range Achievement Test* (4th ed.). Lutz, FL: PAR.

Williams, C. L., & Berry, J. W. (1991). Primary prevention of acculturative stress among refugees. *American Psychologist, 46,* 632–641.

Wilson, M. S., & Reschly, D. J. (1996). Assessment in school psychology training and practice. *School Psychology Review, 25,* 9–23.

Witt, J. C., Daly, E. M., & Noell, G. (2000). *Functional assessments: A step by step guide to solving academic and behavior problems.* Longmont, CO: Sopris West.

Wolery, M., Bailey, D. B., & Sugai, G. M. (1989). *Effective teaching: Applied behavior analysis with exceptional students.* Boston: Allyn & Bacon.

Woodcock, R. W. (1987). *Woodcock Reading Mastery Tests—Revised.* Circle Pines, MN: American Guidance Service.

Woodcock, R. W. (1998). *Woodcock Reading Mastery Tests—Revised: Normative update.* Circle Pines, MN: American Guidance Service.

Woodcock, R. W., McGrew, K. S., & Mather, N. (2001a). *The Woodcock–Johnson III: Tests of achievement.* Itasca, IL: Riverside.

Woodcock, R. W., McGrew, K. S., & Mather, N. (2001b). *The Woodcock–Johnson III: Tests of cognitive abilities.* Itasca, IL: Riverside.

World Health Organization. (1992). *The ICD-10 classification of mental disorders.* Geneva: Author.

Worrell, T. G., Skaggs, G. E., & Brown, M. B. (2006). School psychologists' job satisfaction: A 22-year perspective in the USA. *School Psychology International, 27,* 131–145.

Yansen, E. A., & Shulman, E. L. (1996). Language assessment: Multicultural considerations. In L. A. Suzuki, P. J. Meller, & J. G. Ponterotto (Eds.), *Handbook of multicultural assessment* (pp. 353–393). San Francisco: Jossey-Bass.

Yell, M. (2005). *The law and special education* (2nd ed.). Upper Saddle River, NJ: Prentice Hall.

Ysseldyke, J. (2000). Commentary: Déjà vu all over again: What will it take to solve big instructional problems? *School Psychology Review, 29,* 575–576.

Ysseldyke, J., Dawson, P., Lehr, C., Reschly, D., Reynolds, M., & Telzrow, C. (1997). *School psychology: A blueprint for training and practice—II.* Bethesda, MD: National Association of School Psychologists.

Ysseldyke, J. E., Algozzine, B., & Epps, S. (1983). A logical and empirical analysis of current practice in classifying students as handicapped. *Exceptional Children, 50,* 160–166.

Ysseldyke, J. E., Burns, M., Dawson, P., Kelley, B., Morrison, D., Ortiz, S., et al. (2006). *School psychology: A blueprint for training and practice III.* Bethesda, MD: National Association of School Psychologists.

Ysseldyke, J. E., Christenson, S. L., Thurlow, M. L., & Bakewell, D. (1989). Are different kinds of instructional tasks used by different categories of students in different settings? *School Psychology Review, 18,* 98–111.

Ysseldyke, J. E., & Thurlow, M. L. (1984). Assessment practices in special education: Adequacy and appropriateness. *Educational Psychologist, 19,* 123–136.

Zhang, D., & Katsiyannis, A. (2002). Minority representation in special education: A persistent challenge. *Remedial and Special Education, 25,* 180–187.

Zhou, Z., Bray, M. A., Kehle, T. J., Theodore, L. A., Clark, E., & Jenson, W. R. (2004). Achieving ethnic minority parity in school psychology. *Psychology in the Schools, 41,* 443–450.

Index

An *f* following a page number indicates a figure; a *t* following a page number indicates a table.